**Orthopedic Research and Therapy**

**Neurosurgery Research Progress**

nova
Medicine & Health
New York

# Orthopedic Research and Therapy

**Musculoskeletal Pain (Common Clinical Presentations)**
Mehmet Cenk Turgut, MD (Editor)
Serdar Toy, MD (Editor)
2021. ISBN: 978-1-68507-410-4 (Hardcover)
2022. ISBN: 978-1-68507-482-1 (eBook)

**Total Hip Arthroplasty: Procedures and Potential Complications**
Nemandra Amir Sandiford, MRCS, MRCS Ed, MSc, MFSEM, FFSEM, FRCS (Editor)
2022. ISBN: 978-1-68507-146-2 (Hardcover)
2022. ISBN: 978-1-68507-342-8978 (eBook)

More information about this series can be found at https://novapublishers.com/product-category/series/orthopedic-research-and-therapy/

# Neurosurgery Research Progress

**Reticular Concept of Nervous System Physiology**
Oleg Sotnikov, PhD (Editors)
2022. ISBN: 978-1-68507-996-3 (Hardcover)
2022. ISBN: 979-8-88697-350-1 (eBook)

**Neuroscience and Technology Transform the Educational Ecosystem**
Franco F. Orsucci (Editor)
Nicoletta Sala (Editor)
2022. ISBN: 979-8-88697-157-6 (Hardcover)
2022. ISBN: 979-8-88697-248-1 (eBook)

More information about this series can be found at https://novapublishers.com/product-category/series/neurosurgery-research-progress/

**Ahmed Majid Heydar**
Editor

# Early Onset Scoliosis

## A Comprehensive Approach

nova
Medicine & Health
New York

DOI: https://doi.org/10.52305/EAKK2104



## NOTICE TO THE READER

The Publisher has taken reasonable care in the preparation of this book but makes no expressed or implied warranty of any kind and assumes no responsibility for any errors or omissions. No liability is assumed for incidental or consequential damages in connection with or arising out of information contained in this book. The Publisher shall not be liable for any special, consequential, or exemplary damages resulting, in whole or in part, from the readers' use of, or reliance upon, this material. Any parts of this book based on government reports are so indicated and copyright is claimed for those parts to the extent applicable to compilations of such works.

Independent verification should be sought for any data, advice or recommendations contained in this book. In addition, no responsibility is assumed by the Publisher for any injury and/or damage to persons or property arising from any methods, products, instructions, ideas or otherwise contained in this publication.

This publication is designed to provide accurate and authoritative information with regards to the subject matter covered herein. It is sold with the clear understanding that the Publisher is not engaged in rendering legal or any other professional services. If legal or any other expert assistance is required, the services of a competent person should be sought. FROM A DECLARATION OF PARTICIPANTS JOINTLY ADOPTED BY A COMMITTEE OF THE AMERICAN BAR ASSOCIATION AND A COMMITTEE OF PUBLISHERS.

**Library of Congress Cataloging-in-Publication Data**

ISBN: 979-8-89113-600-7 (hardcover)
ISBN: 979-8-89113-702-8 (e-book)

Published by Nova Science Publishers, Inc. † New York

# Contents

# Preface

In the ever-changing world of medical science, the management and understanding of Early Onset Scoliosis have experienced a profound transformation. As we navigate the complex landscape of spinal health, the book "Early Onset Scoliosis: A Comprehensive Approach" aims to serve as a comprehensive guide to the current approaches in diagnosis, treatment, and research of the deformity affecting this crucial aspect of pediatric health.

Our journey through the intricacies of pediatric spines unveils a narrative that intertwines the latest advancements in medical technology, evolving treatment paradigms, and deeper comprehension of the underlying biomechanical mechanisms. This book is not just a collection of facts, but a testament to the collaborative efforts of dedicated professionals, contributing to the mosaic of knowledge shaping contemporary understanding of pediatric spine health.

We delve into the spectrum of pediatric scoliosis, from normal physiological development to advanced deformities, focusing on evidence-based practices and patient-centric care. The multidisciplinary nature of our exploration reflects the collaborative spirit required to address the complexities inherent in Early Onset Scoliosis. Radiologists, surgeons, physiatrists, and other healthcare professionals play a vital role in the intricate ballet of diagnosis and treatment, and their insights are interwoven throughout the book.

As we embark on this exploration, it is crucial to acknowledge the evolving nature of medical knowledge. What stands as the gold standard today might transform into a steppingstone for future innovations. Therefore, this book is not a static repository of information but rather a dynamic platform that encourages critical thinking, continuous learning, and adaptation to emerging trends in pediatric spine health management.

Ahmed Majid Heydar, MD
Department of Orthopedics and Traumatology
Bahçelievler Memorial Hospital, İstanbul, Turkey

## Chapter 1

# Definition and Epidemiology of Early-Onset Scoliosis

**Yusuf Sait Durak***, **MD**
Department of Orthopedics and Traumatology, Kurtalan State Hospital, Siirt, Turkiye

### Abstract

Early-onset scoliosis is diagnosed for various reasons up to the age of ten and has many subtypes. These are infantile (0-3 years old), juvenile (4-10 years old), congenital scoliosis, neuromuscular scoliosis, and syndromic scoliosis types. Although its prevalence is not completely known, studies in some developed countries shed light on the epidemiology of early-onset scoliosis. Thoracic insufficiency syndrome is known as the most significant complication of EOS, and one of the treatment goals is to prevent and delay its development.

**Keywords:** early-onset scoliosis, thoracic insufficiency syndrome, complications, idiopathic cases, congenital scoliosis

## Introduction

Scoliosis takes its origin from the ancient Greek word 'scoliosis,' which means the spine bending sideways. The normal structure of the spine was first described by Hippocrates in the 4$^{th}$ century BC. Hippocrates called changes in the structure of the spine 'ithiscolosis.' Galen described scoliosis as bending in

---

* Corresponding Author's Email: yusufsaiddurak@gmail.com.

In: Early Onset Scoliosis
Editor: Ahmed Majid Heydar
ISBN: 979-8-89113-600-7

the coronal plane. Scoliosis represents the most common spinal disorder in children and adolescents (Grivas et al., 2009). During this period, Ibn Sina applied the traction method in the treatment of spinal curvature and conducted biomechanical studies on the spine. Spinal curvatures, traumas, and sciatica are mentioned in the surgical book written by Şerafeddin Sabuncuoğlu in the 15th century (Naderi et al., 2002a, 2002b; Tolo, 1983).

Scoliosis patients are classified into different types according to the age of onset, etiology, severity, and type of curve. Early-onset scoliosis (EOS) is defined as any spinal deformity present before the age of ten, regardless of its etiology (Ruiz et al., 2022). In another definition, it is described as a spinal curvature of 10° and more in the coronal plane until the age of ten. This deformity should be evaluated according to the relationship between the spine and the lungs, among the organs of the thorax. During the critical growth period of the lungs, children with EOS are at risk of developing pulmonary function because the spine creates pressure on the lungs. Since there are early-onset curves in EOS, it has cardiorespiratory problems, increased morbidity and mortality due to the risk of progression. The growth of the lungs is the period from birth to 5 years of age, corresponding to the period of the fastest growth of the thoracic cage. The bronchial tree and alveolar structure develop at a maximum of 8 years of age, and the volume of the chest reaches 50% of the expected volume of adult by 10 years. Furthermore, the progression of the deformity can cause thoracic insufficiency syndrome since the thorax with a curve cannot support normal respiratory function or lung growth.

## Epidemiology

In 1950, Ponseti and Friedman used the term EOS to describe idiopathic scoliosis in patients younger than ten years of age (Ponseti & Friedman, 1950).

In 1954, James et al. divided idiopathic scoliosis into three subgroups: infantile (≤3 years), juvenile (4-9 years), and adolescent (from 10 years to maturity) (James et al., 1959).

A study conducted in Japan between 2000 and 2020 included a total of 2,295,929 children under the age of ten, including 1,170,149 (51.0%) males and 1,125,780 (49.0%) females. The annual incidence of early-onset scoliosis was 0.019% (95% CI: 0.015-0.023%) and the prevalence was 0.077% (95% CI) in a total of 469 patients, 227 (48.4%) males and 242 (51.6%) females. The most common age at which the first application was made was six years old. It was more common in females (51.6%) than in males (48.4%), and left-sided curves (54.2%) were observed more frequently than right-sided curves (45.8%), the majority of which were unilateral thoracic curves (38.2%). Whereas the scoliosis curve did not progress in 44.3% of the cases, it progressed in 38%. Follow-up was inadequate to determine the progression status in 17.7% of the cases. Neuromuscular etiology was the most common cause with 40.1%, and 83.5% of them had cerebral palsy (AlNouri et al., 2022).

The true prevalence of EOS is unknown. It varies depending on the etiology. The incidence of EOS is four times higher in Europe (1-2 per 10,000) than in the United States. It is believed to be much higher in Asia, particularly in southern India (Vidyadhara & Shatty, 2015).

Only 1% of the idiopathic scoliosis population is infantile idiopathic scoliosis (Reamy & Slakey, 2001). Spontaneous recovery rates between 20% and 80% have been reported in the literature. James et al. studied 212 patients with infantile idiopathic scoliosis and reported spontaneous resolution in 31% of children. Of the 212 children, 135 (69%) had aggressive curve progression; 50 children developed >70 degrees of curve, and 26 children developed >100 degrees of deformity (James et al., 1959). It was observed that juvenile idiopathic scoliosis constituted 12% to 21% of idiopathic scoliosis (Robinson & McMaster, 1996; Ponseti & Friedman, 1950; Ji, 1954).

It tends to be more common in females. A right-sided thoracic curve and a double main curve predominate. In 55% to 71% of patients, the juvenile-onset curves progress. The rate of progression varies from slow to moderate. The age of onset of scoliosis and large-angle curves are recorded when the patient presents. Congenital scoliosis is the most common among all EOS causes. The prevalence of congenital scoliosis is approximately 1 in 1000 live births. It is more common in females. The type and location of the abnormality and the child's growth potential determine the progression of congenital scoliosis (Giampietro et al., 2003).

Block vertebrae and bilateral segmentation disorder were accepted as benign anomaly forms. Wedge vertebrae, hemivertebrae, and unilateral non-segmented bars were revealed to cause more severe deformities, respectively. The incidence of scoliosis ranges from 15% to 28% among children with cerebral palsy, and hospitalized patients, children with spastic quadriplegic CP, and limited motor function are impacted most frequently. A study from Sweden comparing mortality rates in patients followed up with scoliosis demonstrated that the mortality rate was more than twice in patients up to 40 years of age (Vidyadhara & Shatty, 2015). Upon comparing EOS with the general population, Pehrsson et al. reported that the mortality rate in patients with untreated scoliosis was the highest in infantile-onset scoliosis, followed by juvenile-onset scoliosis (Pehrsson et al., 1992a; Pehrsson et al., 1992b). Respiratory failure (40%) was the main cause of death. The mean age at death was 54, but some patients died at the age of 16. When the patients were examined after death, it was seen that the number of alveoli was significantly reduced and the patients had very small lungs. As a result, the basic principle of EOS treatment is to promote normal respiratory development and maximize spinal growth while preventing additional deformities that may cause thoracic insufficiency syndrome (Ruiz et al., 2022).

## Definition and Types of Early-Onset Scoliosis

A holistic approach must be followed, which also considers the patient's psychology and quality of life, in the treatment management of EOS. Growth-friendly surgical techniques have failed to meet expectations, such as correcting scoliotic deformity, supporting thoracic growth, and improving pulmonary function. There is no disease; there are patients, that is, not all patients with EOS are the same. Whereas some cases are idiopathic, others have pathology associated with an underlying condition that may impact the patient's treatment. While it is impossible to review all different types of EOS, it is helpful to categorize patients when discussing treatment.

These categories are presented below:

- Idiopathic cases infantile (0-3 years old) or juvenile (4-10 years old)
- Congenital scoliosis
- Neuromuscular cases (those associated with a neuromuscular condition such as spinal muscular atrophy)
- Syndromic cases (associated with an underlying disease, such as Marfan syndrome or Ehlers-Danlos syndrome)
- Sometimes, it may be associated with previous surgeries such as heart surgery.
- Sometimes congenital scoliosis can be observed, in which the bones do not normally form, causing a spinal curvature. There may also be associated abnormalities in the thoracic cage (LeFever & Menger, 2022).

## Infantile Idiopathic Scoliosis

Juvenile idiopathic scoliosis is a type of scoliosis first diagnosed in children between birth and three years of age. The term "idiopathic" means that the cause is not known, and the child is healthy except for the presence of a spinal defect. Congenital abnormalities of the spinal column (amorphous and fused vertebrae) are also commonly diagnosed during this time period, but they are not included in the category of infantile idiopathic. Left-sided curves in the thoracic region are most common in infantile idiopathic scoliosis. It is more likely to be seen in females than in males. Many infants with infantile idiopathic scoliosis are healthy and normal and have only a slight curve in their spine. However, in some patients, there is an increased association with hip dysplasia, mental retardation, and congenital heart disease (Lenke & Dobbs, 2007).

In the prognosis of infantile idiopathic scoliosis, many infantile curves resolve without treatment. Treatment is required in children with significant curves with proven or expected progression. Nowadays, the wide range of interventions available allows for an individualized therapeutic approach (Trobisch et al., 2010).

## Juvenile Idiopathic Scoliosis

Juvenile idiopathic scoliosis is a type of scoliosis that is diagnosed for the first time between the ages of four and ten. Approximately 10% to 15% of all cases of idiopathic scoliosis in children fall into this category. At the younger end of the spectrum, males are slightly more affected than females. The curve is usually on the left side. Toward the upper end of the age spectrum, the situation more closely resembles adolescent idiopathic scoliosis, with a predominance of females and right-sided curves. MRI may be required in juvenile idiopathic scoliosis, as described in infantile scoliosis. The decision in question depends on the condition of the curve, the findings of the physical examination, and the properties of the X-rays (Konieczny et al., 2013).

In the prognosis of juvenile idiopathic scoliosis, juvenile curves that reach 25°-30° tend to worsen if untreated. Support is usually used to manage these curves, but many young children need surgical treatment (Coillard et al., 2010).

## Congenital Scoliosis

“Congenital scoliosis” refers to a spinal deformity caused by the improper formation of the vertebrae. This occurs during the very early periods of intrauterine development, during the first six weeks of embryonic development, before the mother even realizes that she is pregnant. The cause of congenital scoliosis is unknown. Research has demonstrated that congenital scoliosis is not hereditary. Genetic studies performed to date have not provided clear evidence that this condition may be hereditary. Congenital scoliosis is frequently associated with other malformations, such as congenital heart disease, spinal cord dysraphism, or renal malformations. Although congenital scoliosis is often noticed in infancy or toddlerhood, it may not be recognized in some children until adolescence (Arlet et al., 2003).

## Neuromuscular Scoliosis

The vertebrae are affected by many neuromuscular diseases. These include neuropathic (nervous system related) disorders such as cerebral palsy (CP), spinal muscular atrophy (SMA), or spinal cord trauma. Myopathic disorders (muscle related) include muscular dystrophy, poliomyelitis, or arthrogryposis. Depending on the degree of involvement, children with spina bifida may develop different types of spinal deformities. The deformity can impact different parts of the vertebra, depending on the neuromuscular disease and the level of the neurological defect. There may be predominantly scoliosis, kyphosis, lordosis, or a combination of these. Unlike other types of scoliosis, the treatment of neuromuscular scoliosis is difficult to predict since the progression of curves varies according to the diagnosis of neuromuscular disease.

The prognosis of patients is very variable, and the pathophysiology of scoliosis is also diverse. However, predisposing conditions have several common features in many patients, although not in everyone.

Children with neuromuscular scoliosis do not usually feel any pain caused by the condition, and the curve may progress. The earlier the curve develops in neuromuscular scoliosis, the more likely it is to progress. Similarly, the more severe the curve is at the time of first detection, the more likely it is that the curve will progress. Pelvic tilt is often caused by neuromuscular curves. This is a condition in which the child's pelvis tilts unevenly, making sitting difficult for patients who cannot walk. Many children with neuromuscular scoliosis have poor balance and coordination of the neck, trunk, and head. Moreover, it may be accompanied by kyphosis. Curves in different conditions have a high rate of progression, and hence, many patients require surgery (Berven & Bradford, 2002; McCarthy, 1999).

### Syndromic Scoliosis

There are some syndromes involving scoliosis deformity. The syndromes mentioned above include neurofibromatosis, Noonan syndrome, VATER syndrome, Angelman syndrome, Rett syndrome, Marfan syndrome, Ehlers-Danlos syndrome, osteochondrodystrophy (dwarfism), and some other syndromes.

Screening for scoliosis will begin quite early once a child is diagnosed with one of these syndromes. Since syndromes are different, it has been seen that their effects on the spine also differ and curvatures progress at different rates (Levy et al., 2015).

### Thoracic Insufficiency Syndrome

Thoracic insufficiency syndrome is common in patients with EOS since spinal deformity considerably limits lung development. For the optimal respiratory function of the thoracic cage, it must have the ideal volume for age, the ribs must be symmetrical for smooth movement, and the diaphragm muscle must be properly fixed to the chest base. Numerous methods are being developed to prevent and delay thoracic insufficiency syndrome, and new treatment studies are ongoing for early-onset scoliosis (Mayer et al., 2016).

## Conclusion

The definition of early-onset scoliosis has historically varied, and its prevalence is not exactly known. In such cases, children must be followed up with a good examination from birth. Although there are data on early-onset scoliosis in some developed countries, there are not sufficient data on EOS in many countries. In the future, we can reach more data and statistics with new data and new research.

## References

AlNouri, M., Wada, K., Kumagai, G., Asari, T., Nitobe, Y., Morishima, T., Uesato, R., Aoki, M., & Ishibashi, Y. (2022). The incidence and prevalence of early-onset scoliosis: A regional multicenter epidemiological study. *The Spine Journal: Official Journal of the North American Spine Society, 22*(9), 1540-1550. https://doi.org/10.1016/j.spinee.2022.03.016.

Arlet, V., Odent, T., & Aebi, M. (2003). Congenital scoliosis. *European Spine Journal, 12*(5), 456-463. https://doi.org/10.1007/s00586-003-0555-6.

Berven, S., & Bradford, D. S. (2002). Neuromuscular scoliosis: Causes of deformity and principles for evaluation and management. *Seminars in Neurology, 22*(2), 167-178. https://doi.org/10.1055/s-2002-36540.

Robinson, C. M., & McMaster, M. J. (1996). Juvenile idiopathic scoliosis. Curve patterns and prognosis in one hundred and nine patients. *JBJS, 78*(8), 1140-1148. https://doi.org/10.2106/00004623-199608000-00003.

Coillard, C., Circo, A. B., & Rivard, C. H. (2010). SpineCor treatment for Juvenile Idiopathic Scoliosis: SOSORT award 2010 winner. *Scoliosis, 5*(1), 25. https://doi.org/10.1186/1748-7161-5-25.

Giampietro, P. F., Blank, R. D., Raggio, C. L., Merchant, S., Jacobsen, F. S., Faciszewski, T., Shukla, S. K., Greenlee, A. R., Reynolds, C., Schowalter, D. B. (2003). Congenital and Idiopathic Scoliosis: Clinical and Genetic Aspects. *Clinical Medicine & Research, 1*(2), 125–136. https://www.ncbi.nlm.nih.gov/pmc/articles/PMC1069035/.

Grivas, T., Vasiliadis, E., Chatziargiropoulos, T., Polyzois, V., & Gatos, K. (2009). The effect of a modified Boston brace with anti-rotatory blades on the progression of curves in idiopathic scoliosis: Aetiologic implications. *Pediatric Rehabilitation, 6*, 237-242. https://doi.org/10.1080/13638490310001636808.

Ponseti, I. V., & Friedman, B. (1950). Prognosis in idiopathic scoliosis. *JBJS, 32*(2), 381-395.

James, J. I. P., Lloyd-Roberts, G. C., & Pilcher, M. F. (1959). Infantile structural scoliosis. *The Journal of Bone and Joint Surgery. British Volume, 41*(4), 719-735.

Ji, J. (1954). Idiopathic scoliosis; the prognosis, diagnosis, and operative indications related to curve patterns and the age at onset. *The Journal of Bone and Joint Surgery. British Volume, 36-B*(1). https://doi.org/10.1302/0301-620X.36B1.36.

Konieczny, M. R., Senyurt, H., & Krauspe, R. (2013). Epidemiology of adolescent idiopathic scoliosis. *Journal of Children's Orthopaedics, 7*(1), 3-9. https://doi.org/10.1007/s11832-012-0457-4.

LeFever, D., & Menger, R. P. (2022). Infantile and Juvenile Scoliosis. In *StatPearls*. StatPearls Publishing. http://www.ncbi.nlm.nih.gov/books/NBK519498/.

Lenke, L. G., & Dobbs, M. B. (2007). Management of Juvenile Idiopathic Scoliosis. *JBJS, 89*(suppl_1), 55. https://doi.org/10.2106/JBJS.F.00644.

Levy, B. J., Schulz, J. F., Fornari, E. D., & Wollowick, A. L. (2015). Complications associated with surgical repair of syndromic scoliosis. *Scoliosis, 10*(1), 14. https://doi.org/10.1186/s13013-015-0035-x.

Mayer, O., Campbell, R., Cahill, P., & Redding, G. (2016). Thoracic Insufficiency Syndrome. *Current Problems in Pediatric and Adolescent Health Care, 46*(3), 72-97. https://doi.org/10.1016/j.cppeds.2015.11.001.

McCarthy, R. E. (1999). Management of Neuromuscular Scolıosıs. *Orthopedic Clinics of North America, 30*(3), 435-449. https://doi.org/10.1016/S0030-5898(05)70096-1.

Naderi, S., Acar, F., & Arda, M. N. (2002a). History of spinal disorders and Cerrahiyetül Haniye (Imperial Surgery): A review of a Turkish treatise written by Serefeddin Sabuncuoğlu in the 15th century. *Journal of Neurosurgery, 96*(3 Suppl), 352-356.

Naderi, S., Acar, F., & Arda, M. N. (2002b). History of spinal disorders and Cerrahiyetül Haniye (Imperial Surgery): A review of a Turkish treatise written by Serefeddin Sabuncuoğlu in the 15th century. *Journal of Neurosurgery, 96*(3 Suppl), 352-356.

Pehrsson, K., Larsson, S., Oden, A., & Nachemson, A. (1992a). Long-term follow-up of patients with untreated scoliosis. A study of mortality, causes of death, and symptoms. *Spine, 17*(9), 1091-1096. https://doi.org/10.1097/00007632-199209000-00014.

Pehrsson, K., Nachemson, A., Olofson, J., Ström, K., & Larsson, S. (1992b). Respiratory failure in scoliosis and other thoracic deformities. A survey of patients with home oxygen or ventilator therapy in Sweden. *Spine, 17*(6), 714-718. https://doi.org/10.1097/00007632-199206000-00012.

Reamy, B. V., & Slakey, J. B. (2001). Adolescent Idiopathic Scoliosis: Review and Current Concepts. *American Family Physician, 64*(1), 111-117.

Ruiz, G., Torres-Lugo, N. J., Marrero-Ortiz, P., Guzmán, H., Olivella, G., & Ramírez, N. (2022). Early-onset scoliosis: A narrative review. *EFORT Open Reviews, 7*(8), 599-610. https://doi.org/10.1530/EOR-22-0040.

Tolo, V. T. (1983). Progression in scoliosis. A 360 degrees change in 75 years. *Spine, 8*(4), 373-377. https://doi.org/10.1097/00007632-198305000-00006.

Trobisch, P., Suess, O., & Schwab, F. (2010). Idiopathic Scoliosis. *Deutsches Ärzteblatt International, 107*(49), 875-884. https://doi.org/10.3238/arztebl.2010.0875.

Vidyadhara, S. & Shetty, A. P. (2015). Epidemiology, Classification, and Natural History. In: Nnandi, C. (Ed.), *Early Onset Scoliosis: A Comprehensive Guide from the Oxford Meetings*. Thieme.

## Chapter 2

# Normal Growth and Development of the Spine and Thoracic Cage

**Bilal Karabak*, MD**
Department of Orthopedics and Traumatology, Erzurum City Hospital, Erzurum, Turkiye

## Abstract

The normal growth and development of the spine and thoracic cage represent a complex integrity of intertwined events affected by numerous anatomical, biomechanical, biochemical, and genetic factors. The said complex events are affected by signaling pathways, genes, and metabolic processes. The growth of the spine and thoracic cage is nicely synchronized, forming a compatible skeletal structure. There is a sequential order of complex events in the spine growth. Deteriorations in this order lead to deformities. With the increasing severity of spinal deformities, the severity of deformities of the thoracic cage also increases. This condition between spinal and thoracic deformities creates a domino effect. Thoracic deformities can also cause cardiac and lung problems. All these conditions can even cause death.

Knowing the normal growth of the spine and thoracic cage and the parameters that influence this growth enables pathological changes in the spine and thoracic cage to be more easily identified and directed. Mastering normal growth provides the physician the opportunity to intervene at the correct time.

**Keywords:** scoliosis, early-onset scoliosis, spine, infantile scoliosis, spine and thoracic growth

---

* Corresponding Author's Email: bilal_karabak@hotmail.com.

In: Early Onset Scoliosis
Editor: Ahmed Majid Heydar
ISBN: 979-8-89113-600-7

## Introduction

Spine growth is characterized by the harmonious growth of more than 130 growth plates. Spinal deformities and accompanying thoracic cage deformities, cardiac problems, lung problems, and even fatal conditions may develop in the case of irregularities and asymmetrical forces in the growth plates. The regular synchronization of complex events ensures spine growth. Signaling pathways, genes, and metabolic and mechanical processes are programmed in harmony with spine growth. Deterioration in any of these processes leads to deformities and functional disorders. Spine growth begins in the third month of the intrauterine period and ends in the second decade. Spine growth is a dynamic process with periods of acceleration and deceleration. Spine growth is basically divided into three periods. The periods are between birth and 5 years of age, between 5 and 10 years of age, and between 10 years of age and the end of skeletal maturation.

The cervical, thoracic, and lumbar spines grow at various rates in relation to each other. The anterior and posterior sides of the vertebrae also grow at various rates. The posterior sides of the thoracic spines lengthen faster than the anterior, whereas the anterior sides of the lumbar spines lengthen faster than the posterior. This allows the gradual regulation of the relationship of the spinal column with the spinal cord.

The ideal method to evaluate spine growth is the measurement of sitting height. About 60% of the sitting height is the spinal height. The remaining 20% is the head and 20% is the height of the pelvis. The loss in sitting height and proportion is associated with the severity of the deformity.

The younger the patient, the higher the risk of progression of the spinal deformity. It is crucial to intervene in these deformities in a timely and correct manner. Otherwise, irreversible conditions may develop.

## Embryology

Spinal development begins between the 20th and 35th days of embryogenesis, i.e., the 3rd week of gestation. Somite pairs are formed from the paraxial mesoderm. Sclerotome plaques are formed from somite pairs and vertebrae are formed from them. As of the 6th week, the vertebral distresses begin to turn into cartilage tissue. The cartilaginous spinal column becomes integrated in the 8th week. This spinal column becomes ossified at the end of the age of 25. The vertebrae in the neonatal period consist of 3 parts connected by cartilage tissues. The parts begin to ossify and fuse in the first 5 years of life. The fusion that starts from the vertebrae in the lower back progresses in the cranial and caudal directions. The physis at the junction of the pedicle and the vertebral body in the spine is named neurocentral synchondrosis. The joints, called neurocentral synchondrosis, ensure the adaptation of the vertebrae to the spinal cord canal. Neurocentral *synchondrosis* joints ossify and disappear between the ages of approximately 6 and 9 (Moore et al., 2013; Nordin & Frankel, 2001; Tekelioğlu, 1992).

Lordosis occurs in the cervical region as the infant starts to hold his/her head on the straight spine during birth. Afterward, lumbar lordosis occurs when the infant begins to sit and stand up. There is kyphosis, which is a primary curvature, in the thoracic and sacral regions. With the growth of children, these angles also increase and reach their normal values. A normal adult individual has the following physiological curvatures: 30°-50° lordosis in the cervical region, 20°-50° kyphosis in the thoracic region, 40°-80° lordosis in the lumbar region, and 40°-60° kyphosis in the sacral region (Moore et al., 2013).

## Spine Growth

Spine growth begins in the third month of the intrauterine period and ends in the second decade. Spine growth represents a dynamic process with periods of acceleration and deceleration. Spine growth is basically divided into three periods, which are between birth and 5 years of age, between 5 and 10 years of age, and between 10 years of age and the end of skeletal maturation.

## Spine Growth from Birth to 5 Years of Age

Spine growth starts in the intrauterine period. The spine growth during this period is equal to the sum of the spine growth in the other two periods. This is the period when growth is the greatest. The sitting height, which is approximately 35 cm at birth, constitutes 37% of the adult sitting height. The sitting height is about 60 cm at the age of five years. A significant increase of approximately 27-30 cm occurs in the sitting height during this period. The sitting height increases by about 60% in the first two years of life. The sitting height increases by 12 cm in the first year, 5.3 cm in the second year, 3.3 cm in the 3rd year, 3.2 cm in the 4th year, and 2.8 cm in the 5th year. Growth tends to slow down after the first year of life. Nevertheless, growth is still quite fast. During this period, cartilage tissue mostly constitutes the spinal structure. In this period, 30-40% of the spine is ossified. The predominance of cartilage tissue makes the spine vulnerable to deformities. The fastest development of the thoracolumbar spine occurs during this period and adolescence (Akbarnia et al., 2022; Cheng et al., 1998; Khurjekar & Kardile, 2019; Dimeglio, 2001; Jarzem & Gledhill, 1993).

## Spine Growth Between 5 and 10 Years of Age

The period in question is also called the period between five years of age and the pre-puberty period. Spine growth tends to slow in this period. The period between five and ten years of age is the period when spine growth tends to slow. The increase in height is about 5.5 cm/year. One-third of this growth (2.3 cm) is in the sitting height. The increase in the sitting height during this period is about 2.5 cm/year. The T1-S1 spine segment is approximately 1.2 cm/year. The sitting height of males increases by approximately 20% (17 cm) during this period. In the female gender, the sitting height increases by approximately 17% (13 cm). The sitting height is about 60 cm at the age of 5 years. Sixty cm make up 66% of the final height. The growth of 26-30 cm will occur after 5 years of age (Canavese & Dimeglio, 2013; Cheng et al., 1998; Dimeglio, 2001; Dimeglio & Canavese, 2020; Jarzem & Gledhill, 1993; Yang et al., 2016).

## Spine Growth between 10 Years of Age and Skeletal Maturation

This period can also be called the puberty period. The spine enters the rapid growth phase at the beginning of this period. Then it enters the deceleration phase. The sitting height increases by approximately 12 cm during this period. Two-thirds of the growth during this period take place in the rapid growth phase. When the deceleration phase starts, the amount of growth in the sitting height is, on average, 4 cm in the male gender and 3.5 cm in the female gender (Bess & Line, 2022; Canavese & Dimeglio, 2013; Dimeglio, 2001; Yang et al., 2016).

The highest growth rate occurs between the ages of 13-15 in males and between the ages of 11-13 in females. The rapid growth phase during this period takes an important place in the worsening of scoliosis. Puberty is a critical period for orthopedics. Hence, it is essential to identify this period. It would be misleading to identify this period according to the age of the patient. The rapid increase in height, changes in body morphology, the appearance of secondary sexual characteristics, and proportional changes in the upper and lower parts of the body are among the characteristics of this period. Concerning the male gender, the Risser sign is zero at the beginning of puberty, and the triradiate cartilage is open and has 13% of the remaining growth. The sitting height has a growth potential of 12.5 cm. In females, the Risser sign is zero at the beginning of puberty, the triradiate cartilage is open and has 12% of the remaining growth. The sitting height has a growth potential of 11.5 cm (Bess & Line, 2022; Canavese & Dimeglio, 2013; Dimeglio et al., 2016; Yang et al., 2016).

## Growth of the Cervical Spine

The length of the cervical region at birth is 3.7 cm. The growth of the cervical spine approximately doubles in the first 6 years of age. A further growth of 3.5 cm occurs after the growth spurt of puberty. The final length of the cervical spine reaches 13 cm. Between C1-S1 of the cervical spine corresponds to 22% of the height and 16% of the sitting height (Bess & Line, 2022; Canavese & Dimeglio, 2013; Dimeglio, 2001).

## Growth of the Thoracic Spine

T1-T12 is the segment connected to the thoracic cage. This segment is about 12 cm at birth, 18 cm at five years of age, and 27 cm at skeletal maturity. The growth of the thoracic spine is approximately 7.3 cm with 1.3 cm/year in the first five years of age and is the rapid growth phase. It grows 3.8 cm with 0.7 cm/year between 5 and 10 years of age and is a slow growth phase. It grows by 7 cm with 1.1 cm/year during puberty and is characterized by rapid growth. The spinal length of T1-T12 corresponds to 30% of the sitting height (Bess & Line, 2022; Canavese & Dimeglio, 2013; Dimeglio, 2001).

## Growth of the Lumbar Spine

This region is approximately 7 cm at birth. The final length of the lumbar spine is approximately 16 cm. The lumbar spine grows approximately 3 cm in the first five years of age and is in the rapid growth phase. It grows to 2 cm between the ages of five and ten, which is a slow growth phase. It grows by 3 cm during puberty and is characterized by rapid growth. The lumbar spine reaches 90% of its mature length at the age of 10. The L1-L5 spinal length corresponds to 18% of the sitting height (Bess & Line, 2022; Canavese & Dimeglio, 2013; Dimeglio, 2001; Yang et al., 2016).

## Growth of the Thoracic Cage

The growth of the thoracic cage is related to the growth of the spine. The growth of the thoracic cage can be examined in three periods, just as the growth of the spine. The periods in question are between birth and five years of age, between five and ten years of age, and between ten years of age and the end of skeletal maturation.

### Growth of the Thoracic Cage from Birth to 5 Years of Age

At birth, the circumference of the thoracic cage is approximately 32 cm, and the volume of the thoracic cage represents 6% of its final volume. The circumference of the thoracic cage reaches approximately 63% of its final size at the age of 5. At the age of 5, the trunk height reaches 66% of its final form, but the chest volume reaches only 30% of its final state. The growth of the thoracic cage is rapid during this period and adolescence. The circumference of the chest corresponds to approximately 93% of the sitting height. The shape of the thoracic cage at birth is oval compared to its adult form (Akbarnia et al., 2022; Bess & Line, 2022; Canavese & Dimeglio, 2013).

### Growth of the Thoracic Cage between Five and Ten Years of Age

Whereas the volume of the thoracic cage is 3% at the age of five, it reaches 50% at the age of ten.

The growth of the thoracic cage during this period is slower compared to other periods. The chest circumference during this period grows by about 2 cm/year. The chest circumference increases by approximately 10 cm per year during this period (Bess & Line, 2022; Canavese & Dimeglio, 2013; Yang et al., 2016).

## Growth of the Thoracic Cage between Ten Years of Age and Skeletal Maturation

This period is also named the pubertal growth spurt. The growth of the thoracic cage is rapid before five years of age and during adolescence. The volume of the thoracic cage doubles during this period and reaches its final maturity. The shape of the thoracic cage turns into an ellipse during this period (Canavese & Dimeglio, 2013; Dimeglio et al., 2016; Yang et al., 2016).

## Rib-Vertebral-Sternal Complex (RVSC)

The thoracic cage is part of the rib-vertebral-sternal complex (RVSC). This complex represents an elastic three-dimensional complex that sits cube-shaped in the thoracic cavity. The thoracic cage changes from an oval to an ellipse from birth to skeletal maturity (Khurjekar & Kardile, 2019; Dimeglio, 2001; Dimeglio et al., 2016).

## Growth of the Spinal Column

At birth, the thoracic and cervical regions are longer compared to the lumbosacral region. Nevertheless, the lumbosacral region grows faster in the first year after birth. The lumbar vertebrae with their discs grow at a rate of 2 mm/year, and the thoracic vertebrae with their discs grow at a rate of 1 mm/year between the ages of three to 15. The anterior and posterior sides of the vertebrae also grow at various rates. The posterior sides of the thoracic spines grow faster than the anterior ones, whereas the anterior sides of the lumbar spines grow faster than the posterior ones. This enables the gradual regulation of the relationship of the spinal column with the spinal cord (Dimeglio et al., 2016).

The physis at the junction of the pedicle and the vertebral body in the spine is named neurocentral synchondrosis. The joints, called neurocentral synchondrosis, ensure the adaptation of the vertebrae to the spinal cord canal.

This physis is responsible for the ossification of 30% of the vertebral body and a significant part of the posterior arch of the vertebra. Neurocentral synchondrosis joints ossify and disappear between approximately six to nine years of age (Dimeglio et al., 2016).

The spine is approximately 24 cm at birth. The spine is approximately 67 cm in adults. The adult spine height is three times more than that of neonates. In adults, the cervical spine is approximately 11 cm, the thoracic spine is approximately 27 cm, the lumbar spine is approximately 17 cm, and the sacrum is approximately 12 cm (Akbarnia et al., 2022; Dimeglio et al., 2016).

## Conclusion

Knowing the normal growth of the spine and thoracic cage determines the intervention, the time of intervention, and the mode of intervention for the patient with scoliosis. It is possible to consider the growth of the thoracic cage independently of the growth of the spine. The thoracic cage and spine should be considered as a three-dimensional complex. It should be known that spinal and thoracic cage deformities can cause cardiac and lung problems. Knowing when and how the spine will grow is an indispensable part of treatment.

## References

Akbarnia, B. A., Thompson, G. H., Yazici, M., & El-Hawary, R. (Ed.). (2022). *The Growing Spine: Management of Spinal Disorders in Young Children*. Springer International Publishing. https://doi.org/10.1007/978-3-030-84393-9.

Bess, S., & Line, B. (2022). Embryology and anatomy: Spine/spinal cord. In *The Growing Spine: Management of Spinal Disorders in Young Children* (pp. 3-12). Springer.

Canavese, F., & Dimeglio, A. (2013). Normal and abnormal spine and thoracic cage development. *World Journal of Orthopedics*, *4*(4), 167-174. https://doi.org/10.5312/wjo.v4.i4.167.

Cheng, J. C., Leung, S. S. F., Chiu, B. S. K., Tse, P. W. T., Lee, C. W. Y., Chan, A. K. H., Xia, G., Leung, A. K. L., & Xu, Y. Y. Y. (1998). Can we predict body height from segmental bone length measurements? A study of 3,647 children. *Journal of Pediatric Orthopaedics*, *18*(3), 387-393.

Dimeglio, A. (2001). Growth in pediatric orthopaedics. *Journal of Pediatric Orthopaedics*, *21*(4), 549-555.

Dimeglio, A., & Canavese, F. (2020). The immature spine: Growth and idiopathic scoliosis. *Annals of Translational Medicine*, *8*(2), Article 2. https://doi.org/10.21037/atm.2019.11.134.

Dimeglio, A., Canavese, F., & Bonnel, F. (2016). Normal growth of the spine and thorax. *The growing spine: management of spinal disorders in young children*, 47-82.

Jarzem, P. F., & Gledhill, R. B. (1993). Predicting height from arm measurements. *Journal of Pediatric Orthopaedics, 13*(6), 761-765.

Khurjekar, K., & Kardile, M. (2019). Development of the Vertebral Column in EOS. In *The ASSI Monographs* (1st Edition). Thieme Verlag. https://doi.org/10.1055/b-0042-187399.

Moore, K. L., Dalley, A. F., & Agur, A. M. (2013). *Clinically oriented anatomy*. Lippincott Williams & Wilkins.

Nordin, M., & Frankel, V. H. (2001). *Basic biomechanics of the musculoskeletal system*. Lippincott Williams & Wilkins.

Tekelioğlu, M. (1992). Vertebra embriyolojisi. *Vertebra Ankara (Ege R): Türk Hava Kurumu Basımevi*, 15-19.

Yang, S., Andras, L. M., Redding, G. J., & Skaggs, D. L. (2016). Early-Onset Scoliosis: A Review of History, Current Treatment, and Future Directions. *Pediatrics, 137*(1). https://doi.org/10.1542/peds.2015-0709.

# Chapter 3

# Pathogenesis of EOS

**Ali Can Çiçek**[*]**, MD**
Department of Orthopedics and Traumatology, Agri Education and Research Hospital, Agri, Turkiye

## Abstract

Early-onset scoliosis is a disease characterized by lateral curvature of the spine diagnosed before the age of ten. The disease is divided into many subtypes such as congenital, syndromic, neuromuscular, and idiopathic. There is no definitively accepted theory that fully explains the pathogenesis of EOS. Connective tissue diseases, muscle and bone diseases, central and peripheral nervous system disorders, genetic disorders, molecular biological disorders, and platelet disorders may accompany EOS. Although the pathogenesis of EOS is not fully known, the multifactorial pathogenesis remains the most commonly view focused on. Melatonin deficiency, calmodulin deficiency, growth hormone deficiency, platelet disorders, central and peripheral nervous system maturation disorders, connective tissue disorders, low leptin levels, and musculoskeletal system diseases are listed among the most frequently accused multifactorial causes.

**Keywords:** pathogenesis, early-onset scoliosis, etiology

---

[*] Corresponding Author's Email: alicancicek36@hotmail.com.

In: Early Onset Scoliosis
Editor: Ahmed Majid Heydar
ISBN: 979-8-89113-600-7

## Introduction

Early-onset scoliosis (EOS) is a disease characterized by lateral curvature of the spine diagnosed before the age of ten. There may or may not be an underlying cause that triggers EOS. While thoracic curvature is seen in women, lumbar and thoracolumbar curvatures are common in men. When we look at the direction of the curve, the left side in the infantile period, the equal side in the juvenile period, and the right side in the adolescence period are dominant. Therefore, it is examined by dividing it into many subtypes. Although it is not possible to review all subtypes of the disease, it would be useful to categorize treatment modalities while being discussed.

Subtypes:

- Idiopathic (infantile (0-3 years), juvenile (4-10 years), adolescent (10 years or older))
- Congenital
- Syndromic (such as underlying connective tissue diseases)
- Neuromuscular (such as Spinal Muscular Atrophy)

There is no definitively accepted theory that fully explains the pathogenesis of EOS. The view that the disease is due to multifactorial causes is at the forefront. The role of genetic transition in the development of the disease among multifactorial causes cannot be ignored. EOS can be seen with many anomalies. There is no definitive judgment on whether EOS develops primary or secondary (Miller et al., 2005). Connective tissue diseases, muscle and bone diseases, central and peripheral nervous system disorders, genetic disorders, molecular biological disorders, and platelet disorders may accompany EOS (Dayer et al., 2013).

## Etiopathogenesis

### Idiopathic Scoliosis

Many studies on EOS have revealed genetic factors associated with the disease. Studies in twin patients with EOS showed significantly greater concordance with EOS in monozygotic patients than in dizygotic. In addition, while the risk of EOS in first-degree relatives of EOS patients is 11%, this risk decreases to 2% in second-degree relatives and 1% in third-degree relatives (Riseborough and Wynne-Davies, 1973). EOS is more common in girls than in boys. Therefore, it has been thought that the disease is associated with the X chromosome (Konieczny et al., 2013). It has been stated that it is related not only to the X chromosome, but also to chromosomes 6, 9, 16, and 17, which are autosomal genes. In addition, it is known that the family history of patients with EOS is 97% positive (Miller et al., 2005).

Melatonin, secreted by the pineal gland located in the middle region of the brain, is the hormone that regulates the sleep cycle and circadian rhythm. In a study on chickens, pinealectomized chickens had a scoliotic deformity and when melatonin supplementation was given, the rate of scoliosis decreased to 20%. It has been suggested that melatonin is not only responsible for the sleep cycle but also has an effect on the development of scoliosis. Furthermore, it has been observed in prospective clinical studies that melatonin deficiency negatively affects the prognosis of EOS (Machida et al., 1995; Machida et al., 2009).

Calmodulin is a biological molecule involved in muscle contractility, which is thought to play an important role in the etiopathology of EOS. In studies on calmodulin, the level calmodulin was found to be significantly higher in the paraspinal muscles located on the convex side of the deformity compared to the other side (Acaroglu et al., 2009).

Retinoic acid, a derivative of vitamin A, plays an important role in somitogenesis, apart from visual function, cell proliferation and differentiation, growth of bone tissue, immune function, and tumor suppressor gene activation. It is thought that its deficiency may be an important factor in the development of EOS as a result of disruption in the steps of somitogenesis (Dayer et al., 2013).

There are data showing that low leptin levels affect the central nervous system of patients with EOS, especially affecting the growth of the neural and resulting in deformities in the spine as a result of tensions (Clark et al., 2014).

The biomechanical basis of EOS etiopathogenesis is explained by the Hueter-Volkmann law. While the mechanical compression force acting on the growth plates impairs skeletal growth, skeletal growth increases in the case of a decrease in the mechanical compression force. The other biomechanical condition is anterior spinal overgrowth, which can further aggravate pre-existing curvature due to the effect of gravity. It also accelerates the progression of primary curvature, intervertebral disc disorders, and increased stiffness of the intervertebral disc (Drevelle et al., 2010).

According to Wolff's law, it has been proven that bone tissue remodels over time in response to mechanical loads. Bone density is proportional to the magnitude of stress. Trabecular bone orientation is associated with stress orbits. When bone tissue is subjected to forces above or below the normal range of stress and strain, bone tissue remodels in response to stress. While increasing stress/tension stimulates bone formation when it increases, it causes bone destruction when it decreases. For example, osteopenia is observed in the vertebral bodies in cases with rigid posterior spinal instrumentation. As a result of the stress force resulting from soft tissue deformation in scoliosis, it causes asymmetric growth in the vertebral body and intervertebral discs (Akbarnia et al., 2022).

In his study, Stokes suggested that the progression of spinal deformity takes the form of a vicious circle, causing wedging in the vertebral body due to asymmetric stress forces applied on the apophyseal endplates (Stokes, 2007).

In the study by Will et al., while the intervertebral disc and endplates are responsible for the deformity in the spine during the high growth potential period of the skeleton, the bone tissue is held responsible at the end of growth. From this study, the amount of correction made by growth modulation depends on the remaining growth potential at each vertebral level (Will et al., 2009). Based on these data, a mathematical system was developed that estimates the annual growth per level used to calculate the number of vertebral levels and the time required to correct the spinal deformity using asymmetric spine growth (Dimeglio and Canavese, 2020).

Dorsal tension forces acting on the spine are blamed for the formation of rotational instability. In a study on pigs with open-growth cartilage, asymmetric growths in the cartilage around the neuronal center of the vertebrae cause spinal curvatures similar to EOS (Castelein et al., 2005).

When the spinal curvature mechanism is activated, the bone mass of the vertebrae is affected for multifactorial reasons. Vitamin D deficiency, calcium deficiency, disorders in melatonin secretion, anomalies in calmodulin levels, and many other unspecified causes further increase the curvature of the spine (Machida et al., 2009).

When the etiopathogenesis of EOS cases is examined, there are studies that systematically explain the multifactorial causes that interact with each other and that are claimed to have effects on the development of the deformity, apart from biomechanical and genetic causes. There are studies showing that low-fat mass, low non-fat body mass, low leptin level, and high adiponectin level are effective in the formation of spinal curvature.

The low leptin level observed in the blood level as a result of low-fat mass in late childhood causes an independent and irregular growth of the neurological system and skeletal system. As a result, it causes a decrease in the joint range of motion due to axonal stresses and adhesion. In addition, leptin plays an important role in brain development outside of the spinal canal. In many studies investigating the effect of leptin on brain development, mice with small brain sizes have shown improvements in brain size after leptin administration. As it is known, leptin is also involved in myelination. It has been suggested that the thickness of the cerebral cortex is thinner than the normal morphology in adolescents with low leptin levels (Chu et al., 2008; Clark et al., 2014; Hashimoto et al., 2013; Stephan and Swick, 1999).

When the bone and neurological parts of the central nervous systems of patients with EOS were examined, differences were found compared to the normal morphology. When brain structures were examined, volumetric differences in the brain were observed in the MRI images. In the study, where the balance system was also affected, it was observed that especially the cerebellar tonsils were more caudal than the normal morphology. In addition, bone differences such as wider foramen magnum were detected. It was observed that the ratio of the spinal cord to vertebral column widths, which is used to evaluate the disproportionate growth of the spinal canal and spinal will, was lower than normal values. Changes detected in this ratio indicate that neuro-osseous growth is an irregular and disproportionate growth. Therefore, it can cause tension or compression in the vertebral canal (Dayer et al., 2013).

## Congenital Scoliosis

The embryological damage that occurs between the 4th and 8th weeks of intrauterine is blamed for the etiology of congenital scoliosis (Arlet et al., 2003). In the intrauterine 4th week, the precartilage, which is the first of the 3 main steps of ossification in the formation of the vertebral body, migrates to form mesenchymal roots (Blevins et al., 2018). The growth of the last stage of ossification continues until the age of 25, and the development of the vertebral column begins and completes its elongation. The formation of spinal development and the segmentation of the intrauterine embryo are in a permanent state against teratogens during these periods. Damages occurring in this period may result in postpartum scoliosis (Blevins et al., 2018).

Congenital scoliosis (CS) is an early-onset scoliosis subtype that is congenital and includes the malformation of the vertebrae. It is seen at a rate of 1/1000 in the population and is mostly sporadic (Hedequist and Emans, 2007). It is clinically examined as three subtypes; formation failure (type I), segmentation failure (type II), and combined form (type III) (Hedequist and Emans, 2007). Especially kyphoscoliosis arising from the hemi vertebrae and localized anterior defects of the vertebral bodies are usually sporadic (Wynne-Davies, 1975).

In a study examining familial transmission, it was shown that the risk of neural tube defects increased in families with CS (Connor et al., 1987). In a large-scale study of 1250 patients with CS, only 13 patients were found to have vertebral defects in their first- or second-degree relatives (Winter 1988). Considering these studies, it is thought that the etiology of CS is due to multifactorial causes including genetic and/or environmental factors.

Considering the genetic causes, it has been shown that the interaction of signaling pathways such as vertebral bodies, FGF, Wnt, and Notch develops in the embryo (Pourquie, 2011). In a study on mice, it was found that it can increase the development of CS through abnormal FGF signaling as a result of pregnancy hypoxia (Sparrow et al., 2006).

It has also been determined that Notch pathway genes such as MESP2, LFNG, HES7, and JAG1 are involved in normal vertebral development and segmentation (Pourquie, 2011). Spondylocostal dysostosis (SCD) associated with mutations in these genes, congenital vertebral malformations, scoliosis (Sparrow et al., 2006; Whittock et al., 2004; Sparrow et al., 2010), and Alagille syndrome (L. Li et al., 1997).

Again, in studies on the gene, single nucleotide polymorphisms (SNPs) in the PAX1, DLL3, and TBX6 genes were found to be associated with CS (Erol et al., 2004; Fei et al., 2010; Giampietro et al., 2005; Giampietro et al., 2006).

In addition to genetic causes such as polymorphism, 16p11.2 deletion has been described. Of all the genes covered by the 16p11.2 region, which has an important role in somitogenesis, TBX6 was suspected to be the driver gene for the CS phenotype. An increased risk of CS has been shown in cases with heterozygosity for 16p11.2 deletion or TBX6 null mutations (Wu et al., 2015).

Besides deletion 16p11.2, deletion 17p11.2 (Z. Li et al., 2015), deletion 20p11 (Williams et al., 2011) and deletion 22q11.2 (Homans et al., 2020), and other genetic changes have been shown to be associated with CS.

## Syndromic Scoliosis

Connective tissue disorders such as Marfan syndrome (MFS) and Ehlers-Danlos syndrome (EDS) and neurofibromatosis, Prader-Willi syndrome, other skeletal dysplasias are early-onset scoliosis-associated mendelian transition syndromes.

Marfan syndrome, autosomal dominant, including skeletal system disorders (tall, disproportionately long limbs, mild to moderate joint laxity, anterior chest wall deformity, and scoliosis), cardiovascular system disorders (aortic root dilatation and dissection), and ocular system disorders (ectopia lentis). It is a hereditary disease. It occurs as a result of a mutation of FBN1 encoding Fibrillin-1. There are two variants; protein-truncating variants and missense variants (Sakai et al., 2016).

In particular, Marfanoid-progeroid-lipodystrophy syndrome (MPLS) is a rare subtype of MFS with severe lipodystrophy in addition to its typical phenotype. MPLS occurs due to heterozygous mutations affecting exon 65/66 of the FBN1 gene. These mutations perform the potential dominant-negative mechanism in which the mutated allele disrupts the normal allele's function (Lin et al., 2020).

Ehlers-Danlos syndrome is a heterogeneous connective tissue disorder characterized by skin hyper extensibility, joint hypermobility, and tissue fragility. There are 13 EDS subtypes (Malfait et al., 2017). Genetic testing and identification of variants are required to confirm the diagnosis of its subtypes. Kyphoscoliotic EDS, the most common subtype of EDS, is clinically associated with individuals with scoliosis as a result of bi-allelic loss of function of PLOD1, a gene encoding the lysyl hydroxylase enzyme required for collagen formation (Dembure et al., 1984).

In addition, EOS, Down syndrome (21 trisomy) (Sherman et al., 2007), DiGeorge syndrome (22q11.2 deletion) (Kobrynski and Sullivan, 2007), and Prader-Willi syndrome (15q11 deletion) (Holm et al., 1993) and may accompany chromosomal disorders and microdeletion/microduplication syndromes.

## Neuromuscular Scoliosis

Scoliosis commonly accompanies various neuromuscular diseases such as muscular dystrophy, cerebral palsy, and myelodysplasia. Neuromuscular scoliosis causes insufficiency in the muscles stabilizing the spinal canal as a result of the insufficiency of the upper or lower motor neurons, and as a result, deformities occur in the spine (Reames et al., 2011). We can examine the diseases that cause neuromuscular scoliosis as a group, as in the Table 1. In these neuromuscular diseases, scoliosis occurs at an early age and progresses rapidly during or after growth. NMS is associated with a significantly higher rate of complication and economic burden than other types of scoliosis (Murphy et al., 2006).

**Table 1.** Neuromuscular scoliosis: common associated disorders

| Category | Disease |
|---|---|
| Upper Motor Neuron | Cerebral palsy<br>Friedreich's ataxia<br>Charcot-Marie-Tooth disease<br>Roussy-Le´vy disease<br>Trauma<br>Syringomyelia |
| Lower Motor Neuron | Poliomyelitis<br>Werdnig-Hoffmann disease<br>Spinal muscular atrophy<br>Trauma<br>Kugelberg-Welander disease<br>Riley-Day syndrome (dysautonomia) |
| Mixed | Myelodysplasia<br>Myelomeningocele<br>Medullary lesion |
| Myopathy | Duchenne muscular dystrophy<br>Facioscapulohumeral dystrophy<br>Limb-girdle dystrophy<br>Arthrogryposis<br>Congenital hypotonia |

Although a disorder, injury, or neuromuscular disease is generally blamed for the etiology, its exact pathophysiology has not yet been scientifically proven (McCarthy, 1999). Damage to the tone or sensory feedback mechanism along the spinal nerve tract causes biomechanical muscle imbalances. As a result, deformation occurs in the spine. For example, asymmetric paraplegia is common in myelodysplasia and cerebral palsy due to imbalances in muscle strength (McCarthy, 1999). Imbalances in the paraspinal muscles enable the rapid development and progression of deformities in the spine. Spinal deformities can be seen not only as a result of the disease but also after the treatment. For example, in the treatment of spasticity in patients with cerebral palsy, the spinal deformity may develop after the selective removal of abnormal sensory nerve fibers that transmit information from the skeletal muscle to the spinal cord (Turi and Kalen, 2000).

In the treatment of NMS, the only non-surgical treatment option is the brace, except in exceptional cases. Exceptionally, steroids are used in non-surgical treatment to prevent the onset and progression of scoliosis in patients with Duchenne muscular dystrophy caused by a mutation in the DMD gene (Alman et al., 2004). Duchenne muscular dystrophy occurs as a result of homozygous or hemizygous mutation of DMD, an X chromosome-located gene encoding dystrophin. The result of a deficit in dystrophin protein causes muscle wasting and severe muscle weakness. As a result, pseudo hypertrophy occurs, which leads to progressive scoliosis. In a study conducted on these patients, it was proven that glucocorticoid corticosteroid therapy provides a short-term improvement in muscle strength and function (Manzur et al., 2008). Improvement in muscle strength may reduce the progression of scoliosis and the need for spinal surgery (Alman et al., 2004). In addition to steroid therapy, Vyondys 53 (golodirsen), an antisense oligonucleotide of phosphorodiamidate morpholino oligomer, has been used in the treatment of DMD (Heo, 2020).

Another disease that is caused by RYR1 mutations and clinically associated with scoliosis characterized by muscle weakness is the central core disease. These patients may develop malignant hyperthermia after general anesthesia and result in death (Manning et al., 1998).

In addition to myopathies, scoliosis can be seen in many neurological disorders. For example, Charcot-Marie-Tooth (CMT) disease, which is an inherited neuropathy and scoliosis, is seen in approximately 30% of cases (Karol and Elerson, 2007). Its subtypes have been associated with many genes, and the combinatorial effects of these genes increase the burden of the disease (Gonzaga-Jauregui et al., 2015). Mutations such as homozygous duplication of CMT1A and heterozygous triplication of CMT1A increase the probability of EOS (Matsunami et al., 1992).

## Conclusion

EOS is a common disease among spinal diseases and is more prevalent in women than in men. While thoracic curvature is seen in women, lumbar and thoracolumbar curvatures are common in men. When we look at the direction of the curve, the left side in the infantile period, the equal side in the juvenile period, and the right side in the adolescence period are dominant. Although the pathogenesis of EOS is not fully known, multifactorial pathogenesis remains the most commonly view focused on. Melatonin deficiency, calmodulin deficiency, growth hormone deficiency, platelet disorders, central and peripheral nervous system maturation disorders, connective tissue disorders, low leptin levels, and musculoskeletal system diseases are listed among the most frequently accused multifactorial causes.

## References

Acaroglu, E. A., Akel, I., Alanay, A., Yazici, M., & Marcıcio, R. I. (2009). Comparison of the melatonin and calmodulin in paravertebral muscle and platelets of patients with or without adolescent idiopathic scoliosis. *Spine (Phila Pa 1976)*, 34(18), 659-663. https://doi.org/10.1097/brs.0b013e3181a3c7a2.

Akbarnia, B. A., Thompson, G. H., Yazici, M., & El-Hawary, R. (2022). *The Growing Spine* (3rd ed., p. 36). Springer Nature Switzerland AG. https://doi.org/10.1007/978-3-030-84393-9.

Alman, B. A., Raza, S. N., & Biggar, W. D. (2004). Steroid treatment and the development of scoliosis in males with Duchenne muscular dystrophy. *J Bone Joint Surg Am*, 86(3), 519–24. https://doi.org/10.2106/00004623-200403000-00009.

Arlet, V., Odent, T., & Aebi, M. (2003). Congenital scoliosis. *Eur Spine J*, 12, 456–63. https://doi.org/10.1007/s00586-003-0555-6.

Blevins, K., Battenberg, A., & Beck, A. (2018). Management of Scoliosis. *Adv Pediatr*, 65(1), 249-266. https://doi.org/10.1016/j.yapd.2018.04.013.

Castelein, R. M., Van Dieen, J. H., & Smit, T. H. (2005). The role of dorsal shear forces in the pathogenesis of adolescent idiopathic scoliosis: A hypothesis. *Med Hypotheses*, 65(3), 501-508. https://doi.org/10.1016/j.mehy.2005.03.025.

Chu, E. C., Lam, W. M., Ng, B. K., Tze-Ping, L., Lee, K. M., Guo, X., Cheng, J. C., Burwell, R. G., Dangerfield, P. H., Jaspan, T. (2008). Relative shortening and functional tethering of the spinal cord in adolescent scoliosis: Results of asynchronous neuro-osseous growth, summary of an electronic focus group debate of the IBSE. *Scoliosis*, 3, 8. https://doi.org/10.1186/1748-7161-3-8.

Clark, E. M. T., Harding, I., Hutchinson, J., Nelson, I., Deanfield, J. E. (2014). Association between components of body composition and scoliosis: A prospective cohort study reporting differences identifiable before the onset of scoliosis. *J Bone Miner Res*, 29(8), 1729–1736. https://doi.org/10.1002/jbmr.2207.

Connor, J. M., Connor, A. N., Connor, R. A., Tolmie, J. L., Yeung, B., Goudie, D. (1987). Genetic aspects of early childhood scoliosis. *Am J Med Genet*, 27(2), 19–24. https://doi.org/10.1002/ajmg.1320270220.

Dayer, R., Haumont, T., Belaieff, W., Lascombes, P. (2013). Idiopathic scoliosis: Etiological concepts and hypotheses. *J Child Orthop*, 7(1), 11-16. https://doi.org/10.1007/s11832-012-0458-3.

Dembure, P. P., Priest, J. H., Snoddy, S. C., Elsas, L. J. (1984). Genotyping and prenatal assessment of collagen lysyl hydroxylase deficiency in a family with Ehlers-Danlos syndrome type VI. *Am J Hum Genet*, 36(4), 783–790. https://doi.org/10.1016/0026-0495(87)90155-7.

Dimeglio, A., & Canavese, F. (2020). The immature spine: Growth and idiopathic scoliosis. *Ann Transl Med*, 8(2), 22. https://doi.org/10.21037/atm.2019.11.134.

Drevelle, X., Lafon, Y., Ebermeyer, E., Dubousset, J., & Skalli, W. (2010). Analysis of idiopathic scoliosis progression by using numerical simulation. *Spine*, 35(10), 407-412. https://doi.org/10.1097/brs.0b013e3181cb46d6.

Erol, B., Tracy, M. R., Dormans, J. P., Zackai, E. H., Maisenbacher, M. K., O'Brien, M. L., Turnpenny, P. D., Kusumi, K. (2004). Congenital scoliosis and vertebral malformations: Characterization of segmental defects for genetic analysis. *J Pediatr Orthop*, 24(6), 674–82. https://doi.org/10.1097/01241398-200411000-00015.

Fei, Q., Wu, Z., Wang, H., Zhou, X., Wang, N., Ding, Y., Wang, Y., Qiu, G. (2010). The association analysis of TBX6 polymorphism with susceptibility to congenital scoliosis in a Chinese Han population. *Spine (Phila Pa 1976)*, 35(9), 983–9888. https://doi.org/10.1097/brs.0b013e3181bc963c.

Giampietro, P. F., Raggio, C. L., Reynolds, C. E., Ghebranious, N., Burmester, J. K., Glurich, I., Rasmussen, K., McPherson, E., Pauli, R. M., Shukla, S. K., Merchant, S., Jacobsen, F. S., Faciszewski, T., Blank, R. D. (2006). DLL3 as a candidate gene for vertebral malformations. *Am J Med Genet A*, 140(22), 2447–2453. https://doi.org/10.1002/ajmg.a.31509.

Giampietro, P. F., Raggio, C. L., Reynolds, C. E., Shukla, S. K., McPherson, E., Ghebranious, N., Jacobsen, F. S., Kumar, V., Faciszewski, T., Pauli, R. M., Rasmussen, K., Burmester, J. K., Zaleski, C., Merchant, S., David, D., Weber, J. L., Glurich, I., Blank, R. D. (2005). An analysis of PAX1 in the development of vertebral malformations. *Clin Genet*, 68(5), 448–453. https://doi.org/10.1111/j.1399-0004.2005.00520.x.

Gonzaga-Jauregui, C., Harel, T., Gambin, T., Kousi, M., Griffin, L. B., Francescatto, L., Ozes, B., Karaca, E., Jhangiani, S. N., Bainbridge, M. N., Lawson, K. S., Pehlivan, D., Okamoto, Y., Mancias, M., Slavotinek, A., Reitnauer, P. J., Goksungur, M. T., Thomas, S. M., Crawford, O., Koenig, M., Willer, J., Flores, B. N., Pediaditrakis, I., Wojciech, O. U. Wiszniewski, W., Parman, Y., Antonellis, A., Muzny, D. M., Katsanis, N., Battaloglu, E., Boerwinkle, E., Gibbs, R. A., Lupski, J. R. (2015). Exome sequence analysis suggests that genetic burden contributes to phenotypic variability and complex neuropathy. *Cell Rep*, 12(7), 1169–1183. https://doi.org/10.1016/j.celrep.2015.07.023.

Hashimoto, R., Matsumoto, A., Udagawa, J., Hioki, K., Otani, H. (2013). Effect of leptin administration on myelination in ob/ob mouse cerebrum after birth. *Neuroreport*, 24(1), 22-29. https://doi.org/10.1097/wnr.0b013e32835ba875.

Hedequist, D., Emans, J. (2007). Congenital scoliosis: A review and update. *J Pediatr Orthop*, 27(1), 106–116. https://doi.org/10.1097/bpo.0b013e31802b4993.

Heo, Y. A. (2020). Golodirsen: First approval. *Drugs*, 80(3), 329–333. https://doi.org/10.1007/s40265-020-01267-2.

Holm, V. A., Cassidy, S. B., Butler, M. G., Hanchett, J. M., Greenswag, L. R., Whitman, B. Y., Greenberg, F. (1993). Prader-Willi syndrome: Consensus diagnostic criteria. *Pediatrics*, 91(2), 398–402. https://doi.org/10.1542/peds.91.2.398.

Homans, J. F., de Reuver, S., Heung, T., Silversides, C. K., Houben, M. L., McDonald-McGinn, D. M., Kruyt, M. C., Castelein, R. M., Bassett, A. S. (2020). The role of 22q11.2 deletion syndrome in the relationship between congenital heart disease and scoliosis. *Spine J*, 20, 956. https://doi.org/10.1016/j.spinee.2020.01.006.

Karol, L. A., Elerson, E. (2007). Scoliosis in patients with Charcot-Marie-Tooth disease. *J Bone Joint Surg Am*, 89(7), 1504–1510. https://doi.org/10.2106/jbjs.f.01161.

Kobrynski, L. J., Sullivan, K. E. (2007). Velocardiofacial syndrome, DiGeorge syndrome: The chromosome 22q11.2 deletion syndromes. *Lancet*, 370(9596), 1443–1452. https://doi.org/10.1016/s0140-6736(07)61601-8.

Konieczny, M. R., Senyurt, H., & Krauspe, R. (2013). Epidemiology of adolescent idiopathic scoliosis. *J Child Orthop*, 7(1), 3-9. https://doi.org/10.1007/s11832-012-0457-4.

Li, L., Krantz, I. D., Deng, Y., Genin, A., Banta, A. B., Collins, C. C., Qi, M., Trask, B. J., Kuo, W. L., Cochran, J., Costa, T., Pierpont, M. E. M., Rand, E. B., Piccoli, D. A., Hood, L., Spinner, N. B. (1997). Alagille syndrome is caused by mutations in human Jagged1, which encodes a ligand for Notch1. *Nat Genet*, 16(3), 243–251. https://doi.org/10.1038/ng0797-243.

Li, Z., Shen, J., Liang, J., Sheng, L. (2015). Congenital scoliosis in Smith-Magenis syndrome: A case report and review of the literature. *Medicine (Baltimore)*, 94(17), e705. https://doi.org/10.1097/md.0000000000000705.

Lin, M., Liu, Z., Liu, G., Zhao, S., Li, C., Chen, W., Akdemir, Z. C., Lin, J., Song, X., Wang, S., Xu, Q., Zhao, Y., Wang, L., Zhang, Y., Yan, Z., Liu, S., Chen, Y., Zuo, Y., Yang, X., Sun, T., Yang, X. Z., Niu, Y., Li, X., You, W., Qiu, B., Ding, C., Liu, P., Zhang, S., Carvalho, C. M. B., Posey, J. E., Qiu, G., Lupski, J. R., Wu, Z., Zhang, J., Wu, N. (2020). Genetic and molecular mechanism for distinct clinical phenotypes conveyed by allelic truncating mutations implicated in FBN1. *Mol Genet Genomic Med*, 08(1), 1023. https://doi.org/10.1002/mgg3.1023.

Machida, M., Dubousset, J., Imamura, Y., Iwaya, T., Yamada, T., Kimura, J. (1995). Role of melatonin deficiency in the development of scoliosis in pinealectomised chickens. *J Bone Joint Surg*, 77(1), 134-1138. https://doi.org/10.1302/0301-620x.77b1.7822371.

Machida, M., Dubousset, J., Yamada, T., Kimura, J. (2009). Serum melatonin levels in adolescent idiopathic scoliosis prediction and prevention for curve progression- a prospective study. *J Pineal Res*, 46(3), 344-348. https://doi.org/10.1111/j.1600-079x.2009.00669.

Malfait, F., Francomano, C., Byers, P., Belmont, J., Berglund, B., Black, J., Bloom, L., Bowen, J. M., Brady, A. F., Burrows, N. P., Castori, M., Cohen, H., Colombi, M., Demirdas, S., De Backer, J., De Paepe, A., Fournel-Gigleux, S., Frank, M., Ghali, N., Giunta, C., Grahame, R., Hakim, A., Jeunemaitre, X., Johnson, D., Juul-Kristensen, B., Kapferer-Seebacher, I., Kazkaz, H., Kosho, T., Lavallee, M. E., Levy, H., Mendoza-Londono, R., Pepin, M., Pope, F. M., Reinstein, E., Robert, L., Rohrbach, M., Sanders, L., Sobey, G. J., Van Damme, T., Vandersteen, A., Van Mourik, C.,

Voermans, N., Wheeldon, N., Zschocke, J., Tinkle, B. (2017). The 2017 international classification of the Ehlers-Danlos syndromes. *Am J Med Genet C Semin Med Genet*, 175(1), 8–26. https://doi.org/10.1002/ajmg.c.31552.

Manning, B. M., Quane, K. A., Ording, H., Urwyler, A., Tegazzin, V., Lehane, M., O'Halloran, J., Hartung, E., Giblin, L. M., Vaughan, P., Censier, K., Bendixen, D., Comi, G., Heytens, L., Monsieurs, K., Fagerlund, T., Wolz, W., Heffron, J. J. A., Muller, C. R., McCarthy, T. V. (1998). Identification of novel mutations in the ryanodine-receptor gene (RYR1) in malignant hyperthermia: Genotype-phenotype correlation. *Am J Hum Genet*, 62(3), 599–609. https://doi.org/10.1086/301748.

Manzur, A. Y., Kuntzer, T., Pike, M., Swan, A. (2008). Glucocorticoid corticosteroids for Duchenne muscular dystrophy. *Cochrane Database Syst Rev*, 1, CD003725. https://doi.org/10.1002/14651858.cd003725.pub2.

Matsunami, N., Smith, B., Ballard, L., Lensch, M. W., Robertson, M., Albertsen, H., Hanemann, C. O., Muller, H. V., Bird, T. D., White, R., Chance, P. F. (1992). Peripheral myelin protein-22 gene maps in the duplication in chromosome 17p11.2 associated with Charcot-Marie-Tooth 1A. *Nat Genet*, 176-179. https://doi.org/10.1038/ng0692-176.

McCarthy, R. E. (1999). Management of neuromuscular scoliosis. *Orthop Clin North Am*, 30, 435–449. https://doi.org/10.1016/s0030-5898(05)70096-1.

Miller, N. H., Justice, C. M., Marosy, B., Doheny, K. F., Pugh, E., Zhang, J., Dietz, H. C. 3rd, Wilson, A. F. (2005). Identification of candidate regions for familial idiopathic scoliosis. *Spine*, 30(10), 1181-1187. https://doi.org/10.1097/01.brs.0000162282.46160.0a.

Murphy, N. A., Firth, S., Jorgensen, T., Young, P. C. (2006). Spinal surgery in children with idiopathic and neuromuscular scoliosis. What's the difference? *J Pediatr Orthop*, 26(2), 216–20. https://doi.org/10.1097/01.bpo.0000206516.61706.6e.

Pourquie, O. (2011). Vertebrate segmentation: From cyclic gene networks to scoliosis. *Cell*, 145(5), 650–663. https://doi.org/10.1016/j.cell.2011.05.011.

Reames, D. L., Smith, J. S., Fu, K.-M. G., Polly, D. W., Ames, C. P., Berven, S. H., Perra, J. H., Glassman, S. D., McCarthy, R. E., Knapp, D. R., Heary, R., Shaffrey, C. I. (2011). Complications in the surgical treatment of 19,360 cases of pediatric scoliosis: A review of the Scoliosis Research Society Morbidity and Mortality database. *Spine*, 36, 1484–1491. https://doi.org/10.1097/brs.0b013e3181f3a326.

Riseborough, E. J., & Wynne-Davies, R. (1973). A genetic survey of idiopathic scoliosis in Boston, Massachusetts. *J Bone Joint Surg*, 55(5), 974-982. https://doi.org/10.2106/00004623-197355050-00006.

Sakai, L. Y., Keene, D. R., Renard, M., De Backer, J. (2016). FBN1: The disease-causing gene for Marfan syndrome and other genetic disorders. *Gene*, 591(1), 279–921. https://doi.org/10.1016/j.gene.2016.07.033.

Sherman, S. L., Allen, E. G., Bean, L. H., Freeman, S. B. (2007). Epidemiology of down syndrome. *Ment Retard Dev Disabil Res Rev*, 13(3), 221–227. https://doi.org/10.1002/mrdd.20157.

Sparrow, D. B., Sillence, D., Wouters, M. A., Turnpenny, P. D., Dunwoodie, S. L. (2006). Mutation of the LUNATIC FRINGE gene in humans causes spondylocostal dysostosis with a severe vertebral phenotype. *Am J Hum Genet*, 78, 28–37. https://doi.org/10.1086/498879.

Sparrow, D. B., Sillence, D., Wouters, M. A., Turnpenny, P. D., Dunwoodie, S. L. (2010). Two novel missense mutations in HAIRY-AND-ENHANCER-OF-SPLIT-7 in a family with spondylocostal dysostosis. *Eur J Hum Genet*, 18(6), 674-649. https://doi.org/10.1038/ejhg.2009.241.

Stephan, C. M., Swick, A. G. (1999). A role for leptin in brain development. *Biochem Biophys Res Commun*, 256(3), 600-602. https://doi.org/10.1006/bbrc.1999.0382.

Stokes, I. A. (2007). Analysis and simulation of progressive adolescent scoliosis by biomechanical growth modulation. *Eur Spine J*, 16(10), 1621–1628. https://doi.org/10.1007/s00586-007-0442-7.

Turi, M., & Kalen, V. (2000). The risk of spinal deformity after selective dorsal rhizotomy. *J Pediatr Orthop*, 20, 104–107. https://doi.org/10.1097/01241398-200001000-00021.

Whittock, N. V., Sparrow, D. B., Wouters, M. A., Sillence, D., Ellard, S., Dunwoodie, S. L., Turnpenny, P. D. (2004). Mutated MESP2 causes spondylocostal dysostosis in humans. *Am J Hum Genet*, 74(6), 1249–54. https://doi.org/10.1086/421053.

Will, R. E., Stokes, I. A., Qiu, X., Walker, M. R., Sanders, J. O. (2009). Cobb angle progression in adolescent scoliosis begins at the intervertebral disc. *Spine (Phila Pa 1976)*, 34(25), 2782–2786. https://doi.org/10.1097/BRS.0b013e3181c11853.

Williams, P. G., Wetherbee, J. J., Rosenfeld, J. A., Hersh, J. H. (2011). 20p11 deletion in a female child with panhypopituitarism, cleft lip and palate, dysmorphic facial features, global developmental delay, and seizure disorder. *Am J Med Genet A*, 155(1), 186–191. https://doi.org/10.1002/ajmg.a.33763.

Winter, R. B. (1988). Congenital scoliosis. *Orthop Clin North Am*, 19(2), 395–408. https://doi.org/10.1016/s0030-5898(20)30319-9.

Wu, N., Ming, X., Xiao, J., Wu, Z., Chen, X., Shinawi, M., Shen, Y., Yu, G., Liu, J., Xie, H., Gucev, Z. S., Liu, S., Yang, N., Al-Kateb, H., Chen, J., Zhang, J., Hauser, N., Zhang, T., Tasic, V., Liu, P., Su, X., Pan, X., Liu, C., Wang, L., Shen, J., Shen, J., Chen, Y., Zhang, T., Zhang, J., Choy, K. W., Wang, J., Wang, Q., Li, S., Zhou, W., Guo, J., Wang, Y., Zhang, C., Zhao, H., An, Y., Zhao, Y., Wang, J., Liu, Z., Zuo, Y., Tian, Y., Weng, X., Sutton, V. R., Wang, H., Ming, Y., Kulkarni, S., Zhong, T. P., Giampietro, P. F., Dunwoodie, S. L., Cheung, S. W., Zhang, X., Jin, L., Lupski, J. R., Qiu, G., Zhang, F. (2015). TBX6 null variants and a common hypomorphic allele in congenital scoliosis. *N Engl J Med*, 372(4), 341–350. https://doi.org/10.1056/nejmoa1406829.

Wynne-Davies, R. (1975). Congenital vertebral anomalies: Aetiology and relationship to spina bifida cystica. *J Med Genet*, 12(3), 280–288. https://doi.org/10.1136/jmg.12.3.280.

# Chapter 4

# Classification of Early - Onset Scoliosis (C-EOS)

**Anar Alakbarov[1,*], MD**
**and Vusala Garayeva[2], MD**
[1]Department of Orthopedics and Traumatology, Nakhchivan Diagnostic-Treatment Center, Nakhchivan, Azerbaijan
[2]Department of Radiology, Nakhchivan Diagnostic-Treatment Center, Nakhchivan, Azerbaijan

## Abstract

Early-onset scoliosis (EOS) is a spinal deformity that may be idiopathic or derived from congenital anomalies, syndromes, or neuro-muscular disorders. A multi-center group containing experienced spine surgeons developed a classification for early-onset scoliosis. The group defines early onset scoliosis as "scoliosis with onset less than the age of ten years, regardless of etiology." The participants were evaluated and commentated on some variables such as cobb angle, etiology, kyphosis, age, progression, curve flexibility, chest wall abnormalities, other co-morbidities, pulmonary function, nutritional status, ambulatory ability, mental function, and bone quality to determine valid variables to make classification more accurate. After the overall evaluation, they decided that five parameters would be best for classification. *1- Age* (as continuous prefix), *2- Etiology* (as congenital/structural – C, neuromuscular – M, Syndromic – S, and Idiopathic –I), *3- Major curve angle* (up to 20 degrees, 20-50, 51-90 and more than 90 degrees), *4- Kyphosis* (up to 20 degrees, 20-50 and more than 50 degrees) and *5- Annual progression ratio (APR)* (up to 10 degrees, 10-20 and more than

* Corresponding Author's Email: opr.dr.anar@hotmail.com.

In: Early Onset Scoliosis
Editor: Ahmed Majid Heydar
ISBN: 979-8-89113-600-7

20 degrees). This is a recent classification, but it still has two significant 'phases' to complete and become a reliable and valid classification system.

**Keywords:** classification, early-onset scoliosis, vertebral deformity, abnormal spinal curve

## Introduction

To understand and classify early-onset scoliosis (EOS), it is necessary to have an overview of the historical and chronological flow of the subject of scoliosis.

The term "scoliosis" in rough meaning connotes "bending" in the Ancient Greek language. It is one of the oldest known medical conditions as a vertebral deformity with abnormal spinal curves (Figure 1). Hippocrates described the normal curves of the spine in an understandable manner in his books *On articulations* and *Mochlikon*. He also classified five groups of spine disease due to etiology, the clinical manifestations, and gave recommendations for the management of the disease in his treatise On Articulations. Hippocrates introduces five groups of spinal diseases as:

- Concussion ("seisis"), which means burst fractures,
- Fractures of the spinous processes
- Dislocations of the vertebrae
- Kyphosis as a result of the disease (non-traumatic) or spinal injury (traumatic), and
- Scoliosis (Withington et al., 1927).

Hippocrates described most of the spinal diseases, but he did not classify scoliosis.

Many classification systems on scoliosis and on this topic have been developed since his time.

According to etiological factors, scoliosis is classified as Idiopathic, Paralytic, and Congenital (Figure 2). Idiopathic scoliosis means (idios "one's own" and pathos "suffering," idiopathy means approximately "a disease of its own kind") its pathogenesis is poorly understood and accepted genetic and hereditary causes expose scoliosis (Shakil et al., 2014).

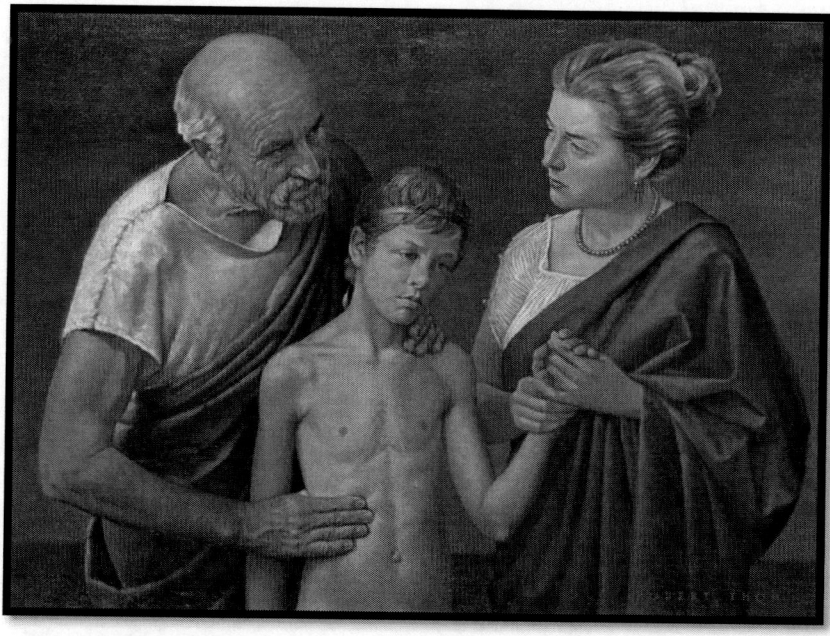

**Figure 1.** Painting of Hippocrates – "Father of Medicine" (examining the inclined head on the left-side and the right lower thoracal bump) by Robert A. THOM in 1958.

| | |
|---|---|
| Idiopathic | Infantile (0 to 3 years) |
| | Juvenile (3 to 10 years) |
| | Adolescent (10 to 18 years) |
| | Adult (above 18 years) |
| Congenital | Osteopathic |
| | Neuropathic |
| Paralytic | Neuropathic |
| | Myopathic |

**Figure 2.** Etiological classification of scoliosis (types and subtypes), (Shakil et al., 2014).

Initially, in 1950, Ponseti and Friedman used "the Early Onset Scoliosis – EOS" term to describe idiopathic scoliosis in patients less than 10 years of age

(Ponseti & Friedman, 1950). The authors determined that the prognosis is worse under 10 years of age than older patients. James sub-classified idiopathic scoliosis into age groups infantile (≤3 years), juvenile (4–9 years), and adolescent (10 years to maturity) in 1954 (James et al., 1959). In other words, early-onset scoliosis contains the infantile and juvenile part of idiopathic scoliosis.

Patients with EOS carry the risk of pulmonary dysfunction, even causing death due to the high risk of spinal deformity progression. The EOS treatment is highly complicated and challenging because children with EOS are heterogeneous, often have a complex medical condition, and need multiple continuous surgeries. Early vertebral fusion surgery was performed until recently for severe progressive EOS that corrected scoliosis, but spinal growth restriction resulted in poor respiratory outcomes. The current treatment goal of EOS is to provide relatively normal growth of the open vertebral epiphyses by controlling the spinal deformity to maintain normal lung development and pulmonary function. To reach a consensus on the treatment of EOS, patients need to be classified and performed acceptable interventions (Yang et al., 2016).

In 2014, the Children Spine Study Group (CSSG) and the Growing Spine Study Group (GSSG) described EOS as any deformity of the spine that begins before ten years old, regardless of etiology. Highly experienced spinal surgeons in pediatric spine surgery of those study groups also published the Classification of EOS (C-EOS) in the same year as the Scoliosis Research Society (SRS) (Williams et al., 2014; Vitale et al., 2016).

Classification systems have many advantages for physicians that guide management and treatment, facilitate research projects and are precious tools because the constitution is a common language for optimizing communication between physicians.

For adult and adolescent idiopathic scoliosis, many classification systems have been described in the literature. But the complexity of pathology seen in –early-onset scoliosis does not allow the classification of the disease. Moreover, current classification systems do not let us evaluate the outcomes of treatment without or with arthrodesis. Doing surgery not based on any classification and detrimental treatment outcomes has been convincing spine surgeons to avoid arthrodesis in the immature individual's spine. The scientific world and the orthopedic literature needed a classification system designed exclusively for the immature spine that adapted to the growing spine associated with clinical development. Eventually, this classification was designed and published, but the –development and maturation 'phases' of the system still continue (Williams et al., 2014).

## Classification

The Children Spine Study Group (CSSG), Growing Spine Study Group (GSSG), and the Scoliosis Research Society (SRS) groups were using the fracture classification framework of Audige et al. for creating the classification of EOS (Audigé et al., 2005). A three-phase development framework was created (Figure 3). Fifteen surgeons from thirteen institutions with at least ten years of EOS patient treating experience were chosen to contribute to EOS classification creation. The geographic spread of the participants and the complexity of early-onset scoliosis were the most challenging part of preparing the classification system. The research group has solved these obstacles with live Internet webinars, e-mail discussions, and in-person group meetings (Williams et al., 2014).

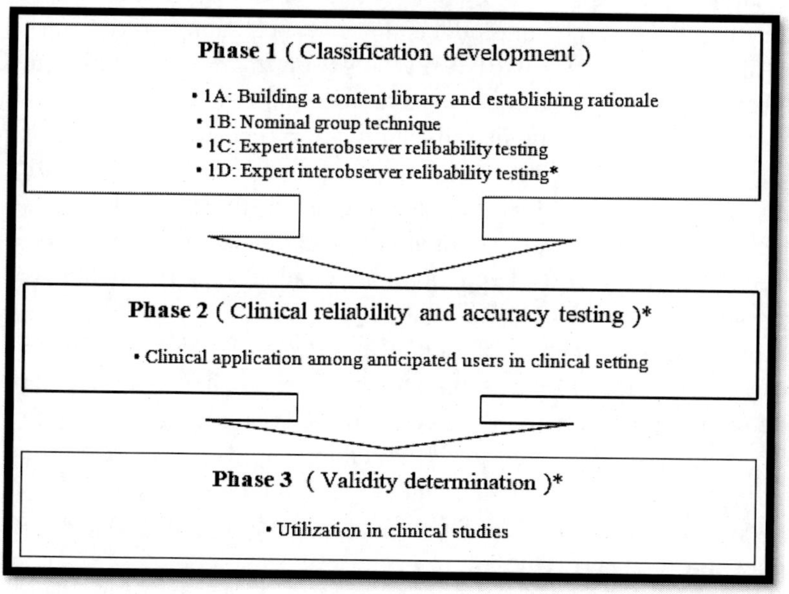


*Future studies will describe the remaining phase of the classification system (Reprinted and redisigned from Vitale et al., 2016).

**Figure 3.** Developmental framework and validation of the C-EOS.

Participants completed a survey of Phase 1 A variables and rated them from number 0 to 3 according to the Likert scale. To determine group-wide importance, each variable content validity ratio was calculated (Figure 4).

| Variable | Not Useful | Useful | Essential | CVR |
|---|---|---|---|---|
| Major curve angle | 0 | 1 | 13 | 0.86 |
| Etiology | 0 | 3 | 11 | 0.57 |
| Kyphosis | 0 | 3 | 11 | 0.57 |
| Age | 5 | 0 | 9 | 0.29 |
| Progression | 3 | 5 | 6 | −0.14 |
| Curve flexibility | 3 | 6 | 5 | −0.29 |
| Chest wall abnormalities | 2 | 8 | 4 | −0.43 |
| Other comorbidities | 3 | 8 | 3 | −0.57 |
| Pulmonary function | 3 | 8 | 3 | −0.57 |
| Nutritional status | 5 | 7 | 2 | −0.71 |
| Ability to walk | 2 | 11 | 1 | −0.86 |
| Mental function | 9 | 5 | 0 | −1.00 |
| Bone quality | 10 | 4 | 0 | −1.00 |

**Figure 4.** The table shows Variable Content Validity Rankings (CVR).

For all variables, the content validity ratio (CVR) was calculated and determined how essential an item is. In the primary survey, significant CVRs were major curve angle (0.86), etiology (0.57), and kyphosis (0.57), which satisfies the 5% level (i.e., exceed the chance expectation) (see Figure 4). The fourth highest-ranking CVR (0.29) was age, but there is no sufficient CVR significance threshold. Further discussions determined that age should be considered as a continuous classification prefix because age has important implications regarding patient management and outcomes. Flexibility and curve progression also did not meet the CVR threshold, but these two parameters were deemed important at the second meeting. Curve progression and flexibility were considered optional modifiers to be included at the discretion of the provider (Vitale et al., 2016).

When the classification of EOS was developed, 13 potential variables were identified; age, progression rate, kyphosis, cobb angle, and etiology ranked highest in relevance. It has been decided that the classification system should include a maximum of 4 variables. Spine progression rate and flexibility are optional modifiers, whereas age should be a continuous prefix. The group members decided on five factors in the ongoing evaluations and subsequent meetings (Figure 5).

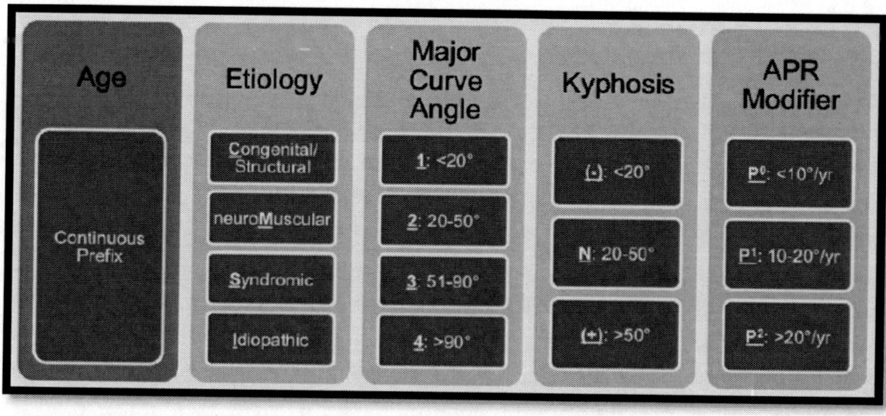


**Figure 5.** The classification of early-onset scoliosis (C-EOS) scheme developed by Williams et al., 2014.

## Age

It is as clear as glass that age has an important impact on the decision-making on treatment and the prognosis of patients with EOS. For now, participants decided to keep age as a continuous prefix, due to the variety of variables with EOS and the lack of studies in multiple age groups. We hope better evidence will be provided by future research for the structure of subgroups for the age prefix (Williams et al., 2014).

## Etiology

To guess EOS treatment outcomes and management of complications are directly related to etiology. The response to treatment and the severity of EOS are often determined by specific factors in a diagnosis. There are four types of etiologic factors that affect the destiny of EOS. The first factor is the congenital/structural etiology. It is marked as the letter 'C' in the classification system. The second is the neuromuscular factor, marked as 'M.' The third etiology is the syndromic factor, which is shown as 'S.' The fourth and last one is the idiopathic factor and is marked as 'I' in the classification system. In prioritized order, etiologic factors are listed from highest value to lowest value. The etiologic assignments should be listed from top to bottom when the etiology is mixed and unclear (Vitale et al., 2016).

## Major Curve Angle

The major curve of a deformed spine should be measured in the standing position radiography for gravity's effect on spine deformity. Firstly, cut points for subgroups based on the spine's major curve range were taken as a value for the management of early-onset scoliosis. After a group discussion, the value modification was performed for EOS. While the evaluation process, a consensus was accepted for the following ranges: 1st Group as below 20°, 2nd Group as between 20° - 50°, 3rd Group between 51° - 90°, and 4th Group above 90°. In addition, to provide a rough guideline for surgical or conservative management, the classification system developer group believes these subgroups may correlate with the outcomes various strategies in the treatment scoliosis. This hypothesis may be tested by future studies structured with the C-EOS (Williams et al., 2014, Vitale et al., 2016).

## Kyphosis

The C-EOS developer group defines kyphosis as the highest curve -Cobb angle on a sagittal plane between two levels. The group members also have a consensus that one of the essential factors is kyphosis in the early-onset scoliosis patients' evaluation. The literature shows that pediatric kyphosis measures differ from the angle of the adult and generally increase with age. According to this, the 20–50° range was selected as normokyphotic (*N*), with hyperkyphosis (+) and hypokyphosis (−) falling on either side. Also, note that hyperkyphosis is important in EOS patients because of the need to undergo growing-rod surgery. The next studies will investigate and validate the impact of kyphosis on the C-EOS schema and the effect on treatment results (Williams et al., 2014).

## Annual Progression Ratio (APR) Modifier (Optional)

The progression rate calculations between times t1 and t2 should be spaced at least six months apart.

$$APR\text{: } \{(\text{major curve at } t2) - (\text{major curve at } t1)\} \times \{12 \text{ months}/(t2 - t1)\}$$

## A Case Example of the C-EOS

A 5-year-old girl presents to the orthopedic clinic with congenital myopathy and at a presentation she had a 25° major spinal curve with 30° kyphosis. When she reached 9 years of age (48 months later), her main spinal curve had reached 73° with 45° kyphosis. The beginning C-EOS of the patient would be 5M2N. After 4 years of follow-up, her C-EOS would be *9M3NP*$_1$ (Annual Progression Rate: 48°/48 months = about 12° per year) (Doak, 2018).

## Conclusion

The classification of a medical condition (classification systems) guides physicians in categorizing pathology and determining treatment. Also, valid and updated classification systems are essential and critical components of the research project beyond providing a common language for physicians. Physicians may research and publish reliable and robust articles for evidence-based treatment guidelines in light of well-designed classification systems. Although many issues about idiopathic scoliosis are not well understood, many classifications have been developed for scoliosis. But there still needs to be a reliable classification of EOS, which is a relatively new concept in the literature. The current classification system was designed and developed recently but will come of age after completing the remaining phases and as long as sufficient research is done and articles are written on this subject. Additionally, it also has limitations; although formal consensus-building methods were used to create a classification system with content validity and reliability, the elements and cut-points included in the classification system are still largely based on the consensus of expert opinion because more data is needed to guide these decisions.

## References

Audigé, L., Bhandari, M., Hanson, B., & Kellam, J. (2005). A concept for the validation of fracture classifications. *Journal of Orthopaedic Trauma*, *19*(6), 404-409. https://doi.org/10.1097/01.bot.0000155310.04886.37.

Doak, J. (2018). Classification of Early-Onset Scoliosis. *Early Onset Scoliosis: A Clinical Casebook* (pp. 9-15). Springer. https://doi.org/10.1007/978-3-319-71580-3_2.

James, J. I. P., Lloyd-Roberts, G. C., & Pilcher, M. F. (1959). Infantile structural scoliosis. *The Journal of Bone and Joint Surgery. British volume*, *41*(4), 719-735. https://doi.org/10.1302/0301-620X.41B4.719.

Ponseti, I. V., & Friedman, B. (1950). Prognosis in idiopathic scoliosis. *JBJS*, *32*(2), 381-395.

Shakil, H., Iqbal, Z. A., & Al-Ghadir, A. H. (2014). Scoliosis: review of types of curves, etiological theories and conservative treatment. *Journal of back and musculoskeletal rehabilitation*, *27*(2), 111-115. https://doi.org/10.3233/bmr-130438.

Thom, R. A. (1958). *Hippocrates: medicine becomes a science*. [Detroit] Parke, Davis&Company 1958. Retrieved from https://collections.nlm.nih.gov/catalog/nlm:nlmuid-101651450-img.

Vitale, M. G., & Trupia, E. (2016). Classification of Early-Onset Scoliosis. In *The Growing Spine* (pp. 113 –121). Springer. https://doi.org/10.1007/978-3-662-48284-1_7.

Williams, B. A., Matsumoto, Hiroko, M. A., McCalla, D. J., Akbarnia, B. A., Blakemore, L. C., Betz, R. R., Flynn, J. M., Johnston, C. E., McCarthy, R. E., Roye, D. P., Skaggs, D. L., Smith, J. T., Snyder, B. D., Sponseller, P. D., Sturm, P. F., Thompson, G. H., Yazici, M., & Vitale, M. G. (2014). Development and initial validation of the Classification of Early-Onset Scoliosis (C-EOS). *JBJS*, *96*(16), 1359-1367. https://doi.org/10.2106/jbjs.m.00253.

Withington, E. T., Potter, P., & Smith, W. D. (Eds.). (1927). *Hippocrates Volume III* (Vol. 3). Loeb Classical Library.

Yang, S., Andras, L. M., Redding, G. J., & Skaggs, D. L. (2016). Early-onset scoliosis: a review of history, current treatment, and future directions. *Pediatrics*, *137*(1). https://doi.org10.1542/peds.2015-0709.

# Chapter 5

# Idiopathic Early - Onset Scoliosis

**Barış Can Kuzuca*, MD**
Department of Orthopedics and Traumatology, Çerkezköy State Hospital, Tekirdağ, Turkiye

## Abstract

Early-onset scoliosis (EOS) is a subgroup of scoliosis that is seen in patients between the 0-10 years old. 0-4 years cases are called infantile EOS and 4-10 years cases as juvenile EOS. EOS is the pathology of the growing spine. It can be caused by neuromuscular, congenital, or syndromic disorders. Idiopathic EOS is an exclusive diagnostic type and has no association with any causal agents or other diseases. The exact pathophysiology is not enlightened, and multifactorial causes are being held responsible for idiopathic cases. The incidence is higher in the male population and the curvature is mostly seen in the low-thoracic spine and on the left-sided. Restriction of the intra-thoracic cavity is the most important cause of morbidity and cor pulmonale and right heart failure is the most common cause of death. Mehta classification and Cobb angles are important in determining the treatment option. Treatments include bracing and casting for mild cases and surgery for severe cases. Surgery options include Distraction Based systems (Growing Rods), Vertical Expandable Prosthetic Titanium Rib (VEPTR) devices, Guided Growth, and Compression Based implants. Currently, the gold standard surgery is the growing rods. The most important complications are mechanical, deterioration of spinal balance, infection, and neurological.

**Keywords:** idiopathic early onset scoliosis, growing spine, growing rods

---

* Corresponding Author's Email: dr.bariskuzuca@gmail.com.

In: Early Onset Scoliosis
Editor: Ahmed Majid Heydar
ISBN: 979-8-89113-600-7

## Introduction

Early-onset scoliosis (EOS) is a complex pathology for the curvature of the spine. It is a general term for a medical condition which affects the growth of the spine. It was first described by Ponseti and Friedman in 1950 for patients younger than 10 years of age. In 1954, it is categorized by James according to age of onset: infantile (≤3 years), juvenile (4-9 years), and adolescent (over 10 years) (Ruiz et al., 2022). Dickson also sub-grouped idiopathic scoliosis into early-onset (0-5 years) and late-onset (over 5 years). These age groups were formulated according to increases in growth velocity periods. EOS has been used for children younger than 5 years of age. Patients with scoliosis and younger than 5 years of age has higher risk for complications, especially cardiothoracic problems (Samdani & Betz, 2009).

Infantile EOS is a structural deformity of the spine in which the spine has apical malrotation and wedging. Patients present with in first 3 years. Infantile cases represent %1 of idiopathic scoliosis. The male to female ratio is approximately 3. Curves are usually left-sided (Samdani & Betz, 2009). The curve in the low thoracic region is mostly observed. The rate of left-sided convexity varies between %56 to %93 (Fernandes & Weinstein, 2007). Intrauterine molding and postnatal pressure are held responsible for pathogenesis. Juvenile EOS occurs between 4-10 years of age. The prevalence is estimated between %8-16 of EOS. The male to female ratio is changed from 2-4. Curves are also left-sided.

In 2014, Vitale also categorized the ethology besides the age of onset as idiopathic, neuromuscular, congenital and syndromic. Neuromuscular scoliosis is caused by nervous system disorders such as cerebral palsy, spinal cord trauma, Rett syndrome, Freidrich's ataxia, and myopathic scoliosis is seen in muscular dystrophy or arthrogryposis. Congenital scoliosis is caused by at least one bony anomaly of the spine, which is present at birth, such as hemivertebrae, wedged vertebrae, block vertebrae or unilateral bars. Congenital malformation conditions such as asphyxiating, thoracic dysplasia (Jeune's syndrome) and spondylocostal dysostosis (Jarcho-Levin syndrome) also cause scoliosis. Syndromic scoliosis is observed in genetically disordered individuals such as Marfan's, Ehlers-Danlos, Down Syndrome, Prader-Willi, Neurofibromatosis, etc. (El-Hawary & Akbarnia, 2015).

Idiopathic EOS is a spinal deformity with no causal agents or associations with other diseases (Williams et al., 2014). The exact pathophysiology is not enlightened, and multifactorial causes are being held responsible for idiopathic cases.

## Clinic

A detailed history, physical examination and radiographic assessment are required for an accurate diagnosis and treatment. The onset of symptoms and progression of the curve should be questioned. Prenatal and birth histories should be taken. Family history is important for genetic disorders (Thorsness et al., 2015).

On physical examination, the clinician should evaluate the curve, asymmetry if present, neurologic status, and development of the patient. According to the age, the motor development of the patient should be evaluated and noted. Normal and if present pathological reflexes such as Hoffman and Babinski and general muscle tone should be examined (Thorsness et al., 2015). For syndromic patients, special marks should be examined such as ear, eye, and finger deformities and skin lesions.

For an infant with scoliosis, an anteroposterior and lateral full spine radiograph should be obtained first. Vertebral anomalies may be detected if present. If there are any congenital anomalies, computed tomography should be obtained to observe them in detail. Otherwise, routine direct graphs are adequate for following-up curve progression. The development of compensatory curves is accepted as a poor prognosis. Progressive curves can be thoracic, double major or lumbar. Thoracic curves tend to resolve spontaneously (Fernandes & Weinstein, 2007). In order to avoid misdiagnosing, the same position should be preserved during imaging. In the infant population, Mehta's Rib-Vertebral Angle Difference (RVAD) should be measured. If the difference is ≥20 degrees, the progression of the curve has a high probability (Samdani & Betz, 2009). In a series of 73 patients, %92 resolved cases have RVAD <20° (Ceballos et al., 1980). For juvenile patients, the Cobb angle is used more frequently. For patients with neurological symptoms or candidates for surgical treatment, a spinal cord MRI should be obtained.

In EOS, it is a fact that the early age of onset is correlated with the progression of the final curvature. Progressive curves usually cause significant deformity and these results in cardiopulmonary deterioration that causes increased mortality. Normal development of lungs ends at the average age of 8. Limitation of the thorax cavity before this age causes a depravation of the thorax volume. The increased mortality is explained by restrictive lung diseases and cardiovascular complications. The most important mortality reasons are pulmonary hypertension, cor pulmonale and right heart failure. The compression of the pulmonary tissue finally causes these conditions. Lung hypoplasia and associated vessels and cardiac problems are seen in severe cases. Karol et al. found a direct association between thoracic height and pulmonary function. As the thoracic spine shortens, forced vital capacity (FVC) decreases and the risk of incidence of restrictive pulmonary diseases increases (Karol et al., 2008). It is found that the minimum thoracic height should be 22cm at skeletal maturity in order avoid developing restrictive lung disease (FVC <50%).

## Treatment

Nowadays, the treatment of EOS is mainly surgical. Even though technological advancements provide better surgical techniques and outcomes, non-surgical treatment options are also available. Before the invention of spinal implants, the only treatment choice for EOS was only casting or bracing. However, it was shown that long-term casting causes the deformation of the ribs.

According to Mehta criteria, curves with <25° Cobb angles and <20° Rib-Vertebral Angle Difference (RVAD) have a low risk of advancement. Patients should be followed up conservatively and re-checked every 4 to 6 months. No further bracing or casting is needed for these patients. In a study of 9 patients, curves <20° resolved spontaneously before two years of age (James, 1954).

Bracing is an alternative non-surgical treatment method for mild progressive curves. However, its effectiveness is still not widely accepted in EOS. Serial casting is a growth-preserving technique that does not compromise the thoracic spine growth or pulmonary development (Hardesty et al., 2018). It can be used for cases that curve >25°, with >10° progression or RVAD>20°. Compliance is a significant problem in pediatric patients. Currently, most braces that are used are derived from custom-moulded thoracolumbosacral orthosis. According to Mehta, it is demonstrated that infantile, low magnitudes, and unresolved progressive curves can be resolved with casting. To avoid the risks of surgery and early spine fusion, casting has proven to be a safer method for idiopathic EOS. The cast or brace is applied to the patient under anesthesia and traction. The casts are changed every 8-12 weeks. Casting should be continued until complete correction of the curve is achieved or rib-cage symmetry and derotation of the apical vertebra are restored. If casting cannot control the curve, surgery should be planned (Hardesty et al., 2018). For non-idiopathic EOS, casting is only applied in patients that surgery should be delayed.

For most severe idiopathic EOS, the primary treatment is surgery. The first implant for scoliosis was introduced by Paul Harrington in the 1960s that applies distraction across the concavity of the curve. However, since rods improved curves in a 2-dimensional plane, this technique resulted in flat-back deformity. Furthermore, the complication of implant failure was high.

Historically, the spinal fusion technique was applied after distraction. Early spinal fusion was applied to prevent the progression of curvature. However, it is found that spinal fusion limited intrathoracic volume. In patients with thoracic fusion, mean FVC at adult age decreased by 40% compared with a normal population. Furthermore, fusion caused the crankshaft phenomenon. The crankshaft phenomenon is a rotational deformity caused by the growth of the anterior spinal column, whereas the posterior growth is disturbed surgically.

Nowadays, modern growth-friendly implants are developed for the treatment of EOS. These implants both control curve progression and preserve normal thorax capacity. These implants are classified into 3 groups as distraction-based, guided growth and compression-based types.

Distraction-based implants, which are most commonly used in the treatment of EOS, apply traction to the spinal column and expandable rods are mainly used. These allow the growth of the spine and provide stability and deformity correction (Hardesty et al., 2018). The rods are periodically lengthened to maintain the curve correction. In traditional systems, only proximal and distal anchors are used on the spine. The area between the anchors is not fused. This allows growth and motion of the spine. Lengthening is performed every 6 months. In a clinical series of dual-growing rods, mean curve correction is reported from 82° to 38° at first surgery (Akbarnia et al., 2005). Complications are reported up to %58 and increase approximately %24 for each additional surgery (Bess et al., 2010).

Vertical Expandable Prosthetic Titanium Rib (VEPTR) devices are used in patients with primary thoracic insufficiency syndrome. The aim of the surgery is to maximize thoracic volume and correct the asymmetrical and deformed thoracal cavity by lengthening the constricted hemithorax. This is obtained by transverse opening wedge thoracostomy of the concave side (Campbell Jr et al., 2004). In VEPTR, ribs are used as anchors. There are also hybrid systems available that use both ribs and the proximal-distal spine to obtain better stability for implants. These implants avoid fusion at the spines and provide better thoracic expansion. Stress on the spine is also reduced with these systems. In a series of 27 patient, VEPTR corrects scoliosis from 74° to 49° and thoracic spine height increased by a mean of 7,1 mm/year (Campbell

Jr et al., 2004). However, distraction-based implants have high rates of complication. The most common complications are anchor failure and rod breakage. Posterior implants may cause kyphosis. Wound complications are also common. Multiple surgeries to lengthen also cause deep wound infection. The Growing Spine Profiler (GSP) is another distraction system that is used in the treatment of EOS. It does not contain a magnetic mechanism, so it needs consecutive surgery and anesthesia in order to achieve maximum benefit (Figure 1 and Figure 2). New Magnetically Controlled Growing Rods (MAGEC) provide lengthening of rods without the need for surgery. The rods are surgically placed similar to TGR constructs, using screws and/or hooks for fixation. Mean corrections of 27° to 36° have been reported with similar complications between MAGEC and growing rod constructs (Hardesty et al., 2018). In a series of 47 patients, the infection rate was significantly lower due to less need for surgery, although implant-related complications were higher in this group (Teoh et al., 2016).

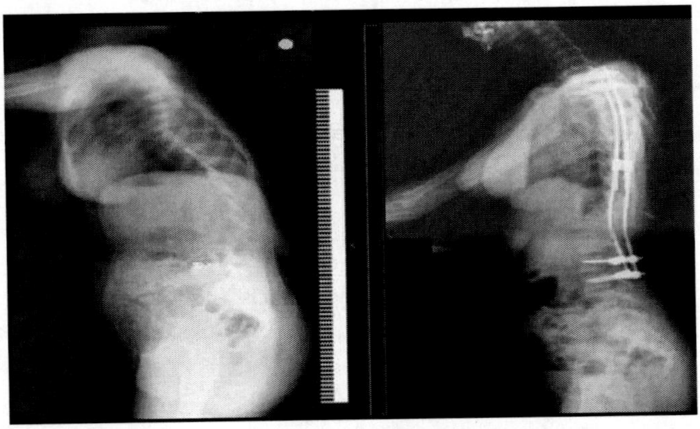

**Figure 1.** Preoperative and postoperative sagittal X-ray of a 9-year-old female patient with EOS.

Guided growth implants provide the growth of the spine along the path of implants. The main benefits of these systems are lower infection rates, hardware failure, less necessity for re-surgery and less exposure to anesthesia (Ruiz et al., 2022). The original guided growth implants used Luque wires wrapped around the lamina of each vertebra, which were wrapped around straight rods. The growth of the vertebra is not limited by the wires sliding along the rods as the vertebra grows. In a 5-patient series, the mean correction rate was reported from 60° to 21° (Ouellet, 2015). A more recent type of guided growth implant has been developed by Richard McCarthy and is called the 'Shilla technique'. In this technique, the pedicle screws are fixed to the apex of the curve with proximal and distal gliding screws. To avoid spontaneous fusion, minimal subperiosteal dissection is used. In a 40-patient series, the mean correction was reported from 69° to 25° at 5 years follow-up (McCarthy & McCullough, 2015).

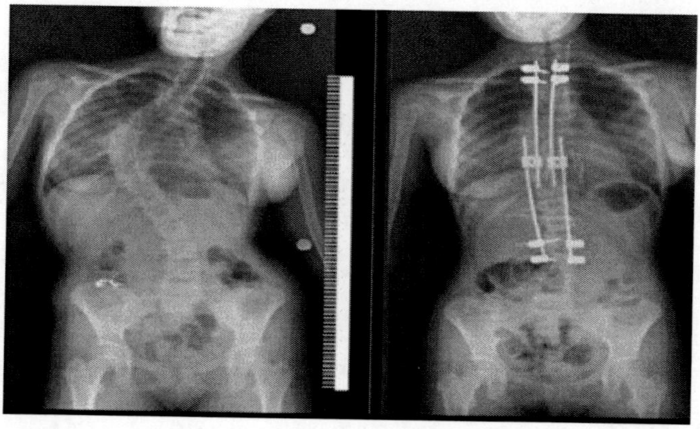

**Figure 2.** Preoperative and postoperative coronal X-ray of a 9-year-old female patient with EOS.

Compression-based implants provide the stopping of the growth of the convex site and correct scoliosis. This correction is accomplished by placing staples, tethers, or other devices across the growth plates of the vertebrae from an anterior approach on the convex side of the scoliosis. In a study of 28 patients, the success rate of stapling was reported as %77,7 for <35° and %85,7 for <20° (Betz et al., 2010). The consensus is that vertebral stapling may be a treatment alternative for mildly idiopathic curves with severity in children with substantial remaining growth (Sturm et al., 2014). In some cases, overcorrection may cause an opposite direction curve development (Yang et al., 2016). Thoracic kyphosis is a contraindication since anterior growth modulation increases kyphosis.

Overall, the main complications are mechanical, deterioration of spinal balance, infection and neurological. Implant failure or rod breakage occurs in at least %15 of cases. It mainly occurs near the connection points and in cases of hyper-kyphosis. The deterioration is mostly seen as Proximal Junctional Kyphosis (PJK). PJK is a non-physiologic, sagittal plane angulation that occurs due to spinal instrumentation. Rib and spine-based systems are more prone to cause PJK. Surgical Site Infection (SSI) is also a common complication in scoliosis surgery due to multiple surgical needs.

Neuromuscular disorders, incontinence, malnutrition and obesity are increased risk factors. The most common responsible microorganisms are the species of *Staphylococcus Aureus* and *Pseudomonas*. With the new technological advancements, the incidence of neurological complications decreased rapidly. Intra-operative monitoring has been recommended mainly during the implantation or changing of rods or instrumentation (Cunin, 2015).

## Conclusion

EOS is a complex pathology for the curvature of the spine which affects the 0-10 year population. It is an important public health issue since it causes both cosmetic and systemic effects in children. EOS can be caused by neuromuscular, congenital, or syndromic disorders. Idiopathic cases have no association with any causal agents or other diseases. The exact pathophysiology is not fully understood, and multifactorial causes are being held responsible. Restriction of the intra-thoracic cavity is the most important cause of morbidity and cor pulmonale and right heart failure is the most common cause of death. So, the most important aim of the treatment is to prepare enough thoracic space for healthy lung development. Treatment modalities include bracing and casting for mild cases and surgery for severe cases. Surgery options include Distraction Based systems (Growing Rods), Vertical Expandable Prosthetic Titanium Rib (VEPTR) devices, Guided Growth and Compression Based implants. the most important complications are mechanical, deterioration of spinal balance, infection and neurological. Under the new technological developments, more effective devices with fewer complications will be introduced.

## References

Akbarnia, B. A., Marks, D. S., Boachie-Adjei, O., Thompson, A. G., & Asher, M. A. (2005). Dual growing rod technique for the treatment of progressive early-onset scoliosis: A multicenter study. *Spine, 30*(17S), S46-S57.

Bess, S., Akbarnia, B. A., Thompson, G. H., Sponseller, P. D., Shah, S. A., El Sebaie, H., Adjei, O. B., Karlin, L. I., Canale, S., Kochert, C. P., & Skaggs, D. L. (2010). Complications of growing-rod treatment for early-onset scoliosis: Analysis of one hundred and forty patients. *JBJS, 92*(15), 2533-2543.

Betz, R. R., Ranade, A., Samdani, A. F., Chafetz, R., D'Andrea, L. P., Gaughan, J. P., Asghar, J., Grewal, H., & Mulcahey, M. J. (2010). Vertebral body stapling: A fusionless treatment option for a growing child with moderate idiopathic scoliosis. *Spine, 35*(2), 169-176.

Campbell Jr, R. M., Smith, M. D., Mayes, T. C., Mangos, J. A., Willey-Courand, D. B., Kose, N., Pinero, R. F., Alder, M. E., Duong, H. L., & Surber, J. L. (2004). The effect of opening wedge thoracostomy on thoracic insufficiency syndrome associated with fused ribs and congenital scoliosis. *JBJS, 86*(8), 1659-1674.

Ceballos, T., Ferrer-Torrelles, M., Castillo, F., & Fernandez-Paredes, E. (1980). Prognosis in infantile idiopathic scoliosis. *JBJS, 62*(6), 863-875.

Cunin, V. (2015). Early-onset scoliosis – current treatment. *Orthopaedics & Traumatology: Surgery & Research, 101*(1), S109-S118. https://doi.org/10.1016/j.otsr.2014.06.032.

El-Hawary, R., & Akbarnia, B. A. (2015). Early onset scoliosis-time for consensus. *Spine Deformity, 2*(3), 105-106. https://doi.org/10.1016/j.jspd.2015.01.003.

Fernandes, P., & Weinstein, S. L. (2007). Natural history of early onset scoliosis. *JBJS, 89*(suppl_1), 21-33. https://doi.org/10.2106/JBJS.F.00754.

Hardesty, C. K., Huang, R. P., El-Hawary, R., Samdani, A., Hermida, P. B., Bas, T., Balioğlu, M. B., Gurd, D., Pawelek, J., McCarthy, R., Zhu, F., Luhmann, S., & Growing Spine Committee of the Scoliosis Research Society. (2018). Early-onset scoliosis: Updated treatment techniques and results. *Spine Deformity, 6*(4), 467-472. https://doi.org/10.1016/j.jspd.2017.12.012.

James, J. I. P. (1954). Idiopathic scoliosis: The prognosis, diagnosis, and operative indications related to curve patterns and the age at onset. *The Journal of Bone and Joint Surgery. British Volume, 36*(1), 36-49.

Karol, L. A., Johnston, C., Mladenov, K., Schochet, P., Walters, P., & Browne, R. H. (2008). Pulmonary function following early thoracic fusion in non-neuromuscular scoliosis. *JBJS, 90*(6), 1272-1281. https://doi.org/10.2106/JBJS.G.00184.

McCarthy, R. E., & McCullough, F. L. (2015). Shilla growth guidance for early-onset scoliosis: Results after a minimum of five years of follow-up. *JBJS, 97*(19), 1578-1584. https://doi.org/10.2106/JBJS.N.01083.

Ouellet, J. (2011). Surgical technique: Modern Luque trolley, a self-growing rod technique. *Clinical Orthopaedics and Related Research®, 469*, 1356-1367. https://doi.org/10.1007/s11999-011-1783-4.

Ruiz, G., Torres-Lugo, N. J., Marrero-Ortiz, P., Guzmán, H., Olivella, G., & Ramírez, N. (2022). Early-onset scoliosis: A narrative review. *EFORT Open Reviews, 7*(8), 599. https://doi.org/10.1530/EOR-22-0040.

Samdani, A. F., & Betz, R. R. (2009). Infantile and juvenile idiopathic scoliosis. In Errico, T. J., Lonner, B. S., Moulton, A. W. (Eds.), *Surgical Management of Spinal Deformities* (pp. 89-96). Philadelphia, PA: WB Saunders/Elsevier. ISBN: 9781437719567.

Sturm, P. F., Anadio, J. M., & Dede, O. (2014). Recent advances in the management of early onset scoliosis. *Orthopedic Clinics, 45*(4), 501-514. https://doi.org/10.1016/j.ocl.2014.06.010.

Teoh, K. H., Winson, D. M., James, S. H., Jones, A., Howes, J., Davies, P. R., & Ahuja, S. (2016). Do magnetic growing rods have lower complication rates compared with conventional growing rods? *The Spine Journal, 16*(4), S40-S44.

Thorsness, R. J., Faust, J. R., Behrend, C. J., & Sanders, J. O. (2015). Nonsurgical management of early-onset scoliosis. *JAAOS-Journal of the American Academy of Orthopaedic Surgeons, 23*(9), 519-528. https://doi.org/10.5435/JAAOS-D-14-00019.

Williams, B. A., Matsumoto, H., McCalla, D. J., Akbarnia, B. A., Blakemore, L. C., Betz, R. R., Flynn, J. M., Johnston, C. E., McCarthy, R. E., Roye jr, D. P., Skaggs, D. L., Smith, J. T., Snyder, B. D., Sponseller, P. D., Sturm, P. F., Thompson, G. H., Yazici, M., & Vitale, M. G. (2014). Development and initial validation of the Classification of Early-Onset Scoliosis (C-EOS). *JBJS, 96*(16), 1359-1367. https://doi.org/10.2106/JBJS.M.00253.

Yang, S., Andras, L. M., Redding, G. J., & Skaggs, D. L. (2016). Early-onset scoliosis: A review of history, current treatment, and future directions. *Pediatrics, 137*(1). https://doi.org/10.1542/peds.2015-0709.

# Chapter 6

# Congenital Scoliosis

**Ömer Cahit Çıtır*, MD**
Department of Orthopedics and Traumatology,
Şırnak Şehit Aydoğan Aydın State Hospital, Şırnak, Turkiye

## Abstract

Deformities that occur as a result of anomalies developing in the spine during the intrauterine period are called congenital scoliosis. Congenital scoliosis is the most common congenital deformity of the spine. It may develop due to an anomaly occurring in one or both of the segmentation and formation stages of the spine developmental stages. Although genetic factors are thought to have an effect on the etiology of congenital scoliosis, it is accepted that many factors have an effect on the process. The diagnosis of the disease is made by physical examination and direct radiographs. However, with the help of developing technology, intrauterine diagnosis is also possible. Congenital scoliosis is classified according to the localization and shape of the deformity. When congenital scoliosis is detected, it is necessary to accurately predict the clinical course of the disease in order to decide on treatment. The probable course of the deformity should be determined, and if progress is expected in the deformity, treatment selection should be made by predicting the rate of progression. Conservative and surgical methods have been described in treatment. The treatment decision should be planned specifically for the patient, taking into account the conditions specific to the patient and the current deformity.

**Keywords:** scoliosis, congenital deformity, spine

---

* Corresponding Author's Email: omrctr@hotmail.com.

In: Early Onset Scoliosis
Editor: Ahmed Majid Heydar
ISBN: 979-8-89113-600-7

## Introduction

Deformities that occur as a result of anomalies developing in the spine during the intrauterine period are called congenital scoliosis. Congenital scoliosis is the most common congenital deformity of the spine (Arlet et al., 2003). It may develop due to an anomaly occurring in one or both of the segmentation and formation stages of the spine developmental stages.

Although the true prevalence of congenital scoliosis is thought to be higher because asymptomatic cases are not diagnosed, it is a common deformity with a known prevalence of 13-51/1000 (Giampietro, 2012). While congenital scoliosis may remain asymptomatic, it may show a course that can lead to severe complications affecting many systems. It may cause neurological, cardiac, pulmonary, and renal complications (Pahys & Guille, 2018).

In the embryological period, the formation of the spine begins with the formation of the notochord. At the end of this stage, somites must fuse properly in front and behind the notochord in order to develop into a healthy vertebra. In later stages, with the formation of intervertebral disc structures, the vertebrae separate, and spinal nerves emerge from between them (Kaplan et al., 2005). An abnormality that may occur at these stages is thought to cause congenital scoliosis. These processes correspond to the 5th and 8th weeks of gestation (Arlet et al., 2003; Grimme & Castillo, 2007). Since an abnormality that develops during the embryological period has the potential to affect the spine as well as other systems, it is possible to see abnormalities in other organ systems together with congenital scoliosis (Pahys & Guille, 2018).

Although genetic factors are thought to have an effect on the etiology of congenital scoliosis, it is accepted that many factors have an effect on the process. It is known that congenital scoliosis is not hereditary (Arlet et al., 2003). In addition to genetic factors, factors such as valproic acid, hyperthermia, alcohol, and hypoxia during pregnancy are effective in the etiology (Grimme & Castillo, 2007; Hedequist & Emans, 2007; Li et al., 2015).

Physical examination and imaging methods are used in the diagnosis of the disease. The treatment algorithm is determined according to the degree of deformity and the possible progression potential (Burnei et al., 2015).

## Diagnosis

The diagnosis of the disease is made by physical examination and direct radiographs. However, with the help of developing technology, intrauterine diagnosis is also possible (Arlet et al., 2003). Computed tomography (CT) is an secondary examination to understand the structure of the spinal bones and deformity in detail (Hedequist & Emans, 2007; 2003). Magnetic resonance imaging (MRI) is used to examine possible spinal anomalies and supporting structures in detail (Pahys & Guille, 2018) (Figure 1).

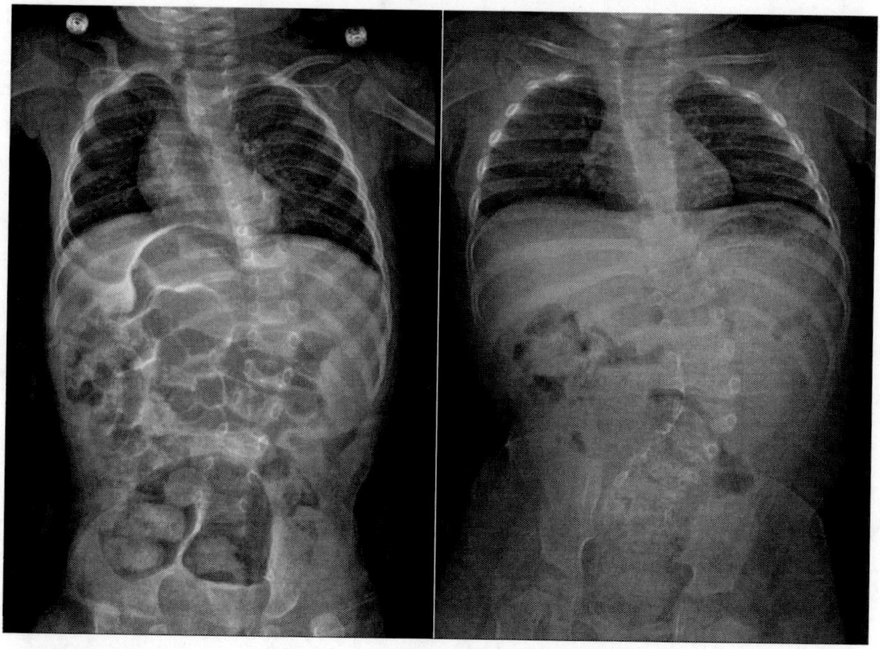

**Figure 1.** Direct X-ray images of two different congenital scoliosis patients aged 2 years.

## Classification

Congenital scoliosis is classified according to the localization and shape of the deformity (Hedequist & Emans, 2007; 2004) (Figure 2). It is observed that segmentation and formation defects often co-occur on the basis of the deformity (Johal et al., 2016).

The formation defect can be seen as complete or incomplete. Wedge vertebra pathology occurs as a result of an incomplete formation defect. As a result of a complete formation defect, hemivertebra pathology is observed. Although there is a bilateral pedicle in the wedge vertebra, there is an asymmetrical height (Hedequist & Emans, 2007). In hemivertebra pathology, there is a single pedicle, half the vertebral body, and half the lamina (Johal et al., 2016). The most common cause of congenital scoliosis is the hemivertebra (Feng et al., 2016). Hemivertebrae are divided into three groups according to the absence, partiality, or completeness of the intervertebral disc structure (Johal et al., 2016; Pahys & Guille, 2018). These are called unsegmented, fully segmented, and partially segmented hemivertebrae. When the formation pathology affects more than one vertebra, the location of the pathological vertebrae determines the prognosis of the deformity. If the hemivertebrae are on the same side of the spine, the potential to progress in the deformity is high, and asymmetrical growth is observed (Hedequist & Emans, 2007). When pathological vertebral structures are on opposite sides of the spine, they show lower progression potential and tend to balance each other. This situation is called hemimetameric shift (Shawen et al., 2002).

In case of segmentation defect, it is important to determine whether the pathology is unilateral or bilateral. Block vertebral pathology is observed when there is a bilateral defect. In the case of unilateral segmentation defect, a unilateral bar structure is formed. While growth is blocked on the side where the bar is formed, curvature develops as growth continues on the opposite side (Hedequist & Emans, 2004).

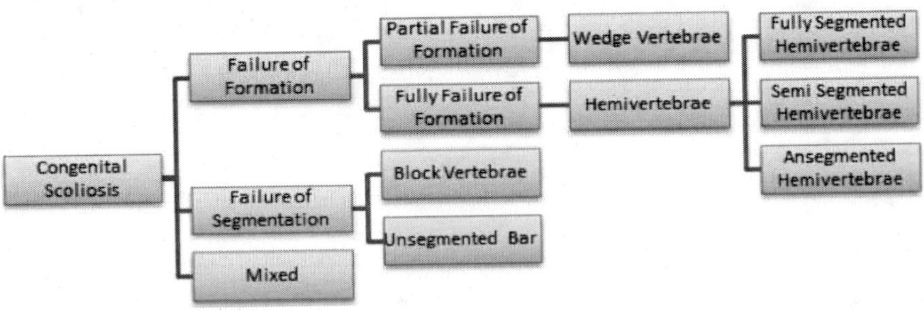


**Figure 2.** Classification of congenital scoliosis.

## Clinic

When congenital scoliosis is detected, the clinical course of the disease must be accurately predicted in order to decide on the treatment. The probable course of the deformity should be determined, and if the deformity is expected to progress, treatment selection should be made by predicting the rate of progression (Tsirikos & McMaster, 2005). There are some basic factors that are considered in the prediction of the prognosis of the deformity. These are the localization of the deformity, the type of vertebral anomaly and the age of the patient (Basu et al., 2002; Pahys & Guille, 2018). The tendency to increase in lumbar and thoracolumbar localized deformities is higher than upper thoracic deformities (Feng et al., 2016; Tsirikos & McMaster, 2005). Considering the general population of congenital patients, it is predicted that the deformity will progress rapidly in 50% of cases, while 25% will have a slow course. It can be thought that the deformity of approximately 25% of patients will be stable (Arlet et al., 2003).

The lowest risk for the progression of the deformity is seen in block vertebral pathology (Giampietro, 2012; Pahys & Guille, 2018). Unilateral bar vertebra, wedge vertebra, and unsegmented hemivertebra deformities are also deformities with low potential to progress. Fully segmented and partially segmented hemivertebrae deformities carry a high risk of progression (Giampietro, 2012; Pahys & Guille, 2018). The risk of progression of the deformity is highest in the case of unilateral bar vertebra and opposite hemivertebra (Burnei et al., 2015; Hedequist & Emans, 2007).

Malforations such as intradural lipoma, syringomyelia, diastometamyelia, tethered spinal cord, and spinal closure may accompany congenital scoliosis (Pahys & Guille, 2018). Spinal and spinal cord abnormalities accompany patients with congenital scoliosis due to an isolated formation defect relatively less than other types. Tethered spinal cord syndrome is the most common spinal anomaly accompanying congenital scoliosis (Pahys & Guille, 2018). Patients with hemivertebrae in the lumbar and thoracolumbar regions should be examined for Klippel-Feil Syndrome (Arlet et al., 2003; Pahys & Guille, 2018). It should also be noted that hemivertebrae may accompany the cervical region in these patients (Arlet et al., 2003; Pahys & Guille, 2018). Since anomalies such as sacral agenesis and caudal regression syndrome can accompany thoracolumbar vertebral deformities, they should be considered when evaluating patients (Balioğlu et al., 2016).

In addition to spine and spinal cord pathologies, abnormalties related to other organ systems may accompany congenital scoliosis. Diseases of the patient's musculoskeletal system, such as Sprengel's deformity and developmental dysplasia of the hip, are frequently associated with congenital scoliosis (Pahys & Guille, 2018). Mixed-type congenital scoliosis cases that cause abnormalities in the thoracic cage and ribs that can progress to thoracic insufficiency can be seen (Hedequist & Emans, 2004; Tsirikos & McMaster, 2005). It should also considered that abnormalities that are associated with congenital scoliosis can be a symptom of syndromic diseases in some cases.

## Treatment

The most successful treatment of congenital scoliosis is treatment with the right timing and the least invasive technique possible (Arlet et al., 2003).

### Follow-up

Follow-up with physical examination and imaging methods applied at regular intervals is called controlled observation. The frequency of follow-up is regulated according to the age of the patient and the type of deformity (Tsirikos & McMaster, 2005). It seems more appropriate to increase the frequency of follow-up during periods of rapid growth, such as adolescence and 0-3 years (Tsirikos & McMaster, 2005).

### Conservative Treatment

Deformities due to congenital scoliosis are mostly rigid deformities. For this reason, corset treatment is generally not appropriate. However, corset application may be required to prevent compensatory deformities (Tsirikos & McMaster, 2005). However, there are publications reporting that deformity progression can be slowed with derotation casting and that surgical intervention can be performed at older ages (Pahys & Guille, 2018).

### Surgical Treatment

There are various methods for the surgical treatment of congenital scoliosis. The oldest of these is in-situ fusion (Hedequist & Emans, 2007). Correction with the limited fusion technique can be combined with hemivertebrectomy in cases of single-level hemivertebrae (Tsirikos & McMaster, 2005). In the presence of complex deformities, treatment can be applied by providing growth regulation with hemiepiphysiodesis (Uzumcugil et al., 2003). Distraction-based systems are also techniques that can be used for complex deformities (Elsbai et al., 2011). These methods can be evaluated and applied on a case-by-case basis, alone or in combination with each other. The posterior approach is frequently used in surgical applications. However, there are combined techniques in which the anterior and posterior approaches are used together. Surgical methods that can be used in the treatment of congenital scoliosis can be listed as:

- In-situ fusion
- Hemivertebrectomy + limited fusion
- Hemiepiphysiodesis
- Distraction-based non-fusion technique
- Directing growth
- Corrective osteotomies.

In the past, gradual treatments were applied in cases where spinal intra-dural pathologies accompanied congeal scoliosis. Thanks to current information and technological possibilities, surgical treatment of both pathologies can be performed safely in the same session (Yilgor et al., 2017). The complication rate in scoliosis surgery has been reported to be 14% in the literature. Congenital scoliosis is the most common type of scoliosis in which neurological complications develop (Weiss & Goodall, 2008).

## Conclusion

Clinical examination is of great importance in the diagnosis and follow-up of congenital spinal deformities. Similarly, clinical examination and comprehensive research are important in terms of abnormalities of the spinal or other organ systems accompanying scoliosis. The main goal in the treatment of scoliosis is to obtain a balanced body without restricting growth. The treatment decision should be planned specifically for the patient, taking into account the conditions specific to the patient and the current deformity.

## References


Arlet, V., Odent, T., & Aebi, M. (2003). Congenital scoliosis. *European Spine Journal, 12*(5), 456-463. https://doi.org/10.1007/s00586-003-0555-6.

Balioğlu, M. B., Akman, Y. E., Ucpunar, H., Albayrak, A., Kargın, D., Atıcı, Y., & Büyük, A. F. (2016). Sacral agenesis: Evaluation of accompanying pathologies in 38 cases, with analysis of long-term outcomes. *Child's Nervous System, 32*(9), 1693-1702. https://doi.org/10.1007/s00381-016-3022-5.

Basu, P. S., Elsebaie, H., & Noordeen, M. (2002). Congenital spinal deformity: A comprehensive assessment at presentation. *Spine, 27*(20), 2255-2259. https://doi.org/10.1097/00007632-200210150-00014.

Burnei, G., Gavriliu, S., Vlad, C., Georgescu, I., Ghita, R., Dughilă, C., Japie, E., & Onilă, A. (2015). Congenital scoliosis: An up-to-date. *Journal of Medicine and Life, 8*(3), 388.

Elsbai, H. B., Yazici, M., Thompson, G. H., Emans JB, Skaggs DL, Crawford AH, Karlin LI, McCarthy RE, Poe-Kochert C, Kostial P, & Akbarnia BA. (2011). Safety and efficacy of growing rod technique for pediatric congenital spinal deformities. *Journal of Pediatric Orthopedics, 31*(1-5). https://doi.org/10.1097/bpo.0b013e318202c1f0.

Feng, Y., Hai, Y., Zhao, S., & Zang, L. (2016). Hemivertebra resection with posterior unilateral intervertebral fusion and transpedicular fixation for congenital scoliosis: Results with at least 3 years of follow-up. *European Spine Journal, 25*, 3274-3281. https://doi.org/10.1007/s00586-016-4556-7.

Giampietro, P. F. (2012). Genetic aspects of congenital and idiopathic scoliosis. *Scientifica, 2012*, 1-16.

Grimme, J. D., & Castillo, M. (2007). Congenital anomalies of the spine. *Neuroimaging Clinics of North America, 17*, 1-16.

Hedequist, D., & Emans, J. (2004). Congenital scoliosis. *Journal of the American Academy of Orthopaedic Surgeons, 12*, 266-275.

Hedequist, D., & Emans, J. (2007). Congenital scoliosis: A review and update. *Journal of Pediatric Orthopaedics, 27*(1), 106-116. https://doi.org/10.1097/bpo.0b013e31802b4993.

Hedequist, D. J., & Emans, J. B. (2003). The correlation of preoperative three-dimensional computed tomography reconstructions with operative findings in congenital scoliosis. *Spine, 28*(22), 2531-2534. https://doi.org/10.1097/01.brs.0000092382.80487.f0.

Johal, J., Loukas, M., Fisahn, C., Chapman, J. R., Oskouian, R. J., & Tubbs, R. S. (2016). Hemivertebrae: A comprehensive review of embryology, imaging, classification, and management. *Child's Nervous System, 32*, 2105-2109. https://doi.org/10.1007/s00381-016-3195-y.

Kaplan, K. M., Spivak, J. M., & Bendo, J. A. (2005). Embryology of the spine and associated congenital abnormalities. *The Spine Journal, 5*(5), 564-576. https://doi.org/10.1016/j.spinee.2004.10.044.

Li, Z., Yu, X., & Shen, J. (2015). Environmental aspects of congenital scoliosis. *Environmental Science and Pollution Research International, 22*, 5751-5755. https://doi.org/10.1007/s11356-015-4144-0.

Pahys, J. M., & Guille, J. T. (2018). What's new in congenital scoliosis? *Journal of Pediatric Orthopaedics, 38*(3), e172-e179. https://doi.org/10.1097/bpo.0000000000000922.

Shawen, S. B., Belmont Jr, P. J., Kuklo, T. R., Owens, B. D., Taylor, K. F., Kruse, R., & Polly Jr, D. W. (2002). Hemimetameric segmental shift: A case series and review. *Spine, 27*(24), E539-E544. https://doi.org/10.1097/00007632-200212150-00025.

Tsirikos, A. I., & McMaster, M. J. (2005). Congenital anomalies of the ribs and chest wall associated with congenital deformities of the spine. *The Journal of Bone and Joint Surgery, 87*(11), 2523-2536. https://doi.org/10.2106/00004623-200511000-00021.

Uzumcugil, A., Cil, A., Yazici, M., Acaroglu, E., Alanay, A., Akalan, N., Ozisik, P., & Surat, A. (2003). The efficacy of convex hemiepiphysiodesis in patients with iatrogenic posterior element deficiency resulting from diastematomyelia excision. *Spine, 28*(8), 799-805. https://doi.org/10.1097/01.brs.0000058942.81012.9f.

Weiss, H. R., & Goodall, D. (2008). Rate of complications in scoliosis surgery–a systematic review of the PubMed literature. *Scoliosis, 3*(1), 9. https://doi.org/10.1186/1748-7161-3-9.

Yilgor, C., Sogunmez, N., & Dalla, M. (2017). Concurrent intradural spinal pathology and pediatric spinal deformity surgery. Turkish Neurosurgery Society 31st Scientific Congress.

# Chapter 7

# Neuromuscular Scoliosis

**Uğur Özdemir[1,*], MD**
**and M. Cemil Gün[2], MD**
[1]Department of Orthopaedics and Traumatology, Bandırma Onyedi Eylül University Faculty of Medicine, Balıkesir, Turkiye
[2]Department of Orthopaedics and Traumatology, Sakarya University Faculty of Medicine, Sakarya, Turkiye

## Abstract

Scoliosis is a common deformity in many types of neuromuscular diseases. Severe spinal curvature can cause difficulty sitting. Conservative and surgical treatment of neuromuscular scoliosis differs from idiopathic scoliosis, being more complex and having a higher rate of complications. Non-surgical measures rarely fully control progressive scoliosis but aim to prevent spinal deformities secondary to muscular hypotonia or contracture. Corrective surgery requires multidisciplinary management and perioperative screening. Pelvic obliquity is commonly associated with neuromuscular scoliosis, making sitting difficult: correction needs to be considered during surgical planning. The goal of surgical correction is to obtain and maintain a well-balanced spine above a well-positioned pelvis. Preoperative multidisciplinary assessment enables potential problems of terrain to be anticipated. Implementing this overall strategic planning can achieve good surgical and functional results in most cases.

**Keywords:** neuromuscular diseases, scoliosis, pelvic obliquity, cerebral palsy, Duchenne muscular dystrophy

---

* Corresponding Author's Email: ugurozdemir.md@gmail.com.

In: Early Onset Scoliosis
Editor: Ahmed Majid Heydar
ISBN: 979-8-89113-600-7

## Introduction

Neuromuscular scoliosis is the most complex form of scoliosis, known as curvatures in the spine. It is the most common form of scoliosis following adolescent idiopathic scoliosis (Roberts and Tsirikos, 2016).

The ligaments and muscles between the vertebrae are supportive structures enabling the spine to stand upright against gravity. Among neuromuscular diseases, scoliosis is a common problem and results from the incompetency observed in the neural units of these muscles.

Neuromuscular scoliosis has a high mortality and morbidity rate because of additional problems caused by the existing neuromuscular disease and complications of deformity treatment, distinguishing it from other types of scoliosis.

All neurological and muscular diseases influencing the trunk muscles may play a role in the etiology (Table 1).

**Table 1.** Etiological classification of neuromuscular scoliosis

| I. Neuropathic | II. Myopathic |
|---|---|
| 1. First Motor Neuron | 1. Arthrogryposis |
| • Cerebral Palsy | 2. Muscular Dystrophy |
| • Spinocerebellar Degeneration | • Duchenne muscular dystrophy |
| 1. Freidreich's Ataxia | • Limb-girdle dystrophy |
| 2. Charcot-Marie-Tooth Disease | • Facioscapulohumeral dystrophy |
| 3. Roussy-Levy Syndrome | 3. Fiber-type disproportion |
| • Syringomyelia | 4. Congenital hypotony |
| • Medulla Spinalis Tumor | 5. Dystrophic myotonia |
| • Medulla Spinalis Trauma | |
| 2. Second Motor Neuron | |
| • Poliomyelitis | |
| • Viral Myelitis | |
| • Trauma | |
| • Spinal Muscular Atrophy | |
| • Werdnig-Hoffmann Disease | |
| • Kugelberg-Welander Disease | |
| • Dysautonomic Disorders (Riley-Day Synd.) | |

Cerebral palsy is the most common cause of neuromuscular scoliosis. The probability of scoliosis development is significantly high, especially in quadriplegic and athetoid cerebral palsy (Halawi et al., 2015). Moreover, neuromuscular scoliosis is often observed in diseases such as spinal muscular atrophies and Duchenne muscular dystrophy.

## Evaluation and Diagnosis

The underlying disease should be identified first in the evaluation of neuromuscular scoliosis because knowing the disease allows you to interpret the character and natural course of the curvature. In these diseases, the trunk muscles that support the spine may be in the flask, spastic, or dyskinetic form. Flask-type curvatures tend to progress faster, whereas dyskinetic-type curvatures tend to progress more slowly. However, the resistance to treatment and complication rates of scoliosis in dyskinetic diseases are higher than those in flask-type curvatures.

It is extremely important to assess the location and severity of curvatures in neuromuscular scoliosis. In this type of scoliosis, curvatures usually cover a large part of the thoracic and lumbar regions. Rib cage and lung development problems are observed in the curvatures of the thoracic region, whereas pelvis and lower extremity problems and resulting walking and sitting balance problems are observed in lumbar region curvatures.

These patients often have back and lower back pain. Physical examination is of great importance in diagnosis. Thoracic deformities, costal gibbosity, trunk balance disorders, and sitting balance should definitely be evaluated. In neuromuscular scoliosis, inadequate compensatory curvature causes spinal and associated trunk imbalance (Mehta and Gibson, 2003). Curvatures are progressive. Even if skeletal development is complete, they can progress (Mehta and Gibson, 2003). This further increases the existing spinal imbalance and causes the formation of pelvic curvature. Therefore, the examination of patients for trunk balance should be carried out standing in patients who can walk and sitting in patients who cannot walk. In patients with neuromuscular scoliosis who can walk, the development of pelvic obliquity may impair the balance of walking over time (Berven and Bradford, 2002). The form of curvature seen in most patients who cannot walk is "C"-shaped thoracolumbar curvatures arising with pelvic obliquity (Mehta and Gibson, 2003). The progressive nature of the deformity and the inclusion of pelvic obliquity in the curvature may also impair the sitting balance in these patients (Berven and Bradford, 2002). In addition to a spinal examination, a hip examination should also be carried out carefully in these patients. In patients with hip muscle involvement, subluxation, and dislocation may develop over time; thus, the balance of walking and sitting may be impaired.

With traction application and bending radiographs, it should be evaluated whether the curvature is flexible in patients with neuromuscular scoliosis. This is extremely important to plan the treatment. Initially, flexible curvatures quickly become rigid, making the treatment quite difficult (Mehta and Gibson, 2003).

The final diagnosis is established by measuring the Cobb angles on the scoliosis radiographs. In patients who cannot walk, a scoliosis radiograph should be taken in the sitting position. In patients with advanced loose neuromuscular units, it may be difficult to take these radiographs even in a sitting position. In these patients, appropriate radiographs should be taken with side supports that will not influence the existing curvature. On radiographs, it should be evaluated whether there is pelvic obliquity, leg height inequality, and hip dislocation. In patients who cannot walk, bending radiographs should be requested to assess the flexibility of curvatures. The probability of neuromuscular scoliosis is high in left thoracic curvatures, rapidly progressive curvatures, and significantly high degree curvatures (Allam and Schwabe, 2013).

## Treatment

The basic principle in the treatment of neuromuscular scoliosis is to prevent the progression of the curvature and optimize the patient's functions. Cosmetic expectations are of secondary importance in this group of patients. In the treatment, it is mainly aimed to obtain a balanced spine that will allow comfortable sitting and/or walking (Drummond, 1996).

Neuromuscular scoliosis is one of the deformities with controversial treatment, and no ideal treatment method has been determined yet. Since it is highly difficult to control the curvature with the use of a corset, conservative treatment is usually unsuccessful. Meanwhile, there are many additional pathologies that technically complicate the surgical treatment and increase complication rates in these patients. In the planning of treatment, the natural course of the underlying disease and the functional level of the patient at the time of admission are noteworthy. Conservative treatment is preferable to surgical treatment for a patient with a progressive deformity whose life expectancy is not so long. For patients with progressive deformities and stable neurological conditions, surgical treatment is the best option.

## Conservative Treatment

The conservative treatment of neuromuscular scoliosis includes corseting and sitting position modifications. Unlike adolescent idiopathic scoliosis, the effectiveness of exercise treatment has not been shown in neuromuscular scoliosis (Lonstein and Akbarnia, 1983).

In corset treatment, it is mainly aimed to slow down the speed of progression, not stopping or improving the progression of the curvature. In this way, the problem of sitting balance disorder and respiratory problems that may develop is prevented and surgical treatment is delayed. A corset is also used to ensure balanced sitting and walking in patients who cannot tolerate surgery. It is more appropriate to use it in flexible and low-level curvatures. TLSO is the most common type of corset.

In corset treatment, the most common complication is a compression wound. Attention should be paid to skin compression, particularly in patients with sensory problems, speech impairment, and intellectual disabilities. In neuromuscular scoliosis, rapid progressions may be observed in curvatures despite the corset treatment. This leads to skin compression. If corset treatment is preferred in these patients, strict follow-up should be carried out, and families should be informed about possible skin compression. In patients with compression wounds, continuing the treatment with corset modification may lead to problems in wound healing. It is more appropriate to take a break from the treatment in these patients.

In patients who cannot be mobilized and use wheelchairs, sitting positon modification is a type of treatment in which sitting balance is ensured with trunk and gluteal region supports (Holmes et al., 2003). In this treatment, skin problems are the most common complications. In recent years, pressure measurement devices and devices with computer analysis, where supports are designed patient-specifically, have been developed to decrease compression wounds (Petito and Young, 2011). However, despite all these technological developments, patients should be followed-up carefully for compression wounds.

## Surgical Treatment

In neuromuscular scoliosis, the success rate of conservative treatment methods is low due to the tendency of curvatures to progress rapidly and the comorbid conditions caused by the underlying disease. Surgical treatment is the only treatment that will fix the deformity and prevent its progression. If rapid progression is observed after the onset of scoliosis in these patients, surgical treatment between 20°-40° is recommended (Olafsson et al., 1999; Mullender et al., 2008). Waiting for further degrees of curvature for surgical treatment may increase the possibility of comorbid problems and the risk of complications. Therefore, sufficient functional surgical correction may not be possible.

In neuromuscular scoliosis, the purpose of surgical treatment is to increase pulmonary functions, obtain a balanced trunk and sitting position, and enhance the patient's comfort in life. However, it should be remembered that, among all types of scoliosis, neuromuscular scoliosis is the type with the highest complication rate due to surgical treatment (Reames et al., 2011). Hence, preoperative evaluation and planning are of great importance in these patients. With the right planning, radical treatment of the patient should be performed in the first surgical operation. Otherwise, the risk of complications, which is already high, increases further with multiple surgical operations. Continued treatment with conservative methods may be more appropriate in patients with a short life expectancy or with a general condition that cannot tolerate surgical treatment.

Since respiratory functions are usually low in neuromuscular diseases, lung problems are frequently observed after surgical operations. The onset of curvature at an early age and the developmental delays of the lungs increase the respiratory problems arising from surgical treatment. Aspirations or retronasal discharges that exist before the operation are risk factors for respiratory complications. Therefore, the respiratory system should be carefully examined in the preoperative assessment. The history of frequent lung infection should be questioned in patients, and it should be evaluated by effective coughing whether the expiratory volume is sufficient or not. In these patients, pneumonia and respiratory failure are often observed after surgery. If they are not treated carefully, mortality rates will be high. Unlike idiopathic scoliosis, thoracic failure and restrictive lung problems are frequently observed in neuromuscular scoliosis (Allam and Schwabe, 2013). It is highly possible for patients with a forced vital capacity of less than 40% to not tolerate surgery (Allam and Schwabe, 2013). In these patients, early surgical treatment should be preferred before respiratory functions worsen, and tracheostomy preparation should also be carried out in the case of non-extubation in the postoperative period.

Cardiomyopathy, which is frequently observed in the myopathic group, should be investigated in detail. In these patients, soft tissue quality is poor and muscles are edematous. This is a serious problem faced even in early deformities. Severe soft tissue contractures arise with the progression of curvatures.

In most patients, blood loss during surgery is an expected problem. Therefore, the clotting function should be evaluated prior to surgery. Even if clotting tests are normal, the use of antiepileptic agents such as valproate should be investigated. Such medications can prolong the bleeding time by disrupting platelet function.

One of the important and unnoticeable problems in these patients is nutritional disorders. Wound healing problems and postoperative infection resulting from the weakening of the immune system are commonly observed in patients with nutritional disorders. These problems are more likely to be seen in patients with serum albumin levels below 3.5 mg/dl (McCarthy, 1999).

## Surgical Technique

In the surgical treatment of neuromuscular scoliosis, it is aimed to obtain a balanced spine and pelvis in the frontal and sagittal planes. The surgical techniques to be preferred may differ depending on the characteristics of the disease, the location, and degree of curvature, whether there is pelvic distortion, and whether the patient can walk or has the potential to walk. Nowadays, posterior surgical interventions are the most preferred and used methods for treatment purposes, and successful results are obtained with fusion techniques extending from the upper thoracic region to the pelvis.

The general principle is to prefer long instrumentation and fusion in this group of patients because it is impossible to compensate for the curvature due to the underlying neuromuscular disease. If the fusion is too short, transition deformities develop below or above the instrumented segment. Therefore, posterior instrumentation and fusion are the approaches that should be preferred most in surgical treatment (Drummond, 1996; Sengupta et al., 2002). Anterior approaches should also be carried out in severe curvatures that cannot be corrected posteriorly alone (Thomson and Banta, 2001). In patients younger than 10 years of age, an anterior approach can also be applied to avoid the "crankshaft" phenomenon. Finally, a combination of anterior-posterior surgery can be performed in patients at high risk of pseudoarthrosis.

In the planning phase of the treatment, one of the main problems is whether the pelvis will take part in instrumentation and fusion. In this decision, the functional level of the patient is important. It is not desired to fix the pelvis in patients who can walk. On the other hand, if a balanced pelvis can be obtained with fusion and instrumentation extending to L5 in patients who cannot walk, there is no need to fix the pelvis. However, if residual deformity will remain in the pelvis, the pelvis should take part in fusion without hesitation (Mubarek et al., 1993; Alman and Kim, 1999; Mehta and Gibson, 2003).

## Planning in Cerebral Palsy

Cerebral palsy is the most common cause of neuromuscular scoliosis, and 25% of these patients have spinal deformities. As the disease worsens, the probability of scoliosis development increases. The probability of scoliosis development is significantly high, especially in quadriplegic and athetoid cerebral palsy (Halawi et al., 2015). Patients usually have high-angle curvatures and fixed pelvic obliquities. Hence, instrumentation and fusion usually involve T2-3 and the pelvis. If adequate correction is not achieved, it is better to prefer a posterior approach after anterior relaxation. Combining approaches also prevent the pseudoarthrosis problem, which is often observed in these patients.

## Planning in Duchenne Muscular Dystrophy

Duchenne muscular dystrophy is the most common cause of myopathic neuromuscular scoliosis. In these patients, spinal deformity arises when patients lose their walking function and become dependent on a wheelchair, in other words, mostly at 11-12 years of age. Scoliosis is rare in patients who can walk. In these patients, the cause of scoliosis is the paralysis of the extensor trunk muscles, and the progression of curvatures above 20° is generally inevitable. The main treatment method in these patients is surgery. On the other hand, recent publications have reported that scoliosis development slows with steroid treatment in Duchenne muscular dystrophy and the need for surgical treatment is delayed (Alman et al., 2004; Yılmaz et al., 2004).

The most controversial point in surgical treatment is the participation of the pelvis in the fusion or stopping at L5. Here, there are two different views: The first suggests that the pelvis does not need to participate in fusion after instrumentation when it stops at L5 and if pelvic obliquity does not exist (Mubarek et al., 1993). However, the second view asserts that the pelvis should always participate in fusion by suggesting that the sitting balance will be impaired in these patients in a later period (Alman and Kim, 1999).

## Conclusion

The basic principle in the treatment of neuromuscular scoliosis is to prevent the progression of the curvature and optimize the patient's functions. Neuromuscular scoliosis is one of the deformities with controversial treatment, and no ideal treatment method has been determined yet. Since it is highly difficult to control the curvature with the use of a corset, conservative treatment is usually unsuccessful. In surgical treatment, it is mainly aimed to obtain a balanced spine that will allow comfortable sitting and/or walking. However, there are many additional pathologies that technically complicate the surgical treatment and increase the complication rates in these patients. Therefore, preoperative evaluation and planning are of great importance to these patients. With proper planning according to the natural course of the underlying disease and the patient's functional level at the time of admission, the complications that may arise due to the treatment can be prevented.

## References

Allam, A. M., & Schwabe, A. L. (2013). Neuromuscular scoliosis. *PM & R: the journal of injury, function, and rehabilitation*, *5*(11), 957–963. https://doi.org/10.1016/j.pmrj.2013.05.015.

Alman, B. A., & Kim, H. K. (1999). Pelvic obliquity after fusion of the spine in Duchenne muscular dystrophy. *The Journal of bone and joint surgery. British volume*, *81*(5), 821–824. https://doi.org/10.1302/0301-620x.81b5.9383.

Alman, B. A., Raza, S. N., & Biggar, W. D. (2004). Steroid treatment and the development of scoliosis in males with duchenne muscular dystrophy. *The Journal of bone and joint surgery. American volume*, *86*(3), 519–524. https://doi.org/10.2106/00004623-200403000-00009.

Berven, S., & Bradford, D. S. (2002). Neuromuscular scoliosis: causes of deformity and principles for evaluation and management. *Seminars in neurology*, *22*(2), 167–178. https://doi.org/10.1055/s-2002-36540.

Drummond, D. S. (1996). Neuromuscular scoliosis: recent concepts. *Journal of pediatric orthopedics*, *16*(3), 281–283. https://doi.org/10.1097/00004694-199605000-00001.

Halawi, M. J., Lark, R. K., & Fitch, R. D. (2015). Neuromuscular Scoliosis: Current Concepts. *Orthopedics*, *38*(6), e452–e456. https://doi.org/10.3928/01477447-20150603-50.

Holmes, K. J., Michael, S. M., Thorpe, S. L., & Solomonidis, S. E. (2003). Management of scoliosis with special seating for the non-ambulant spastic cerebral palsy population--a biomechanical study. *Clinical biomechanics (Bristol, Avon)*, *18*(6), 480–487. https://doi.org/10.1016/s0268-0033(03)00075-5.

Lonstein, J. E., & Akbarnia, A. (1983). Operative treatment of spinal deformities in patients with cerebral palsy or mental retardation. An analysis of one hundred and seven cases. *The Journal of bone and joint surgery. American volume*, *65*(1), 43–55.

McCarthy, R. E. (1999). Management of neuromuscular scoliosis. *The Orthopedic clinics of North America*, *30*(3), 435–viii. https://doi.org/10.1016/s0030-5898(05)70096-1.

Mehta, J. S., & Gibson, M. J. (2003). The treatment of neuromuscular scoliosis. *Curr Orthop*, 17, 313-21.

Mubarak, S. J., Morin, W. D., & Leach, J. (1993). Spinal fusion in Duchenne muscular dystrophy--fixation and fusion to the sacropelvis?. *Journal of pediatric orthopedics*, *13*(6), 752–757. https://doi.org/10.1097/01241398-199311000-00012.

Mullender, M., Blom, N., De Kleuver, M., Fock, J., Hitters, W., Horemans, A., Kalkman, C., Pruijs, J., Timmer, R., Titarsolej, P., Van Haasteren, N., Jager, M. V., Van Vught, A., & Van Royen, B. (2008). A Dutch guideline for the treatment of scoliosis in neuromuscular disorders. *Scoliosis*, *3*, 14. https://doi.org/10.1186/1748-7161-3-14.

Olafsson, Y., Saraste, H., & Al-Dabbagh, Z. (1999). Brace treatment in neuromuscular spine deformity. *Journal of pediatric orthopedics*, *19*(3), 376–379.

Petito, C., & Young, M. H. (2011). Custom molded seating: choosing the right system for your client. *Rehab management*, *24*(2), 22–24.

Reames, D. L., Smith, J. S., Fu, K. M., Polly, D. W., Jr, Ames, C. P., Berven, S. H., Perra, J. H., Glassman, S. D., McCarthy, R. E., Knapp, R. D., Jr, Heary, R., Shaffrey, C. I., & Scoliosis Research Society Morbidity and Mortality Committee (2011). Complications in the surgical treatment of 19,360 cases of pediatric scoliosis: a review of the Scoliosis Research Society Morbidity and Mortality database. *Spine*, *36*(18), 1484–1491. https://doi.org/10.1097/BRS.0b013e3181f3a326.

Roberts, S. B., & Tsirikos, A. I. (2016). Factors influencing the evaluation and management of neuromuscular scoliosis: A review of the literature. *Journal of back and musculoskeletal rehabilitation*, *29*(4), 613–623. https://doi.org/10.3233/BMR-160675.

Sengupta, D. K., Mehdian, S. H., McConnell, J. R., Eisenstein, S. M., & Webb, J. K. (2002). Pelvic or lumbar fixation for the surgical management of scoliosis in duchenne muscular dystrophy. *Spine*, *27*(18), 2072–2079. https://doi.org/10.1097/00007632-200209150-00020.

Thomson, J. D., & Banta, J. V. (2001). Scoliosis in cerebral palsy: an overview and recent results. *Journal of pediatric orthopedics. Part B*, *10*(1), 6–9.

Yilmaz, O., Karaduman, A., & Topaloğlu, H. (2004). Prednisolone therapy in Duchenne muscular dystrophy prolongs ambulation and prevents scoliosis. *European journal of neurology*, *11*(8), 541–544. https://doi.org/10.1111/j.1468-1331.2004.00866.x.

# Chapter 8

# Syndromic Early-Onset Scoliosis

**M. Fatih Serttaş*, MD**
Department of Orthopedics and Traumatology, Sakarya University, Sakarya, Turkiye

## Abstract

Syndromic scoliosis (SS) is an umbrella term that encompasses all scoliosis associated with an underlying systemic disease. Since almost all of these syndromes occur in the first decade of life and affect the spine, almost all syndromic scoliosis falls into the early-onset scoliosis (EOS) group. Scoliotic deformity is a common occurrence in these cases. Since EOS is caused by a wide variety of etiologies, the natural course varies greatly according to the characteristics of the syndrome causing spinal deformity. Unfortunately, as these patients tend to have a greater number of concomitant medical comorbidities, surgical correction of these deformities may incur significant clinical cost. The true prevalence of syndromic EOS is unknown. Curve patterns usually consist of a single long curve that covers the entire spine. Each syndrome may have additional spinal pathologies, which makes surgical implant placement more difficult. Since these syndromes are common diseases in many branches, it should not be forgotten that more predictable and safer surgeries can be performed paying more attention to details with an interdisciplinary approach. Given the rarity of these syndromic cases, it is necessary to establish a common network through which we can follow the results and research.

**Keywords:** early-onset scoliosis, syndromic, marfan, neurofibromatosis

---

* Corresponding Author's Email: mfserttas@gmail.com.

In: Early Onset Scoliosis
Editor: Ahmed Majid Heydar
ISBN: 979-8-89113-600-7

## Introduction

Syndromic scoliosis (SS) is an umbrella term that encompasses all scoliosis associated with underlying systemic disease (Levy et al., 2015). Since almost all of these syndromes occur in the first decade of life and affect the spine, almost all syndromic scoliosis falls into the early-onset scoliosis (EOS) group. In addition, the term "exotic scoliosis" was coined by Campbell and Smith in 2007. They are named because deformities can be so unusual and devastating that they require an exotic approach for effective treatment. Mesenchymal and connective tissue disorders (Marfan syndrome, Ehler-Danlos syndrome, etc.), skeletal dysplasias (Achondroplasia, etc.), metabolic and endocrine syndromes (Osteogenesis Imperfecta), storage diseases (mucopolysaccharidoses), and rare unclassifiable syndromes (Prader Willi syndrome, etc.) associated spinal deformity is usually included in this spinal deformity category.

Scoliotic deformity is a common occurrence in these cases. Since EOS is caused by a wide variety of etiologies, the natural course varies greatly according to the characteristics of the syndrome causing spinal deformity. For example, the natural history of patients with skeletal dysplasia may depend more on the form of the dysplasia than on the presence and extent of the coronal plane spinal deformity. Similarly, pathologies such as spondylolisthesis may be seen in the spine of a patient with scoliosis due to a connective tissue disorder, depending on the form of the disorder. Knowing the medical and surgical abnormalities associated with various diagnoses in children with EOS is extremely important (Campbell, 2009).

Unfortunately, as these patients tend to have a greater number of concomitant medical comorbidities, surgical correction of these deformities may incur significant clinical cost. The risk of complications during the surgical procedure in syndromic patients is relatively high compared to the idiopathic population (Levy et al., 2015; Milbrandt and Johnston, 2005; Lerman et al., 2003). However, given that these syndromes are rare and rarely undergo spinal surgery, few data are available regarding deformity correction outcomes in this population.

### Syndromes Affecting the Spine

The true prevalence of syndromic early-onset scoliosis is unknown. Curve patterns usually consist of a single long curve that covers the entire spine. Each syndrome may have additional spinal pathologies, making surgical implant placement more difficult (for example, having a dural ectasia accompanying neurofibromatosis) (Yang et al., 2016). During the evaluation of syndromic scoliosis, a specific diagnosis of suspected syndrome to guess the new medical problems that may arise during the genetic study after surgery is crucial, so a referral to the geneticist is mandatory. When a definitive genetic diagnosis is confirmed, the surgeon should explore the literature to learn the fine details of the syndromes underlying the spinal disorder. MRI of the entire spine is monitored preoperatively to detect the spine cord. Occult spinal cord abnormalities may increase the risk of neurologic injury during surgical correction. MRI scans may detect as follows; distal spinal cord tethers, lateral tethers of the proxima, spinal cord, intradural mass lesions, syringomyelia, dural ectasia, Arnold-Chiari malformations, complex bone/cartilage malformations of the spine. In addition, syndromic scoliosis is often associated with a primary chest wall deformity that can lead to thoracic insufficiency syndrome, so it should be included in the evaluation of the chest. These syndromes are 1) Mesenchymal and connective tissue disorders, 2) Skeletal dysplasias, 3) Metabolic and endocrine syndromes, 4) Storage diseases, and 5) Unclassifiable rare syndromes, under 5 main headings (Table 1). Examining closely the spinal involvement of the most common syndromes will help us to gain information about the general character of these diseases.

**Table 1.** Syndromic scoliosis classification

| Syndromic Scoliosis | |
|---|---|
| 1. Mesenchymal and Connective Tissue Disorders | Marfan Syndrome, Ehlers-Danlos Syndrome, Down Syndrome (Trisomy 21), Von Reclinghaussen Syndrome (Neurofibromatosis) |
| 2. Skeletal Dysplasia | Achondroplasia, Hypochondroplasia, Spondyloepiphyseal Dysplasia, Kniest Dysplasia |
| 3. Storage Diseases (Mucopolysaccharidoses) | Hurler Syndrome (MPS I), Morquio Syndrome (MPS IV), Sly Syndrome (MPS VII) |
| 4. Metabolic and Endocrine Syndromes | Osteogenesis Imperfecta |
| 5. Unclassified Rare Syndromes | Escobar Syndrome, Prader Willi Syndrome, Arskol Syndrome, Crisponi Syndrome, Proteus Syndrome, Saethre Chotzen Syndrome |

## Marfan Syndrome

Marfan syndrome, which occurs with the symptoms of many systems in the body, is a connective tissue disease that especially affects the cardiovascular, musculoskeletal, and eye systems. Many radiological findings in the cervical spine have been described in Marfan syndrome. These include loss of cervical lordosis and focal cervical kyphosis. In addition, patients have an increase in basilar distance due to increased odontoid height and subclinical atlantoaxial subluxation in approximately one in five patients (Demetracopoulos and Sponseller, 2007; Place and Enzenauer, 2006; Sponseller et al., 1995). Cervical stenosis is very rare. Scoliosis is seen in 2/3 of patients with Marfan syndrome (Di Silvestre et al., 2005; Herring, 2014; Jones et al., 2002). Although the clinical findings are similar to adolescent idiopathic scoliosis, they occur earlier in life. Unlike the idiopathic type, it has been shown that the curvature is greater and progresses faster in Marfan scoliosis. Approximately 1/8 of patients require scoliosis surgery. It has been determined that double main curvature is more common and the progression is faster in scoliosis that occurs in the infantile age (Di Silvestre et al., 2005; Herring, 2014; Jones et al., 2002). Spontaneous mutations are usually seen in such patients, while other system involvements are more common. The incidence of sagittal plane deformities, especially thoracolumbar kyphosis, has increased in patients with Marfan syndrome. The incidence of spondylolisthesis was found to be 6% (Sponseller et al., 1995). Compared to the normal population, the incidence of spondylolisthesis has increased twofold, and the degree of anterior displacement of the spine is higher.

## Ehlers-Danlos Syndrome

Ehlers-Danlos syndrome (EDS) is a genetically inherited, clinically heterogeneous group of connective tissue diseases that occur with defective collagen synthesis. Although clinical findings are predominant in these patients according to the subtypes of the disease, skin hyperelasticity, joint hypermobility, tissue fragility, easy tissue injury, and then atrophic scar tissue are the main findings. Spinal involvement in the syndrome is characteristically seen as kyphoscoliosis (Ainsworth and Aulicino, 1993). Although postural thoracolumbar kyphosis can be seen in infancy, this postural deformity improves as the child grows and their muscles become stronger (Giunta et al., 1999). MacFarlane and Coventry reported cases of EDS with thoracolumbar kyphoscoliosis and wedge-shaped vertebrae (Macfarlane, 1959; Coventry, 1961). Sussman et al. reported two related patients with EDS and stated that these patients had severe scoliosis and ocular fragility (Sussman et al., 1974). In scoliosis seen early in EDS, the deformity progresses rapidly and becomes rigid with age due to muscle hypotonia and ligamentous laxity. If the deformity is not treated, it can cause serious respiratory and functional problems (Natarajan et al., 2011).

## Neurofibromatosis

Neurofibromatosis (NF) is a multisystemic (neural tissue, soft tissue, bone, skin, kidney, and mediastinum) and autosomal dominant genetic disease involving endoderm, mesoderm, and neuroectoderm. Skeletal complications are usually present early in life. Spinal deformities are less common and the exact cause is unknown. The most common osseous pathology associated with NF-1 is scoliosis. Pathology may be secondary to osteomalacia, bone erosion due to neurofibromas, endocrine disorder, or mesodermal dysplasia. We need to be careful when following these patients. Spinal neuropathophysiology, which we cannot prevent by its nature, can continue throughout life, although it is rare. Scoliosis may occur in the thoracic and/or lumbar region. The deformity may have dystrophic features or be indistinguishable from idiopathic scoliosis. We can say that dystrophic scoliosis is accompanied by more than 3 dystrophic samples such as lateral, anterior, and posterior (most common) vertebral scalloping, rib penciling, vertebral rotation, vertebral wedging, thin transverse processes such as garbage, enlarged intervertebral foramen, narrowed pedicle. We can capture these features more easily by evaluating X-ray, CT, and MR together (Crawford et al., 2012; Tsirikos et al., 2004).

Tsirikos et al. evaluated scalloping in patients with NF-1 using plain X-ray and MRI. Scalloping is seen on either the concave edge of the curve or in an area that is not related to the deformity. Posterior vertebral scalloping is closely associated with dural ectasia. Anterior vertebral scalloping is mostly associated with dural ectasia or neurofibroma. It was found that only 50% of lateral vertebral scalloping cases were associated with dural ectasia or tumor. Only dural ectasia without scalloping was seen in only 10% of these cases. MRI is more sensitive in detecting scalloping (Tsirikos et al., 2004).

Deformity at an early age, high Cobb angle, abnormal kyphosis, vertebral scalloping, severe rotation at the apex of the curve, the apex of the curve in the middle or lower 1/3 of the thoracic region, concave or 1 or more ribs on both sides, 4 or more ribs. Itemization is a risk factor for progression (Figure 1). The progression is almost certain if dystrophic features develop before the age of 7, the presence of 3 rib dentitions, or 3 combined dystrophic features. Patients with rapid progression have a high risk of developing neurological deficits due to lamina fractures due to scalloping (Crawford, 2001).

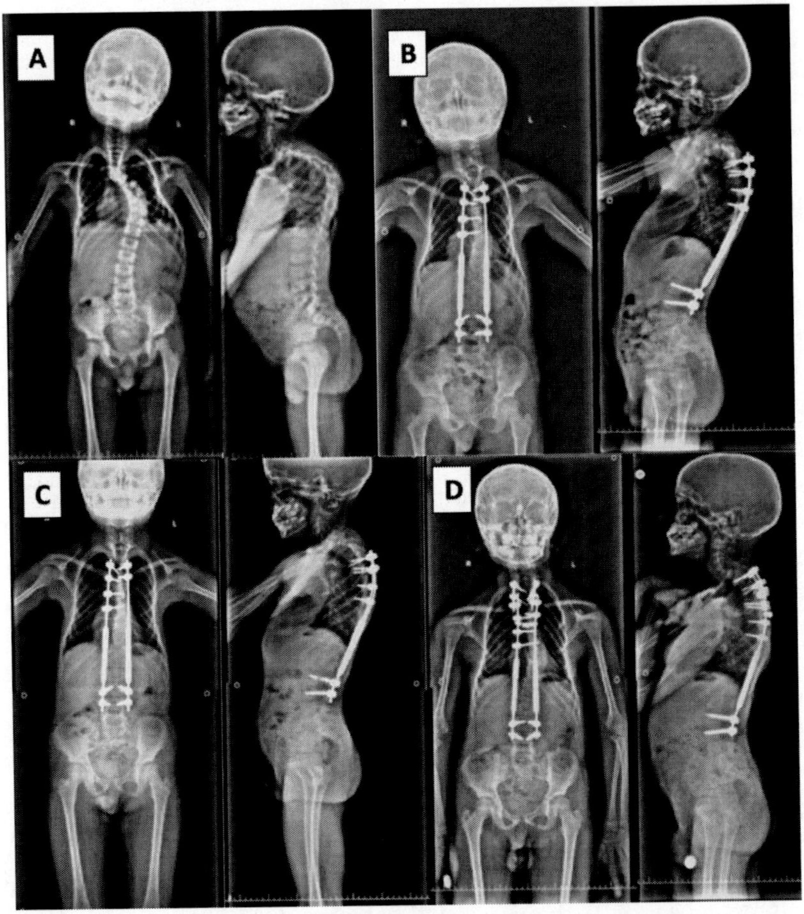


**Figure 1.** Preoperative AP-lateral spine radiographs of a 5-year-old patient diagnosed with NF-1 (A), postoperative 1st-month AP-lateral spine radiographs of the patient who underwent magnetic growing-rod (B), proximal junctional kyphosis (PJK) developed in the 1st postoperative year (C), spine AP-lateral radiographs of the patient who underwent revision after PJK development at the age of 10 (D).

Abubakar et al. stated in their study that the location, edge, width, and gender of the curvature do not affect the shaping of the deformity. If the deformity develops before the age of 7 years, it should be closely followed for the development of dystrophic features. It was stated that the only factor affecting the progress was the penciling in the jeans. He stated that other radiological findings did not contribute to the progression. However, approximately 85% of the patients had three or more dystrophic features of progression (Durrani et al., 2000). Vertebral scalloping and dural ectasia are dystrophic features with the most important individual predictive power (Lykissas et al., 2013).

## Osteogenesis Imperfecta

Osteogenesis imperfecta results from errors in collagen synthesis, either qualitatively or quantitatively. Although osteogenesis imperfecta disease is inherited in an autosomal dominant or recessive manner, it has also been reported that it may occur with spontaneous mutations (Janus et al., 2000). Osteogenesis imperfecta has an incidence of 1/5000 to 10000. The clinics of patients with osteogenesis imperfecta are characterized by bone fragility, osteopenia, joint laxity, dentinogenesis imperfecta, blue sclera, bone deformities, and spinal curvature.

The risk of developing scoliosis increases with the degree of involvement of the disease. There is no consensus on the etiopathogenesis of spinal curvature. However, the theory emphasized that the injury occurs in the vertebral growth plate due to primary multiple vertebral fractures. Hypermobility in the spinal ligaments, abnormalities in the intervertebral disc, leg length inequality, and pelvic tilt are among the causes. Watanabe et al. found a significant relationship between bone Z scoring and scoliosis in their study. It has been reported that the presence of biconcave vertebrae in the presence of radiological osteoporosis is a risk factor for the development of scoliosis (Watanabe et al., 2007). Ishikawa et al. reported that biconcave vertebrae in 6 or more consecutive vertebrae before puberty and having a Cobb angle greater than 50° are risk factors for the development of scoliosis (Hoek, 1975). Although there is controversy about the treatment of spinal curvature, the accepted view should be to stop the progression of the curvature with surgical intervention, since curvatures greater than 50° will adversely affect vital capacity. Follow-up is recommended when spinal deformities occur in patients with osteogenesis and Cobb angles are small.

Poor bone quality in osteogenesis imperfecta cases prevents adequate correction and presents problems related to implant failure. In their study, Chee-Huan et al. achieved a more successful correction with the use of pedicle screws, and no loss of correction was observed in their follow-up (Pan et al., 2006). An increase in the amount of bleeding due to bleeding diathesis should be considered when performing the posterior surgical intervention. In the treatment of scoliosis that occurs in cases of osteogenesis imperfecta, the type of the disease and the Cobb angle of the curvature gain importance in the planning of the treatment. In cases where surgical treatment is planned, the application of bisphosphonates to correct osteoporosis will improve bone quality. Progressive deformities can be treated with posterior surgeries performed with pedicle screws and titanium rod combinations.

## Achondroplasia

Achondroplasia is the most common form of osteochondroplasia characterized by skeletal dysplasias, abnormal shape and size of cartilage and skeleton as a result of impaired enchondral bone formation. It is the most common non-lethal skeletal dysplasia. Its frequency ranges from 1.3 to 15 per 100,000 live births. The gender distribution is equal (Ain et al., 2000). The most important clinical finding of the disease is shortness. This finding can be detected postnatally, and it is diagnosed by measuring the length of the femur on fetal ultrasound. Body length may be normal, but arm distance and standing distance decrease.

Most of the patients are uncomfortable with their vertebral problems. Infants are predisposed to cervical spinal cord compression due to hypoplasia of the foramen magnum. Neurological dysfunction due to thoracolumbar spinal stenosis and scoliosis may also be observed in these patients (Berkowitz et al., 1990). Cervical instability can be seen, albeit infrequently. Posterior fusion is recommended when necessary (Hammerschlag et al. 1988). Thoracolumbar kyphosis and lumbar hyperlordosis are seen in the reduction of the distance between the pedicles and the lower parts of the spine. The type of surgical approach should be determined after the anatomical and clinical evaluation of the patient. Factors such as the presence or absence of thoracolumbar kyphosis, the severity of the stenosis, the duration of clinical findings, and the onset and severity of symptoms should be questioned. Decompression by laminectomy is often recommended and is considered effective in the treatment of neurological symptoms (Stokes et al., 1983). The sooner the decompression is performed after the onset of symptoms, the higher the success rate.

## Hurler Syndrome (Mucopolysaccharidosis I)

Mucopolysaccharidoses (MPS) result from the lysosomal accumulation of partially degraded mucopolysaccharides. Mucopolysaccharides are large molecules that contain a sugar residue and a protein core attached to it, formed by the regular repetition of sulfated hexanoate or hexosamine disaccharide units. The deficiency of one of the specific hydrolases, which degrades sulfate and carbohydrate residues step by step, leads to the incomplete degradation of molecules and the storage of partially degraded products in lysosomes (Dierks et al., 2009).

Hypoplasia is observed on the anterior and upper surfaces of the corpuscles of the lower thoracic and upper lumbar vertebrae, and pecking is observed in the anterior inferior vertebral corpuscles. Dorsal kyphosis or gibbus deformity may develop in patients (Herring, 2002). Orthosis and plaster do not have place during the development of the thoracolumbar and lumbar gibbons. In cases with rapid progression, kyphectomy and posterior fusion can be performed in young children, and additional posterior instrumentation in older children. Since there is severe anterior vertebral body insufficiency, the kyphotic deformity may progress despite the operation, so posterior interventions should be supported with anterior support radiographs. Roberts et al. reported that a 66% correction was achieved by reducing the kyphotic curves, which were on average the thoracolumbar 78°, to 27° with posterior instrumentation, and suggested that posterior fusion supported by anterior support grafting, that is, circumferential fusion, should be applied in order to prevent correction losses (Roberts and Tsirikos, 2015).

## Escobar Syndrome

Escobar syndrome (ES) is a genetically inherited syndrome characterized by reticulated skin structures and joint contractures in the extremities, especially in all flexion and folding regions (knee, elbow, intercrural space, and neck), prominently in the popliteal region. It has been shown that patients with Escobar syndrome have scoliosis and intraspinal abnormalities related to the bone structure of the spine. Sung et al. detected 26° scoliosis in one of the 2 siblings with Escobar syndrome and did not observe any curvature in the other (Sung et al., 2015). The spinal deformity was defined in 14 of 40 patients with confirmed Escobar syndrome with the CHRNG mutation, and significant scoliosis or kyphosis was detected in 11 (Al Kaissi et al., 2013; Hoffmann et al., 2006; Morgan et al., 2006). Tsou showed scoliosis in 29 of 48 patients (60%) (Tsou, 1977). Angsanuntsukh encountered scoliosis in 13 (93%) of 14 ES patients (Angsanuntsukh et al., 2011). These pathologies were seen together with intraspinal anomalies; the tethered cord was detected in 2 patients (14%), and syringomyelia in 1 patient (7%). However, since not all patients have magnetic resonance imaging (MRI) results, an exact ratio is not given. A unilateral unsegmented bar was found in two cases, and the Cobb angle was measured at 39° (20°-75°) in radiological evaluations for scoliosis. Joo et al. reported that scoliosis with vertebral anomalies in children with Escobar syndrome is progressive, and the prevalence of scoliosis is 81% (Joo et al., 2012). He obtained data from 16 out of 19 patients, and they detected between 1969 and 2008, encountered intraspinal anomalies in 8 patients who underwent MRI and detected 13 (81.3%) scoliosis in 16 patients. The age at which scoliosis was first detected was 3.3 ± 2.6 years (1 month to 8.2 years). The baseline Cobb angles were 37.4° ± 18.1° (14°-75°), while an average of 4.0° ± 4.9° annual follow-up was 43.3° ± 19.1° (20°-72°). Progression of the scoliosis curvature was observed (Figure 2). Congenital scoliosis was found in 7 of the patients (unilateral unsegmented bar in 3 cases, the fusion of the cervical vertebrae in 3 cases, and block vertebra in 1 case) and neuromuscular scoliosis in 1 case. The most common radiological finding was defined as a decrease in intervertebral disc space with vertebral height in the thoracic region. Intraspinal anomalies were observed in four patients (3 tethered spinal cords, and 1 syrinx). It was observed that 5 out of 13 patients were able to go to school unaided at their last follow-up. It has been shown that scoliosis is common in MPS, often seen together with cervical fusion, and intraspinal anomalies such as tethered cord and syringomyelia are common together (Joo et al., 2012).

The fusion and unsegmentation of vertebrae are reported in the literature as the most common anomalies in patients with Escobar syndrome (Joo et al., 2012; Ramer et al., 1960; Thompson et al., 1987). However, it is not fully understood what causes these underlying pathologies. It has been tried to be partially explained by decreased fetal movement or fetal akinesia (Hoffmann et al., 2006; Morgan et al., 2006). Formation of the fracture or fibrosis bar is stated as another cause (Tsou, 1977). Contrary to previous studies, fusion or nonsegmentation of the vertebrae has been shown to be widespread anomalies, with narrowing in the intervertebral area, irregularity in the endplates, and a decrease in the height of the vertebrae in the thoracic region found in the patients (Joo et al., 2012).

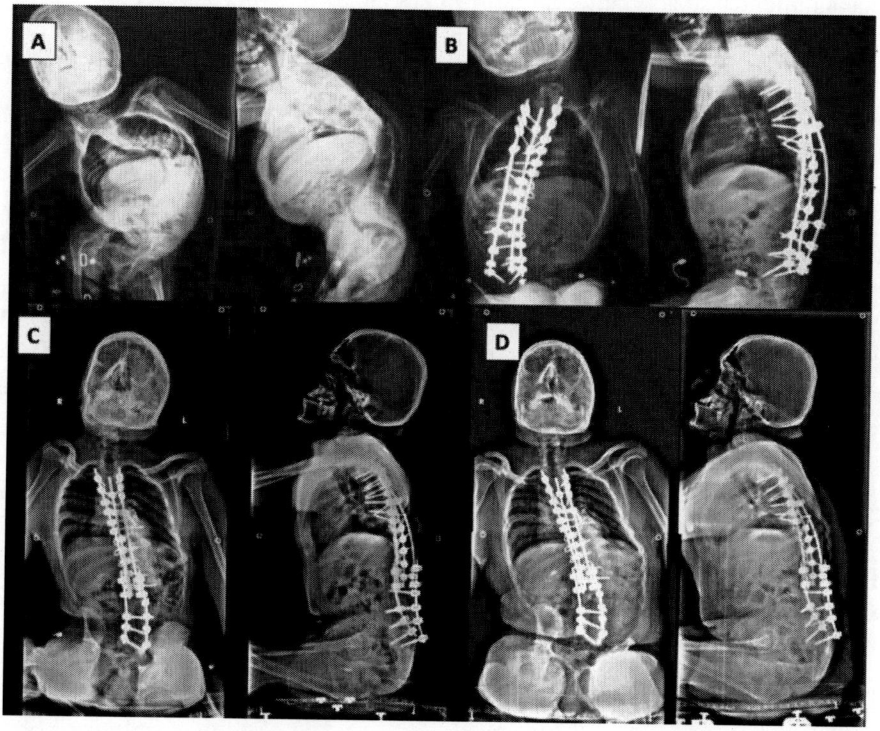


**Figure 2.** 10-year-old AP-lateral spine radiographs of a nonambulatory patient with Escobar syndrome (A), early postoperative spine AP-lateral radiographs (B) after posterior spinal fusion (PSF) postoperative 4-year spine AP-lateral radiographs (C), postoperative 9-year spine AP-lateral radiographs (D).

In particular, MRI studies have shown that the rate of intraspinal anomalies is high in the presence of increased thoracic kyphosis accompanying scoliosis (Eule et al., 2022). The most common intraspinal anomaly seen with scoliosis is syringomyelia with or without Chiari malformation (Davids et al., 2004). the tethered cord, lipoma, diastematomyelia, and fatty phylum are the other most common anomalies. Intraspinal anomaly rates are as high as 20-58% in congenital scoliosis (Belmont et al., 2004; Blake et al., 1986). Joo detected intraspinal pathology in 4 patients (30.8%) with ES (3 tethered cords, 1 syringomyelia) (Joo et al., 2012).

## Conclusion

Beyond the parameters described in this paper, there are numerous management issues when evaluating patients with syndromic scoliosis. For example, dealing with patients with intellectual disabilities, which is common in many of the syndromes mentioned, poses additional challenges in post-operative rehabilitation. The solution to minimize risk in these patients will likely involve a multidisciplinary approach that integrates family, nursing, anesthesia, and other providers into the patient care role. Since these syndromes are common diseases in many branches, it should not be forgotten that more predictable and safer surgeries can be performed paying more attention to details with an interdisciplinary approach.

Given the rarity of these syndromic cases, it is necessary to establish a common network through which we can follow the results and research. More data may be obtained to assist in the management of treatment of other patients with rare spinal abnormalities.

Although the complication rates of syndromic scoliosis surgery are significant, most authors believe that the surgeries are generally beneficial. Given the potential benefits of surgery and the high level of complications in patients with syndromic scoliosis, it is essential to examine the quantity and quality of these complications to pinpoint the source of intraoperative and postoperative difficulties. For this, more prospective studies are needed.

## References

Ain, M. C., Elmaci, I., Hurko, O., Clatterbuck, R. E., Lee, R. R., & Rigamonti, D. (2000). Reoperation for spinal restenosis in achondroplasia. *Journal of spinal disorders*, *13*(2), 168–173. https://doi.org/10.1097/00002517-200004000-00013.

Ainsworth, S. R., & Aulicino, P. L. (1993). A survey of patients with Ehlers-Danlos syndrome. *Clinical orthopedics and related research*, (286), 250–256.

Al Kaissi, A., Kenis, V., Laptiev, S., Ghachem, M. B., Klaushofer, K., Ganger, R., & Grill, F. (2013). Is webbing (pterygia) a constant feature in patients with Escobar syndrome? *Orthopaedic surgery*, *5*(4), 297–301. https://doi.org/10.1111/os.12064.

Angsanuntsukh, C., Oto, M., Holmes, L., Rogers, K. J., King, M. M., Donohoe, M., & Kumar, S. J. (2011). Congenital vertical talus in multiple pterygium syndrome. *Journal of pediatric orthopedics*, *31*(5), 564–569. https://doi.org/10.1097/BPO.0b013e31822108d0.

Belmont, P. J., Jr, Kuklo, T. R., Taylor, K. F., Freedman, B. A., Prahinski, J. R., & Kruse, R. W. (2004). Intraspinal anomalies associated with isolated congenital hemivertebra:

the role of routine magnetic resonance imaging. *The Journal of bone and joint surgery. American volume*, *86*(8), 1704–1710.

Berkowitz, I. D., Raja, S. N., Bender, K. S., & Kopits, S. E. (1990). Dwarfs: pathophysiology and anesthetic implications. *Anesthesiology*, *73*(4), 739–759.

Blake, N. S., Lynch, A. S., & Dowling, F. E. (1986). Spinal cord abnormalities in congenital scoliosis. *Annales de radiologie*, *29*(3-4), 377–379.

Campbell R. M., Jr (2009). Spine deformities in rare congenital syndromes: clinical issues. *Spine*, *34*(17), 1815–1827. https://doi.org/10.1097/BRS.0b013e3181ab64e9.

Coventry M. B. (1961). Some skeletal changes in the Ehlers-Danlos syndrome. A report of two cases. *The Journal of bone and joint surgery. American volume*, *43-A*, 855–860.

Crawford A. H. (2001). Neurofibromatosis. In: Weinstein, S. L. (Ed.), *The pediatric spine: principles and practice* (2nd ed., pp: 471-490). Philadelphia: Lippincott Williams and Wilkins.

Crawford, A. H., Lykissas, M. G., Schorry, E. K., Gaines S., Jain V., Greggi T., & Viskochil D. (2012). Neurofibromatosis: Etiology, Commonly Encountered Spinal Deformities, Common Complications and Pitfalls of Surgical Treatment. *Spine Deform,* 1(Suppl 1), 85–94. https://doi.org/10.1016/j.jspd.2012.04.004.

Davids, J. R., Chamberlin, E., & Blackhurst, D. W. (2004). Indications for magnetic resonance imaging in presumed adolescent idiopathic scoliosis. *The Journal of bone and joint surgery. American volume*, *86*(10), 2187–2195. https://doi.org/10.2106/00004623-200410000-00009.

Demetracopoulos, C. A., & Sponseller, P. D. (2007). Spinal deformities in Marfan syndrome. *The Orthopedic clinics of North America*, *38*(4), 563–vii. https://doi.org/10.1016/j.ocl.2007.04.003.

Di Silvestre, M., Greggi, T., Giacomini, S., Cioni, A., Bakaloudis, G., Lolli, F., & Parisini, P. (2005). Surgical treatment for scoliosis in Marfan syndrome. *Spine*, *30*(20), E597–E604. https://doi.org/10.1097/01.brs.0000182317.33700.08.

Dierks, T., Schlotawa, L., Frese, M. A., Radhakrishnan, K., von Figura, K., & Schmidt, B. (2009). Molecular basis of multiple sulfatase deficiency, mucolipidosis II/III and Niemann-Pick C1 disease - Lysosomal storage disorders caused by defects of non-lysosomal proteins. *Biochimica et biophysica acta*, *1793*(4), 710–725. https://doi.org/10.1016/j.bbamcr.2008.11.015.

Durrani, A. A., Crawford, A. H., Chouhdry, S. N., Saifuddin, A., & Morley, T. R. (2000). Modulation of spinal deformities in patients with neurofibromatosis type 1. *Spine*, *25*(1), 69–75. https://doi.org/10.1097/00007632-200001010-00013.

Eule, J. M., Erickson, M. A., O'Brien, M. F., & Handler, M. (2002). Chiari I malformation associated with syringomyelia and scoliosis: a twenty-year review of surgical and nonsurgical treatment in a pediatric population. *Spine*, *27*(13), 1451–1455. https://doi.org/10.1097/00007632-200207010-00015.

Giunta, C., Superti-Furga, A., Spranger, S., Cole, W. G., & Steinmann, B. (1999). Ehlers-Danlos syndrome type VII: clinical features and molecular defects. *The Journal of bone and joint surgery. American volume*, *81*(2), 225–238. https://doi.org/10.2106/00004623-199902000-00010.

Hammerschlag, W., Ziv, I., Wald, U., Robin, G. C., & Floman, Y. (1988). Cervical instability in an achondroplastic infant. *Journal of pediatric orthopedics*, *8*(4), 481–484. https://doi.org/10.1097/01241398-198807000-00021.

Herring J. A. (Ed.). (2002). Tachdjian's Pediatric Orthopedics. Volume-3, Section IV, Chapter 29, W. B. Saunders, *Philadelphia*; pp: 1575-1575.

Herring J. A. (2014). Orthopaedic Related Syndromes (Chapter 41). In: Herring JA (Ed.), *Tachdjian's Pediatric Orthopaedics* (Fifth Edition, pp: e473-e581). Philadelphia: Elsevier.

Hoek, K. J. (1975). Scoliosis in osteogenesis imperfecta, *J Bone Joint Surg*, 57-A, 136-138.

Hoffmann, K., Muller, J. S., Stricker, S., Megarbane, A., Rajab, A., Lindner, T. H., Cohen, M., Chouery, E., Adaimy, L., Ghanem, I., Delague, V., Boltshauser, E., Talim, B., Horvath, R., Robinson, P. N., Lochmüller, H., Hübner, C., & Mundlos, S. (2006). Escobar syndrome is a prenatal myasthenia caused by disruption of the acetylcholine receptor fetal gamma subunit. *American journal of human genetics*, *79*(2), 303–312. https://doi.org/10.1086/506257.

Janus, G. J., Finidori, G., Engelbert, R. H., Pouliquen, M., & Pruijs, J. E. (2000). Operative treatment of severe scoliosis in osteogenesis imperfecta: results of 20 patients after halo traction and posterior spondylodesis with instrumentation. *European spine journal : official publication of the European Spine Society, the European Spinal Deformity Society, and the European Section of the Cervical Spine Research Society*, *9*(6), 486–491. https://doi.org/10.1007/s005860000165.

Jones, K. B., Erkula, G., Sponseller, P. D., & Dormans, J. P. (2002). Spine deformity correction in Marfan syndrome. *Spine*, *27*(18), 2003–2012. https://doi.org/10.1097/00007632-200209150-00008.

Joo, S., Rogers, K. J., Donohoe, M., King, M. M., & Kumar, S. J. (2012). Prevalence and patterns of scoliosis in children with multiple pterygium syndrome. *Journal of pediatric orthopedics*, *32*(2), 190–195. https://doi.org/10.1097/BPO.0b013e31823ab359.

Lerman, J. A., Emans, J. B., Hall, J. E., & Karlin, L. I. (2003). Spinal arthrodesis for scoliosis in Down syndrome. *Journal of pediatric orthopedics*, *23*(2), 159–161.

Levy, B. J., Schulz, J. F., Fornari, E. D., & Wollowick, A. L. (2015). Complications associated with surgical repair of syndromic scoliosis. *Scoliosis*, *10*, 14. https://doi.org/10.1186/s13013-015-0035-x.

Lykissas M. G., Schorry E. K., Crawford A. H., Gaines S., Rieley M., Jain V. V. (2013). Does the presence of dystrophic features in patients with type 1 neurofibromatosis and spinal deformities increase the risk of surgery? *Spine*; *38*(18), 1595- 601.

Macfarlane, I. L. (1959). Ehlers-Danlos syndrome presents certain unusual features. *The Journal of bone and joint surgery. British volume*, *41-B*, 541–545. https://doi.org/10.1302/0301-620X.41B3.541.

Milbrandt, T. A., & Johnston, C. E., 2nd (2005). Down syndrome and scoliosis: a review of a 50-year experience at one institution. *Spine*, *30*(18), 2051–2055. https://doi.org/10.1097/01.brs.0000179100.54453.72.

Morgan, N. V., Brueton, L. A., Cox, P., Greally, M. T., Tolmie, J., Pasha, S., Aligianis, I. A., van Bokhoven, H., Marton, T., Al-Gazali, L., Morton, J. E., Oley, C., Johnson, C. A.,

Trembath, R. C., Brunner, H. G., & Maher, E. R. (2006). Mutations in the embryonal subunit of the acetylcholine receptor (CHRNG) cause lethal and Escobar variants of multiple pterygium syndrome. *American journal of human genetics*, *79*(2), 390–395. https://doi.org/10.1086/506256.

Natarajan, D., Samartzis, D., Wong, Y. W., Luk, K. D., & Cheung, K. M. (2011). Natural history of spinal deformity in a patient with Ehlers-Danlos syndrome: a case report with 20-year follow-up. *The spine journal: official journal of the North American Spine Society*, *11*(7), e1–e4. https://doi.org/10.1016/j.spinee.2011.02.029.

Pan, C. H., Ma, S. C., Wu, C. T., & Chen, P. Q. (2006). All pedicle screw fixation technique in correcting severe kyphoscoliosis in an osteogenesis imperfecta patient: a case report. *Journal of spinal disorders & techniques*, *19*(5), 368–372. https://doi.org/10.1097/01.bsd.0000208253.06706.42.

Place, H. M., & Enzenauer, R. J. (2006). Cervical spine subluxation in Marfan syndrome. A case report. *The Journal of bone and joint surgery. American volume*, *88*(11), 2479–2482. https://doi.org/10.2106/JBJS.E.00445.

Ramer, J. C., Ladda, R. L., & Demuth, W. W. (1988). Multiple pterygium syndrome. An overview. *American journal of diseases of children (1960)*, *142*(7), 794–798. https://doi.org/10.1001/archpedi.1988.02150070108039.

Roberts, S. B., & Tsirikos, A. I. (2016). Thoracolumbar kyphoscoliosis with unilateral subluxation of the spine and postoperative lumbar spondylolisthesis in Hunter syndrome. *Journal of neurosurgery. Spine*, *24*(3), 402–406. https://doi.org/10.3171/2015.6.SPINE15268.

Sponseller, P. D., Hobbs, W., Riley, L. H., 3rd, & Pyeritz, R. E. (1995). The thoracolumbar spine in Marfan syndrome. *The Journal of bone and joint surgery. American volume*, *77*(6), 867–876. https://doi.org/10.2106/00004623-199506000-00007.

Stokes, D. C., Phillips, J. A., Leonard, C. O., Dorst, J. P., Kopits, S. E., Trojak, J. E., & Brown, D. L. (1983). Respiratory complications of achondroplasia. *The Journal of pediatrics*, *102*(4), 534–541. https://doi.org/10.1016/s0022-3476(83)80180-2.

Sung, K. H., Lee, S. H., Kim, N., & Cho, T. J. (2015). Orthopaedic manifestations and treatment outcome of two siblings with Escobar syndrome and homozygous mutations in the CHRNG gene. *Journal of pediatric orthopedics. Part B*, *24*(3), 262–267. https://doi.org/10.1097/BPB.0000000000000119.

Sussman, M., Lichtenstein, J. R., Nigra, T. P., Martin, G. R., & McKusick, V. A. (1974). Hydroxylysine-deficient skin collagen in a patient with a form of Ehlers-Danlos syndrome. *The Journal of bone and joint surgery. American volume*, *56*(6), 1228–1234.

Thompson, E. M., Donnai, D., Baraitser, M., Hall, C. M., Pembrey, M. E., & Fixsen, J. (1987). Multiple pterygium syndrome: evolution of the phenotype. *Journal of medical genetics*, *24*(12), 733–749. https://doi.org/10.1136/jmg.24.12.733.

Tsirikos, A. I., Ramachandran, M., Lee, J., & Saifuddin, A. (2004). Assessment of vertebral scalloping in neurofibromatosis type 1 with plain radiography and MRI. *Clinical radiology*, *59*(11), 1009–1017. https://doi.org/10.1016/j.crad.2004.04.006.

Tsou, P. M. (1977). Embryology of congenital kyphosis. *Clinical orthopaedics and related research*, (128), 18–25.

Watanabe, G., Kawaguchi, S., Matsuyama, T., & Yamashita, T. (2007). Correlation of scoliotic curvature with Z-score bone mineral density and body mass index in patients with osteogenesis imperfecta. *Spine*, *32*(17), E488–E494. https://doi.org/10.1097/BRS.0b013e31811ec2d9.

Yang, S., Andras, L. M., Redding, G. J., & Skaggs, D. L. (2016). Early-Onset Scoliosis: A Review of History, Current Treatment, and Future Directions. *Pediatrics*, *137*(1), 10.1542/peds.2015-0709. https://doi.org/10.1542/peds.2015-0709.

## Chapter 9

# Clinical Examination of EOS

**Yücel Bilgin[*], MD**
Department of Orthopedics and Traumatology, Bursa Uludag University, Bursa, Turkiye

### Abstract

Early-onset scoliosis (EOS) is defined as scoliosis seen under 10 years of age. Since lung development continues in these patients, diagnosis and treatment planning are different. Clinical evaluation of early-onset scoliosis is performed using the patient's medical history, physical examination, and imaging modalities as needed. This assessment requires an individualized approach based on the patient's age, degree of curvature, symptoms, and general health.

**Keywords:** early-onset scoliosis, idiopathic, clinical examination, neuromuscular, congenital

## Introduction

Although scoliosis is defined as the curvature of the spine in the coronal plane, it is a three-planned deformity of the spine. Early-onset scoliosis (EOS) is defined as scoliosis seen under 10 years of age, regardless of etiology, by the Growing Spine Study Group (GSSG) and the Children's Spine Study Group (CSSG) (El-Hawary & Akbarnia, 2015; Williams et al., 2014). According to the etiology, it can be idiopathic, congenital, neuromuscular, and syndromic. The first step in clinical evaluation is anamnesis and physical examination.

[*] Corresponding Author's Email: dryucelbilgin@gmail.com.

In: Early Onset Scoliosis
Editor: Ahmed Majid Heydar
ISBN: 979-8-89113-600-7

Then, radiological methods are used. Since most of the thorax and lung capacity develops in those under 10 years of age, early diagnosis and application of treatment methods that will not prevent growth are important in the success of treatment.

The aim of this chapter is to discuss in detail the clinical evaluation of early-onset scoliosis. The importance of clinical evaluation, how the process progresses, and what steps should be taken will be explained in detail in the rest of the article.

## Medical History in Early-Onset Scoliosis

In EOS, a medical history is taken about the prenatal, birth, and postpartum periods. Congenital infections, perinatal asphyxia, genetic diseases, etc. are questioned. In addition, additional organ and system diseases are questioned in congenital scoliosis. In particular, cardiac and renal abnormalities may accompany.

Patients can apply with a back curve noticed by their parents, or they can be noticed and directed by the pediatrician during the pediatric examination. It can be noticed during school screenings for separate school-aged children. The complaints of the patients are usually curvature of the back, shoulder asymmetry, pelvic asymmetry, breast asymmetry, and costal prominence. Patients should be questioned about how long this complaint has existed and whether they have pain. Menarche status should be questioned in female patients. It provides information about the growth rate.

The accompanying patients in the medical history guide the diagnosis. Especially neuromuscular scoliosis accompanies neuromuscular diseases such as cerebral palsy, Frederich's ataxia, spinal muscular atrophy, and muscular dystrophies.

A family history must be included in the medical history. There is a genetic predisposition to scoliosis. A history of the patient's growth rate should be taken. Rapid progress can also be seen in scoliosis, especially during periods of rapid growth.

Psychological problems may accompany in patients with advanced curvature scoliosis. This aspect should also be evaluated in the medical anamnesis and support from child psychiatry should be sought when necessary.

## Physical Examination in Early-Onset Scoliosis

The physical examination in EOS begins with a posture examination. Asymmetries are reviewed in the posture of the patient while standing. In order to evaluate the spine, especially in patients with a height difference between the lower extremities, posture should be examined in the sitting position. In EOS, physical examination findings such as scoliosis-related curvature of the back, shoulder asymmetry, pelvic asymmetry, breast asymmetry, and costal prominence are present. Based on the available findings, the type and direction of the scoliotic curvature can be determined. The Adams test is used in the physical examination of scoliosis. The patient leans forward with the knees and hips fully extended. If there is a difference between the costal heights, the test is positive in favor of scoliosis. By using the scoliometer, information about the degree of scoliosis can be obtained at this position. Coronal imbalance is present in scoliosis if the plumb hanging over the C7 verebra spinous process does not pass through the midline of the sacrum.

On physical examination, the patient's height and weight are also recorded. These findings guide the estimation of curvature progression based on the patient's growth rate. A skin examination is performed on the entire body of the patient. Abnormal pigmentation, hairy patches, and skin tags are warning signs of intraspinal pathologies. A detailed neurological examination should be performed. Sensory and motor functions should be evaluated. In addition, superficial, deep tendon, and pathological reflexes should be evaluated.

Depending on the etiology, additional physical examination findings are seen in EOS. In the presence of cafe-u-laut spots on the skin, it may be accompanied by neurofibromatosis (Jett & Friedman, 2010). In the presence of abnormal hyperlaxity, various connective tissue diseases, especially Marfan syndrome, may be associated (Marelli et al., 2023). In neuromuscular scoliosis, the extent of neurologic involvement should be analyzed in detail. Ability to stand, mobilize, use a wheelchair, general physical and mental function, condition of the upper extremities, nutritional and respiratory status should be reviewed and examined. Patients should be classified according to the gross motor function scale. The use of baclofen, antiepileptics, and other drugs should be reviewed. In this group of patients, the family is the only source of useful information. In the presence of Friedreich's ataxia, ataxic gait, loss of balance coordination, weakness in muscle strength, speech problems, and concomitant heart diseases can be detected (Kearney et al., 2016). In the presence of Duchenne muscular dystrophy, loss of muscle strength, loss of motor skills, swaying gait pattern, cardiac problems, and respiratory problems may accompany scoliosis (Chang et al., 2023). Neuromuscular scoliosis can also be seen in patients with spinal muscular atrophy. This group of diseases is caused by the degeneration of motor neurons. On clinical examination; muscle weakness, loss of motor skills, feeding problems, respiratory problems, posture disorders, involuntary movements, loss of reflexes, and muscle atrophy can be detected (Nishio et al., 2023).

In syndromic scoliosis, features of the syndromes can be detected. High foreheads, low ears, short stature, strabismus, and pulmonary stenosis can be detected in Noonan syndrome. In the presence of Di George syndrome, cardiac anomalies, hypocalcemia, hypoplastic thymus, and immune deficiency can be detected (Funato, 2022). Bifid uvula and great vessel aneurysms can be detected in the presence of Loeys Dietz syndrome (Charoenngam et al., 2023; Chung, 2023). Blue sclera, frequent fractures, and hearing loss can be detected in the presence of osteogenesis imperfecta (Yu et al., 2023). In the presence of Klippel-Feil syndrome, low hairline, short neck, restricted neck range of motion, and torticollis may accompany (Frikha, 2020). Beals syndrome is another syndrome in which scoliosis can be detected. In this syndrome, there is a mutation in the fibrillin-2 (FBN-2) gene. The patients have an appearance characterized by arachnodactyly of the fingers and toes, long stature, and elongated extremities. It is typical for the upper ear helix to fold. Another feature is joint contractures. It may be accompanied by cardiovascular and gastrointestinal abnormalities (Callewaert et al., 2009). Neurofibromatosis is a different syndrome in which scoliosis can be detected. In clinical evaluation, macrocephaly, abnormal bone growth, short stature, and skeletal abnormalities such as osteopenia, osteomalacia, dental problems, dysplasia of long bones, and cystic osseous lesions can be seen (Jett & Friedman, 2010). In the presence of Ehlers-Danlos syndrome, hypermobility in the joints, elasticity, and fragile tissue structure can be detected on the clinical examination (Marathe et al., 2022; Scicluna et al., 2022; Yonko et al., 2021). This syndrome is a connective tissue disease that occurs with a defect in collagen synthesis.

Additional findings of physical examination related to intraspinal anomalies accompanying scoliosis can also be detected. In the presence of syrinx, pain, muscle weakness in the upper extremities, bladder dysfunction, and loss of sensation below the level of the lesion can be detected (Köksal, 2023). In the presence of tense cord syndrome, progressive motor and sensory deficits, gait abnormalities, and loss of bladder control can be detected (Köksal, 2023). In the presence of diastematomyelia, depending on the level and location of the pathology, pain, weakness, and neurological deficits can be detected (Köksal, 2023).

## Conclusion

The clinical assessment of this disease is vital for an accurate diagnosis and effective treatment planning. Medical history and physical examination are the first steps to understand the history and symptoms of the patients, while visual assessments and special tests provide important information about the curvature and severity of the spine.

The clinical evaluation of early-onset scoliosis plays a critical role in understanding the individual needs of patients and creating appropriate treatment plans. Imaging modalities are important in monitoring the degree of curvature and progression, and these data are used to support treatment decisions.

In conclusion, the clinical evaluation of early-onset scoliosis is a detailed process performed with a multidisciplinary approach. This evaluation is important in order to positively affect the lives of patients and to control the progression of the disease. This process, which is carried out meticulously by experts, aims to provide the support patients need and to determine the most appropriate treatment strategies.

## References

Callewaert, B. L., Loeys, B. L., Ficcadenti, A., Vermeer, S., Landgren, M., Kroes, H. Y., Yaron, Y., Pope, M., Foulds, N., Boute, O., Galán, F., Kingston, H., Van Der Aa, N., Salcedo, I., Swinkels, M. E., Wallgren-Pettersson, C., Gabrielli, O., De Backer, J., Coucke, P. J., & De Paepe, A. M. (2009). Comprehensive clinical and molecular assessment of 32 probands with congenital contractural arachnodactyly: report of 14 novel mutations and review of the literature. *Human Mutation*, *30*(3), 334–341. https://doi.org/10.1002/HUMU.20854.

Chang, M., Cai, Y., Gao, Z., Chen, X., Liu, B., Zhang, C., Yu, W., Cao, Q., Shen, Y., Yao, X., Chen, X., & Sun, H. (2023). Duchenne muscular dystrophy: pathogenesis and promising therapies. *Journal of Neurology*, *270*(8). https://doi.org/10.1007/S00415-023-11796-X.

Charoenngam, N., Rittiphairoj, T., Ponvilawan, B., Jaroenlapnopparat, A., Waitayangkoon, P., Suppakitjanusant, P., Prasitsumrit, V., Pongchaiyakul, C., & Holick, M. F. (2023). Bone Fragility in Hereditary Connective Tissue Disorders: A Systematic Review and Meta-Analysis. *Endocrine Practice: Official Journal of the American College of*

*Endocrinology and the American Association of Clinical Endocrinologists*, *29*(7), 589–600. https://doi.org/10.1016/J.EPRAC.2023.02.003.

Chung, J. C. Y. (2023). Pathology and pathophysiology of the aortic root. *Annals of Cardiothoracic Surgery*, *12*(3), 159–167. https://doi.org/10.21037/ACS-2023-AVS1-17.

El-Hawary, R., & Akbarnia, B. A. (2015). Early Onset Scoliosis - Time for Consensus. *Spine Deformity*, *3*(2), 105–106. https://doi.org/10.1016/J.JSPD.2015.01.003.

Frikha, R. (2020). Klippel-Feil syndrome: a review of the literature. *Clinical Dysmorphology*, *29*(1), 35–37. https://doi.org/10.1097/MCD.0000000000000301.

Funato, N. (2022). Craniofacial Phenotypes and Genetics of DiGeorge Syndrome. *Journal of Developmental Biology*, *10*(2). https://doi.org/10.3390/JDB10020018/S1.

Jett, K., & Friedman, J. M. (2010). Clinical and genetic aspects of neurofibromatosis 1. *Genetics in Medicine*, *12*(1), 1–11. https://doi.org/10.1097/GIM.0B013E3181BF 15E3.

Kearney, M., Orrell, R. W., Fahey, M., Brassington, R., & Pandolfo, M. (2016). Pharmacological treatments for Friedreich ataxia. *The Cochrane Database of Systematic Reviews*, *2016*(8). https://doi.org/10.1002/14651858.CD007791.PUB4.

Köksal, M. (2023). Skolyoz Klinik Muayenesi. *Journal of Anatolian Medical Research*, *8*(1), 14–20. https://dergipark.org.tr/tr/pub/jamer/issue/76232/1181876.

Marathe, N., Lohkamp, L. N., & Fehlings, M. G. (2022). Spinal manifestations of Ehlers-Danlos syndrome: a scoping review. *Journal of Neurosurgery. Spine*, *37*(6), 783–793. https://doi.org/10.3171/2022.6.SPINE211011.

Marelli, S., Micaglio, E., Taurino, J., Salvi, P., Rurali, E., Perrucci, G. L., Dolci, C., Udugampolage, N. S., Caruso, R., Gentilini, D., Trifiro', G., Callus, E., Frigiola, A., De Vincentiis, C., Pappone, C., Parati, G., & Pini, A. (2023). Marfan Syndrome: Enhanced Diagnostic Tools and Follow-up Management Strategies. *Diagnostics (Basel, Switzerland)*, *13*(13). https://doi.org/10.3390/DIAGNOSTICS13132284.

Nishio, H., Niba, E. T. E., Saito, T., Okamoto, K., Takeshima, Y., & Awano, H. (2023). Spinal Muscular Atrophy: The Past, Present, and Future of Diagnosis and Treatment. *International Journal of Molecular Sciences*, *24*(15). https://doi.org/10.3390/IJMS241511939.

Scicluna, K., Formosa, M. M., Farrugia, R., & Borg, I. (2022). Hypermobile Ehlers-Danlos syndrome: A review and a critical appraisal of published genetic research to date. *Clinical Genetics*, *101*(1), 20–31. https://doi.org/10.1111/CGE.14026.

Williams, B. A., Matsumoto, H., McCalla, D. J., Akbarnia, B. A., Blakemore, L. C., Betz, R. R., Flynn, J. M., Johnston, C. E., McCarthy, R. E., Roye, D. P., Skaggs, D. L., Smith, J. T., Snyder, B. D., Sponseller, P. D., Sturm, P. F., Thompson, G. H., Yazici, M., & Vitale, M. G. (2014). Development and initial validation of the Classification of Early-Onset Scoliosis (C-EOS). *The Journal of Bone and Joint Surgery. American Volume*, *96*(16), 1359–1367. https://doi.org/10.2106/JBJS.M.00253.

Yonko, E. A., LoTurco, H. M., Carter, E. M., & Raggio, C. L. (2021). Orthopedic considerations and surgical outcomes in Ehlers-Danlos syndromes. *American Journal of Medical Genetics. Part C, Seminars in Medical Genetics*, *187*(4), 458–465. https://doi.org/10.1002/AJMG.C.31958.

Yu, H., Li, C., Wu, H., Xia, W., Wang, Y., Zhao, J., & Xu, C. (2023). Pathogenic mechanisms of osteogenesis imperfecta, evidence for classification. *Orphanet Journal of Rare Diseases*, *18*(1), 234. https://doi.org/10.1186/S13023-023-02849-5.

## Chapter 10

# Radiological Examination of Early-Onset Scoliosis

**Alim Can Baymurat***, **MD**
Department of Orthopedics and Traumatology, Gazi University, Faculty of Medicine, Ankara, Turkey

## Abstract

Early-onset scoliosis (EOS) is a progressive childhood spinal disease that can potentially cause severe spinal deformities and respiratory problems. The management of EOS disease is a challenging process for spine surgeons and requires a multidisciplinary approach for EOS patients with accompanying pathologies.

The approach for patients with EOS differs according to the etiology of the disease, the age of the patient, and the extent of the spinal deformity, and radiological examination has an essential place in the diagnosis and treatment of these patients.

The initial assessment of pediatric patients with suspected spinal deformity begins with a detailed history and physical evaluation, and plain radiographs of the spine are performed in the first step of their radiological examinations. On plain radiography, deformities and extents of the spine are assessed in the coronal and sagittal planes. Furthermore, bone maturation and concomitant musculoskeletal pathologies are evaluated. Computed tomography (CT) is used to examine congenital segmentation and formation deformities of the spine. Magnetic resonance imaging (MRI) of the entire spine is recommended for patients with EOS, because of generally associated intraspinal pathologies in

* Corresponding Author's Email: alimcanbaymurat@yahoo.com.

In: Early Onset Scoliosis
Editor: Ahmed Majid Heydar
ISBN: 979-8-89113-600-7

patients with EOS and especially for patients with EOS who are scheduled for surgical treatment.

Current advances in imaging methods in the medical field provide a three-dimensional understanding of the details of EOS deformities, which makes it beneficial in the treatment planning of the disease.

**Keywords:** early-onset scoliosis, radiological examination, Cobb angle, computed tomography, magnetic resonance imaging

## Introduction

EOS is a spinal deformity with a curvature of 10° or more, which is observed in children under the age of 10, regardless of its etiology. Treatment of patients with EOS remains a challenge for spine surgeons because of this age group, the still-growing spine, and additional intraspinal and extraspinal pathologies (Goker and Yazici, 2022). Since the use of X-rays by Wilhelm Roentgen in 1895, imaging techniques have improved a lot in the field of medicine, and it provides a better understanding of pathology by evaluating spinal deformities in three-dimensional (Smith et al. 2016). On radiological examination of the patients, the extent of the spinal deformity and the bone maturation of the patient is evaluated, and the potential for the progression of scoliosis is evaluated. Additionally, radiographic examinations enable us to evaluate the lung capacity and respiratory function of patients.

Generally, patients with EOS are exposed to repeated radiation for many years of radiological follow-up. Some measures are taken to reduce the exposure of patients to X-rays. Furthermore, MRI and the EOS system (EOS Imaging, Paris, France) significantly reduce exposure to X-rays.

EOS patients are separated into types of idiopathic, congenital, neuromuscular, and syndromic in accordance with the etiology, and the treatment and follow-up of patients differ according to the etiology of the disease and the extent of spinal curvature (El-Hawary and Akbarnia, 2015). This section provides an overview of current imaging techniques for the management of children with early-onset scoliosis.

## Imaging Methods in Spine Deformities

### Plain Radiography

The first radiological examination to assess spinal deformity is plain radiography. Radiological examination of spinal deformities is performed on direct radiography standing (patients who cannot stand can sit or lie down), posterior-anterior (PA) radiographs, and lateral coronal and sagittal plane scoliosis radiographs. The PA position reduces the amount of radiation exposure to the cornea, thyroid, breast tissue, and reproductive organs. Additionally, lead plate protections should be used when necessary (Drummond et al., 1983). Scoliosis radiograph should be taken in a way that C1 cervical spines in the cranial area and the pelvis in the caudal area should be visible (Cassar-Pullicino and Eisenstein, 2002). Inequalities in the lower extremities and pelvic obliquities should be considered on standing radiographs. In case of a leg length discrepancy, a lift should be placed under the shorter leg by the length of the leg. Plain radiographs allow evaluation of the etiology of the deformity (idiopathic, congenital, neuromuscular, etc.) and analysis of both coronal and sagittal balance. The degree of curvature can be measured and documented by measuring various curvatures using the Cobb technique. Skeletal maturation is assessed by observing various growth plates, such as the triradiate cartilage of the hip or the iliac apophysis (Risser sign) (Greiner, 2002).

### EOS System

The EOS system (EOS Imaging, Paris, France) reduces radiation exposure to approximately one-tenth and provides a better imagining of spinal deformities and software analysis than X-Ray, but it is used in very few centers because of high costs. The EOS system (EOS Imaging, Paris, France) is a novel development in imaging technology that enables a three-dimensional (3D) assessment of scoliosis deformity through the two-dimensional (2D) images obtained. It requires a standing position for the scan and allows convenient assessment of gravity and posture in accordance with the deformity, but requires patients to stand upright and stable with weight. The EOS system is a powerful imaging method for the 3D assessment of scoliosis deformity (Faria et al., 2013; Glaiser et al., 2012).

## Computed Tomography

Computed tomography (CT) enables the opportunity to examine bone pathologies in more detail, and it is possible to understand complex spinal deformities with three-dimensional CT imaginings in more detail. It gives an opportunity to better understand spinal anomalies in congenital spinal malformations. Its use in the diagnosis and follow-up of idiopathic scoliosis is controversial regarding high radiation risk (Smith et al., 2016).

## Magnetic Resonance Imaging

In suggestive intraspinal pathological symptoms such as unexplained back or headache, asymmetries or absence of abdominal skin reflex, lumbar or sacral hair growth, milky brown skin lesions, changes in foot size, foot cavus deformity, extremity muscle atrophy or loss of motor strength, MRI examination should be performed in patients with early-onset scoliosis. The incidence of intraspinal pathology has been reported to be 20% in patients with early-onset idiopathic scoliosis without clinical findings and 3% to 52% in congenital scoliosis. Therefore, EOS patients, especially those scheduled for surgical treatment, should be evaluated preoperatively with MRI in terms of intraspinal malformation (Smith et al., 2016).

## Early-Onset Idiopathic Scoliosis

EOS patients without a specific etiology are defined as infantile idiopathic scoliosis for children 3 years and younger and juvenile idiopathic scoliosis for children 4-10 years of age. The radiologic evaluation of early-onset idiopathic scoliosis patients is usually performed with plain radiography. If necessary, more radiological examinations are requested.

Plain radiography is a simple and reliable method of radiological evaluation in patients with suspected scoliosis. The initial evaluation should contain posteroanterior (PA) and lateral radiographs of the spine (including the cervical spine and pelvis). Supine position radiographs should be performed for children who are too young to stand. Congenital deformities are eliminated with plain radiographs. Additionally, Cobb angles of the spine in the coronal and sagittal planes are measured. Main curvatures and compensatory curvatures are detected by bending and/or traction radiographs. The treatment plan is based on the progression of the Cobb angle of scoliosis in the first and subsequent follow-ups and Mehta's rib vertebral angle difference (RVAD) (Glaser et al., 2012). Mehta's costal vertebral angle is evaluated to predict the progression of scoliosis on the thoracic curves of patients with infantile idiopathic scoliosis. The costal-vertebral angle is the angle between a line drawn vertically to the apical vertebral end plate and a line drawn through the middle of the costa. Mehta's RVAD is calculated by subtracting the costa-vertebral angle on the concave side from the costa-vertebral angle on the convex side (Figure 1).

While the fact that the RVAD is less than 20° will not progress in 83% of cases, the degree of RVAD of 20° or more is often associated with progression. Additionally, Mehta defined a second radiographic parameter to help estimate the overlap of the rib head and the vertebral body in the apical vertebra (Figure 1). In phase 1, there is no overlap of the costal head with the apical vertebra. Measurement of RVAD is recommended to detect progression in this group of patients. In phase 2, the costal head overlaps the apical vertebra. The progression of the curvature is unavoidable in phase 2, and it has been reported that RVAD does not need to be measured (Glaser et al., 2012; Mehta, 1972).

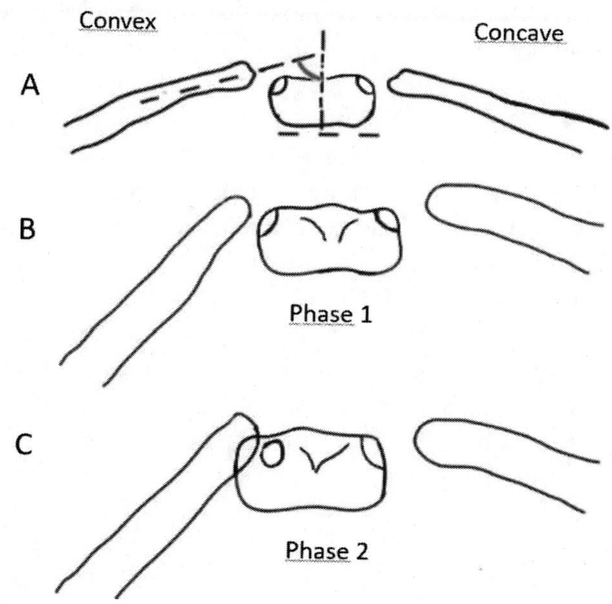


**Figure 1.** A: Rib vertebral angle difference (RVAD); B: Phase of the rib head: phase 1; C. Phase of the rib head: phase 2.

Advanced imaging in infantile and juvenile scoliosis is directly associated with the presence of bone and neural axis abnormalities. CT is useful to evaluate pedicle anatomy and bone anomalies in patients scheduled for surgical treatment. MRI method has been used to evaluate neural axis and soft tissue pathologies.

Neurological abnormalities have been reported at a rate of 20% in patients with idiopathic scoliosis under the age of 10 years (Lewonowski et al., 1992; Diab, 2011). MRI should be performed in patients with infantile and juvenile idiopathic scoliosis and in any suspected cases of spinal dysraphism (left thoracic curvature, painful scoliosis, abnormal neurological examination) (Dubousset, 2022).

## Early-Onset Congenital Scoliosis

Congenital scoliosis (CS) is a spinal deformity in the coronal plane caused by malformations that occur in the early embryonic period. While the formation of somites (precursors of spinal segments) begins between weeks 3 and 5 of pregnancy, segmentation occurs between weeks 6 and 8 of pregnancy. It results in fully segmented hemivertebra, semi-segmented hemivertebra, unsegmented hemivertebra, and incarcerated hemivertebra due to the defect of formation. While the segmentation defect is seen as an unsegmented bar and a unilateral unsegmented bar with contralateral hemivertebra and block vertebra, the formation and segmentation defect can also be seen as mixed (Ruf, 2022). Radiological examination of patients with CS related to mixed congenital bone pathologies requires advanced radiological examinations in addition to plain radiographs.

In the evaluation of CS patients with a direct roentgenogram, standing posterior-anterior and lateral radiographs are performed, and in patients who cannot stand, plain radiographs are performed while lying on their back and side. Cobb angles of spinal deformities in the coronal and sagittal planes are measured. Congenital malformations of the spine are examined. With the help of that, it is possible to specify the type of malformation, the extent of the curvature, and the potential progression of the vertebral anomaly (Facanha-Filho et al., 2001) (Figure 2 a, b).

Initial radiological examination is direct roentgenograms in the radiological evaluation of scoliosis patients. However, complex deformities of the spine in patients with CS may complicate the interpretation of plain radiographs. Advanced imaging techniques are required in patients scheduled for surgical treatment. CT is promising for the examination of osseous structures. Three-dimensional computed tomography is the best radiological method for defining the defect of congenital formation and segmentation of the spine (Newton et al., 2002) (Figure 2 c, d, e, f). It is mostly recommended in the initial evaluation of CS patients and complex deformities of the spine definition in patients scheduled for surgical treatment; however, it is not recommended for routine observation or serial follow-up.

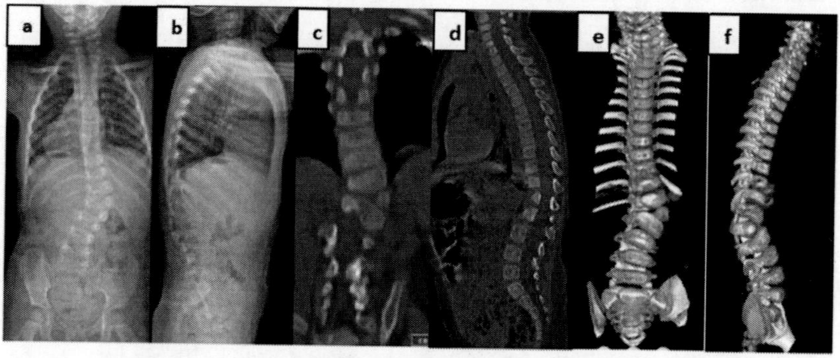


**Figure 2.** a: Posterion-anterior plain radiography of the spine; b: Lateral plain radiography of the spine; c: Computed tomography of the spine in the coronal plane; d: Computed tomography of the spine in the sagittal plane; e: 3D computed tomography of the entire spine in the coronal plane; f: 3D computed tomography of the entire spine in the sagittal plane.

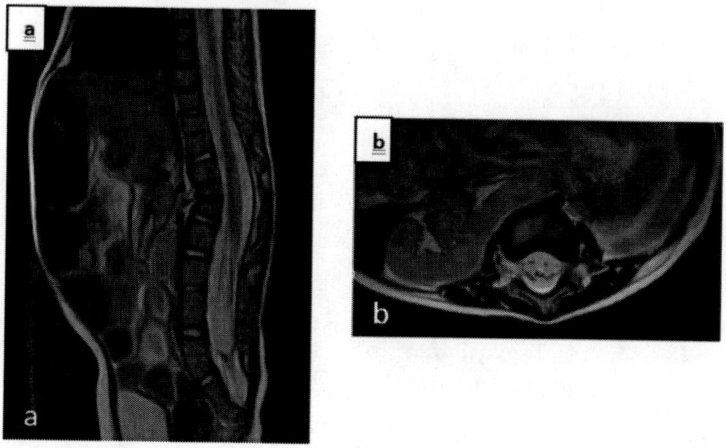


**Figure 3.** MRI images of a patient with congenital kyphoscoliosis in the thoracolumbar spine. a: Sagittal section; b: Axial section.

MRI has been used to evaluate intraspinal pathology (Figure 3 a, b). In case of weakness, loss of sensation, spasticity, and pathological reflexes in the extremities, an MRI of a complete spine should be performed. Additionally, skin pathologies such as pain, dimples, hairy patch, or nevus on the patient's back should be examined with MRI (Bradford et al., 1991).

## Early-Onset Neuromuscular Scoliosis

Neuromuscular scoliosis (NMS) is caused by muscle imbalance according to a neuropathic or myopathic disease, an abnormal biomechanical load on the spine. Neuromuscular scoliosis usually has an early-onset, progresses rapidly, and may continue to progress after skeletal maturation is complete. While NMS progresses as idiopathic scoliosis with preserved ambulation ability, it is sometimes seen as chair-bound or bed-bound patients with a large curvature reaching the sacrum and pelvis (Lonstein and Akbarnia, 1983) (Figure 4).

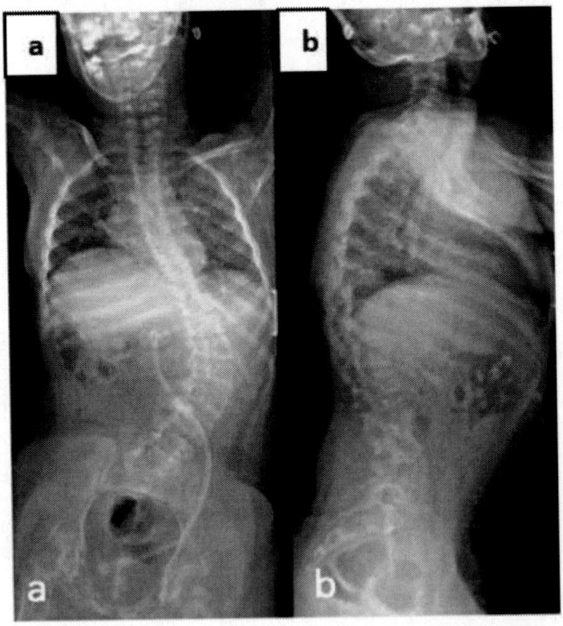


**Figure 4.** Neuromuscular scoliosis 8-year-old girl with cerebral palsy. a: Posterion-anterior plain radiography of the spine; b. Lateral plain radiography of the spine.

For the radiological evaluation of NMS patients, PA and lateral radiographs of the entire spine are performed while standing (it may be necessary to support the head and body by sitting in patients who cannot stand, or in severely affected children with poor truncal control). The type and size of the curvature, the balance of the spine in the coronal and sagittal planes, the pelvic obliquity, and the tilt are evaluated on the radiograph (Shah and Lau, 2016). Advanced imaging examination is usually required to eliminate intraspinal pathologies.

## Early-Onset Syndromic Scoliosis

Syndromic scoliosis is a scoliosis that develops secondary to a more severe underlying disease process. Syndromic scoliosis is usually seen in Marfan syndrome, Ehlers-Danlos syndrome, Loeys-Dietz syndrome, Down syndrome, Rett syndrome, Achondroplasia, Neurofibromatosis, and Prader-Willi syndrome.

Radiographic evaluation of patients with syndromic scoliosis begins with a direct roentgenogram, as in all spinal deformities. It should be evaluated with standing posterior-anterior and lateral radiography in terms of the extent of the deformities and the severity of rotation in the coronal and sagittal planes. If there is no rotational deformity of the spine in the direct roentgenogram of scoliosis patients, an advanced radiological examination should be performed in terms of intraspinal masses, syrinx, or bone tumors. MRI should be performed in patients under 10 years of age, those with neurological deficits, and those with spinal dysraphism. In some patients with syndromic scoliosis, the pedicle width and laminar thickness may be smaller than normal, and the biconcave vertebra, the transitional vertebra and the increased transverse process distance are common. Therefore, it is necessary to examine the CT imaginings of the entire spine in terms of osseous anomalies in patients considered for surgical treatment. The increase in the distance of the anterior atlanto-odontoid is one of the signs of atlantoaxial instability. Asymptomatic atlantoaxial instability is seen in 10%-20% of patients with Down syndrome. Therefore, cervical radiographs should be carefully examined in terms of atlantoaxial instability in patients with syndromic scoliosis (Suresh and Sponseller, 2022) (Figure 5).

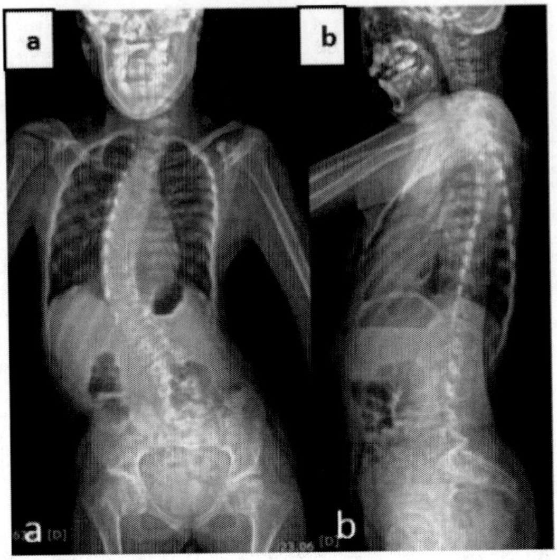


**Figure 5.** a. Syndromic scoliosis. 9-year-old girl with Larsen syndrome. a: Posterion-anterior plain radiography of the spine; b. Lateral plain radiography of the spine.

## Conclusion

The management of early-onset scoliosis continues to be a challenge for spine surgeons despite advances in medicine. By combining advanced imaging methods with detailed anamnesis and examination findings of the patients, it is possible to evaluate the respiratory function and capacity, which are most affected in this disease, in addition to knowledge of the extent, types, and the progression potential of the deformity. Radiological evaluation is an indivisible part of the evaluation method of the disease at all stages, such as diagnosis, differential diagnosis, treatment, and follow-up of EOS patients, and all surgeons who deal with the management deformities in a child with a growing spine should have sufficient knowledge of the radiological evaluation of the spine.

## References

Bradford, D. S., Heithoff, K. B., Cohen, M. (1991). Intraspinal abnormalities and congenital spine deformities: a radiographic and MRI study. *J Pediatr Orthop. 11*(1), 36-41. https://doi.org/10.1097/01241398-199101000-00009.

Cassar-Pullicino, V. N., Eisenstein, S. M. (2002). Imaging in scoliosis: what, why and how? *Clin Radiol. 57*(7), 543-562. https://doi.org/10.1053/crad.2001.0909.

Diab, M., Landman, Z., Lubicky, J., Dormans, J., Erickson, M., Richards, B. S. members of the Spinal Deformity Study Group. (2011). Use and outcome of MRI in the surgical treatment of adolescent idiopathic scoliosis. *Spine (Phila Pa 1976). 36*(8), 667-671. https://doi.org/10.1097/BRS.0b013e3181da218c.

Dubousset, J. (2022). *Essentials of Spine Surgery: Idiopathic Scoliosis.* (Senkoylu,A., Canavese, F. Eds.), Springer Nature Switzerland AG. https://doi.org/10.1007/978-3-030-80356-8.

Drummond, D., Ranallo, F., Lonstein, J., Brooks, H. L., Cameron, J. (1983). Radiation hazards in scoliosis management. *Spine (Phila Pa 1976). 8*(7),741-748. https://doi.org/10.1097/00007632-198310000-00010.

El-Hawary, R., Akbarnia, B. A. (2015). Early onset scoliosis - time for consensus. *Spine Deform, 3*(2), 105-106. https://doi.org/10.1016/j.jspd.2015.01.003.

Facanha-Filho, F. A., Winter, R. B., Lonstein, J. E., Koop, S., Novacheck, T., L'Heureux, Jr. E. A., Noren, C. A. (2001). Measurement accuracy in congenital scoliosis. *J Bone Joint Surg Am.83*(1), 42-45. https://doi.org/10.2106/00004623-200101000-00006.

Faria, R., McKenna, C., Wade, R., Yang, H., Woolacott, N., Sculpher, M. (2013). The EOS 2D/3D X-ray imaging system: a cost-effectiveness analysis quantifying the health benefits from reduced radiation exposure. *Eur J Radiol. 82*(8),342-349. https://doi.org/10.1016/j.ejrad.2013.02.015.

Glaser, D. A., Doan, J., Newton, P. O. (2012). Comparison of 3-dimensional spinal reconstruction accuracy: biplanar radiographs with EOS versus computed tomography. *Spine (Phila Pa 1976). 37*(16),1391-1397. https://doi.org/10.1097/BRS.0b013e3182518a15.

Goker, B., Yazici, M. (2022). *Essentials of spine surgery: early onset idiopathic scoliosis.* Springer.

Greiner, K. A. (2002). Adolescent idiopathic scoliosis: radiologic decision-making. *Am Fam Physician. 65*(9), 1817-1822.

Lewonowski, K., King, J. D., Nelson, M. D. (1992). Routine use of magnetic resonance imaging in idiopathic scoliosis patients less than eleven years of age. *Spine (Phila Pa 1976).17*(6 Suppl). https://doi.org/10.1097/00007632-199206001-00008.

Lonstein, J. E., Akbarnia, A. (1983). Operative treatment of spinal deformities in patients with cerebral palsy or mental retardation. An analysis of one hundred and seven cases. *J Bone Joint Surg Am, 65*(1), 43-55.

Mehta, M. H. (1972). The rib-vertebra angle in the early diagnosis between resolving and progressive infantile scoliosis. *J Bone Joint Surg Br. 54*(2):230-243.

Newton, P. O., Hahn, G. W., Fricka, K. B., Wenger, D. R. (2002). Utility of three-dimensional and multiplanar reformatted computed tomography for evaluation of pediatric congenital spine abnormalities. *Spine (Phila Pa 1976). 27*(8), 844-850. https://doi.org/10.1097/00007632-200204150-00012.

Ruf, M. (2022). *Essentials of Spine Surgery: Congenital Scoliosis.* (Senkoylu,A., Canavese, F. Eds.). Springer Nature Switzerland AG. https://doi.org/10.1007/978-3-030-80356-8.

Shah, S. A., Lau, L. L. (2016). Treatment of spinal deformity in cerebral palsy. In: Akbarnia, B. A., Yazici, M., Thompson, G. H. (Eds.), *The Growing spine. management of spinal disorders in young children* (pp. 191-210). Springer Heidelberg New York Dordrecht London. https://doi.org/10.1007/978-3-662-48284-1.

Smith, J. T., Newton, P. O., Farnsworth, C. L., Parvaresh, K. (2016). *The Growing spine, management of spinal disorders in young children: imaging of the growing spine*. Springer.

Suresh, K. V., Sponseller, P. D. (2022). *Essentials of spine surgery: sendromic scoliosis.* (Senkoylu, A., Canavese, F. Eds.). Springer Nature Switzerland AG. https://doi.org/10.1007/978-3-030-80356-8.

# Chapter 11

# Biomechanics of EOS

**Bilal Yekeler[1,*], MD**
**and Umut Doğu Aktürk[2], MD**
[1]Department of Neurosurgery, Bayburt State Hospital, Bayburt, Turkiye
[2]Department of Neurosurgery, Emsey Hospital, Istanbul, Turkiye

## Abstract

Early-onset scoliosis (EOS), which begins before the age of 10, radiologically lateral Cobb angle (a parameter measuring spinal curvature) is ≥10°, and it is the most common form of structural spinal deformity. EOS is a very challenging case for surgeons. These patients are young patients who have the potential to grow significantly. These patients are likely to have progressive deformities, cosmetic deformities, and cardiopulmonary disorders, and in most cases, early intervention is necessary. Although the beginning of EOS is not fully understood, many studies have been conducted about which factors may be effective at this point. Some of these theories are based on a biomechanical and three-dimensional pathoanatomic basis. The purpose of this chapter is to examine the biomechanical background of this condition and try to better understand the disease.

**Keywords:** biomechanics of EOS, spine biomechanics, scoliosis biomechanics

* Corresponding Author's Email: bilalyekeler@gmail.com.

In: Early Onset Scoliosis
Editor: Ahmed Majid Heydar
ISBN: 979-8-89113-600-7

## Introduction

When considering the biomechanics of the spine, it is composed of connected structures more suitable for deformation, such as intervertebral discs, facet articular cartilages, a number of connective tissues, and considerable rigid segments (vertebrae). The biomechanical role of this complex system is both to withstand loads to ensure constant upright posture and to enable versatile mobility and stability in any position. Another important role is to prevent abnormal intervertebral movement, which can affect nerves (Skalli & Vergari, 2018). The spine is only one part of an integral neuro-muscular system. Other important components of this system are listed as follows:

- Head or cephalic vertebrae weighing 4-5 kg (Vital & Senegas, 1986)
- The pelvis, which is the basis of the structure (called the pelvic vertebra by Jean Dubousset) (Hasegawa & Dubousset, 2022). These base moves show a change in the pelvic tilt angle and a consequent change in the sacral slope angle to ensure postural control.
- The thorax, including the ribs, which protect vital organs in the rib cage (lung and heart) and strengthen the thoracic vertebrae,
- The musculoskeletal system,
- The central nervous system.

This system allows a person to maintain their balance while in an upright posture, under gravitational loadings, with their head above the pelvis and their eyes in a horizontal plane.

Scoliosis is a three-dimensional alteration of the entire spine, with lateral and axial deviations and rotations. Local changes such as vertebral rotation and wedging also occur, especially at the apical level. Perdriolle explained that with degeneration of the vertebral and intervertebral discs in the axial plane, increased torsion in the scoliotic slope causes hyperkyphosis in the thoracic region and rotation in the upper extremity (Perdriolle & Vidal, 1987).

These changes in the growing spine exposed to gravitational loadings determine the local pressure, which affects the biomechanics of the spine and causes bone growths and changes in the disc structure, leading to an increase in the slope (Meir et al., 2007). Furthermore, muscle forces may become asymmetric to provide recovery in posture.

Some biomechanical concepts that cause scoliosis are listed, such as axial rotational instability (Wong, 2015), biomechanical and neuromuscular factors

(Veldhuizen et al., 2000), anterior spinal overgrowth and asynchronous, spinal neuro-osseous growth (the spinal cord cannot grow parallel with the vertebral column, causing the spine to 'bend') (Porter, 2001; Roth, 1981), asymmetric mechanical compression, also known as the Hueter-Volkmann Law, and biomechanical spinal growth modulation as a result of decreased load (Stokes et al., 2006). Examples selected from hypotheses and techniques contain the intrinsic "dorsal shear loads" hypothesis, which is related to the axial rotational instability of the spine caused by bipedalism (Castelein et al., 2005).

The vertical posture of a person is an essential factor in the discussion of the biomechanics of EOS because EOS has not been observed in any species other than humans (Janssen, de Wilde, et al., 2011). The vertical posture of human bipedal (bipedalism) is enabled by carrying the body directly over the pelvis. In other vertebrate species, both bipedal and quadrupedal, the body is carried in front of the pelvis (Cheng et al., 2015).

## Growth and Spine Development

Many anthropometric studies have indicated that children with EOS are taller and thinner than their peers, according to the analysis of body length in children with normal and scoliosis (Siu King Cheung et al., 2003). It was found that the ratio of leg length to body length in scoliotic children is the same as in the normal population, which indicates an overall growth disorder in EOS rather than growth limited to the spine (Nissinen et al., 1993). Therefore, growth has an essential role in the development and progress of EOS. However, the biomechanics of this growth in the development of EOS are not fully understood. Castelein emphasized that human posture is important in the beginning and progress of EOS (Castelein et al., 2005).

Goldberg stated that girls with adolescent idiopathic scoliosis (AIS) had an earlier growth rate and reached their adult height earlier compared to the healthy control group who were not scoliotic (Goldberg et al., 1993; Ylikoski, 1993). According to the authors supporting deviation in the growth pattern, a longer and thinner spine can deviate from the sagittal plane when exposed to the forces of load vectors and can cause early-onset scoliosis (Dickson et al., 1984; Millner & Dickson, 1996). Deacon and Dickson et al. stated that in scoliotic patients, the anterior column height of the apical vertebra is significantly higher than the posterior column height (Deane & Duthie, 1973; Dickson et al., 1984).

In addition to the spine, the periapical ribs in patients with EOS (Normelli et al., 1985), asymmetric growth in other bones, and asymmetric morphology (Burwell et al., 2006). Asymmetric and asynchronous neuro-osseous growth of the spine and spinal cord has been found to be associated with anterior spinal abnormal growth (Chu et al., 2006, 2008).

## Primary and Secondary Biomechanical Factors

Various possible factors have a role in the development of spinal deformity in EOS. After a certain level of asymmetry develops, the progression of this deformity is probably caused by a mechanical disorder of the spinal load distribution. Factors that can lead scoliosis contain conditions such as hyperkyphosis, a 'slender' spine, and abnormal sagittal curvatures. Spines with these characteristics are more sensitive to "bending" in the frontal plane and rotation in the axial plane, which is the maximum at the apex of the spinal curvature (Millner & Dickson, 1996). In the spine with scoliosis and rotation, ligaments, and muscle structures have also been associated with "tethering" (Jarvis et al., 1988). Furthermore, it is possible that neuromuscular anomalies cause asymmetric spinal loading and therefore the onset and progression of scoliosis (Veldhuizen et al., 2000).

Along with studies that investigated how asymmetric loading would cause progressive spinal deformity, and several animal experiments that surgically achieved this loading (Bobyn et al., 2015), it is supported, although the role of biomechanics in the initiation of EOS is unclear (Villemure & Stokes, 2009). Conservative follow-up with a corset on EOS is based on this theory.

In the progression of scoliosis, the "vicious cycle" hypothesis has been asserted that the loads placed on the spine of the lateral slope will be asymmetrically divided, which will cause the vertebral growth to be asymmetric (Roaf, 1960). This asymmetry leads to the progression of the lateral slope according to the Hueter-Volkmann Law, which stated that increasing compression loads reduce growth and decreasing compression loads accelerate growth (Mehlman et al., 1997). This condition can cause the vertebra to wedge. This hypothesis has been supported by experimental studies conducted in various mammalian species that measure the severity of pressure on the convex and concave planes of vertebrae and measure the growth sensitivity and geometric changes of vertebrae under stress in an asymmetric growing spine (I. A. F. Stokes, 2007). According to this analysis, it is predicted that a small curvature in a growing spine can cause the progression of scoliosis.

## Bipedalism

Another theory asserted in the development of EOS is associated with the biomechanics of human bipedalism. Idiopathic scoliosis has only been diagnosed in humans, even though spinal deformities have been observed in animals (Kouwenhoven & Castelein, 2008). The biomechanical load of the human spine is majorly different from that of other species, while the spinal anatomy of humans and other vertebrate species is very similar to each other. Along with a lordotic curvature that develops between the ischial and iliac bones and expands toward the lumbar spine, it places the human center of gravity directly on the pelvis. All other vertebrate species, including bipedal ones, lack these lordotic curvatures, and alternatively, they walk by flexing the hips and knees, placing the center of gravity of the body in front of the hips (Schlösser et al., 2014).

These differences affect humans. For example, by the anatomy of the spine, it can endure axial and anterior loads; however, as a result of the posture, certain areas of the human spine are sloped toward the posterior and are exposed to posterior loads (Castelein et al., 2005; Janssen, Kouwenhoven, et al., 2011). Research has claimed that "dorsal shear loads" can reduce rotational pathology (Castelein et al., 2005; Janssen, Kouwenhoven, et al., 2011; Kouwenhoven & Castelein, 2008). Therefore, the rotational stability depends on whether the vertebrae are loaded in the anterior or posterior direction, and it can also depend on whether the vertebrae are sloped anteriorly or posteriorly in the sagittal plane.

## Dorsal Shear Force

The dorsal shear force affects the growing spine. This condition causes different mechanical stresses in the spine (Kouwenhoven et al., 2007). Resisting axial loads, the spine can carry these loads through its vertebral end plates and elastic discs. The anterior shear load is easily balanced due to the facet joints of the spine and strong posterior ligaments. Increasing the forward loading directed at the spinal segments makes the segment rotationally more stable. However, dorsal shear loads on the growing and undergrowth spine are not properly tolerated mechanically and cause rotational instability (Kouwenhoven et al., 2007). As a result, according to Hueter-Volkmann Law, this condition causes the anterior side of the disc to expand and the bone to extend forward (I. A. Stokes et al., 1996). Stokes indicated that the progression of skeletal deformity during periods of peak growth occurs with asymmetric loading, according to the Hueter-Volkmann Law. The presence of asymmetric loading on the end plates of the vertebrae will result in rotational lordosis induced by rapid growth at the onset of a scoliosis deformity. If the progression of scoliosis is caused by asymmetric loading, it is considered that the dorsal shear load is responsible for this condition (I. A. Stokes, 1997).

## Conclusion

The spine is a very complex organ, and spinal biomechanics is a complex condition. Studies conducted in recent years have contributed to the understanding of the biomechanics of the spine and the pathomechanism of EOS. Additionally, it is still discussed whether between the anterior and posterior elements of the instability growth causing rotational lordosis is the key factor in the pathology or whether asymmetric growth and muscle activity have a primary role. The effect of human-derived upright bipedal posture, which makes the human spine less resistant to rotation and decompensation, on pathomechanism is being researched. All human vertebrae are dependent on these destabilizing loads, but what drives some of them to disorder toward the progressive rotational instability that we call scoliosis is still waiting to be proven. It is obvious that the mechanism is complex and multifactorial.

## References

Bobyn, J. D., Little, D. G., Gray, R., & Schindeler, A. (2015). Animal models of scoliosis. *Journal of Orthopaedic Research: Official Publication of the Orthopaedic Research Society, 33*(4), 458-467. https://doi.org/10.1002/jor.22797.

Burwell, R. G., Aujla, R. K., Freeman, B. J. C., Dangerfield, P. H., Cole, A. A., Kirby, A. S., Pratt, R. K., Webb, J. K., & Moulton, A. (2006). Patterns of Extra-Spinal Left-Right Skeletal Asymmetries in Adolescent Girls with Lower Spine Scoliosis: Relative Lengthening of the Ilium on the Curve Concavity & of Right Lower Limb Segments. In *Research into Spinal Deformities 5* (ss. 57-65). IOS Press. https://ebooks.iospress.nl/publication/9535.

Castelein, R. M., Dieën, J. H. V., & Smit, T. H. (2005). The role of dorsal shear forces in the pathogenesis of adolescent idiopathic scoliosis – A hypothesis. *Medical Hypotheses*, *65*(3), 501-508. https://doi.org/10.1016/j.mehy.2005.03.025.

Cheng, J. C., Castelein, R. M., Chu, W. C., Danielsson, A. J., Dobbs, M. B., Grivas, T. B., Gurnett, C. A., Luk, K. D., Moreau, A., Newton, P. O., Stokes, I. A., Weinstein, S. L., & Burwell, R. G. (2015). Adolescent idiopathic scoliosis. *Nature Reviews. Disease Primers*, *1*, 15030. https://doi.org/10.1038/nrdp.2015.30.

Chu, W. C. W., Lam, W. W. M., Chan, Y.-L., Ng, B. K. W., Lam, T.-P., Lee, K.-M., Guo, X., & Cheng, J. C. Y. (2006). Relative shortening and functional tethering of spinal cord in adolescent idiopathic scoliosis?: Study with multiplanar reformat magnetic resonance imaging and somatosensory evoked potential. *Spine*, *31*(1), E19-25. https://doi.org/10.1097/01.brs.0000193892.20764.51.

Chu, W. C. W., Man, G. C. W., Lam, W. W. M., Yeung, B. H. Y., Chau, W. W., Ng, B. K. W., Lam, T., Lee, K., & Cheng, J. C. Y. (2008). Morphological and functional electrophysiological evidence of relative spinal cord tethering in adolescent idiopathic scoliosis. *Spine*, *33*(6), 673-680. https://doi.org/10.1097/BRS.0b013e318166aa58.

Deane, G., & Duthie, R. B. (1973). A New Projectional Look at Articulated Scoliotic Spines. *Acta Orthopaedica Scandinavica*, *44*(4-5), 351-365. https://doi.org/10.3109/17453677308989071.

Dickson, R., Lawton, J., Archer, I., & Butt, W. (1984). The pathogenesis of idiopathic scoliosis. Biplanar spinal asymmetry. *The Journal of Bone and Joint Surgery. British Volume*, *66-B*(1), 8-15. https://doi.org/10.1302/0301-620X.66B1.6693483.

Goldberg, C. J., Dowling, F. E., & Fogarty, E. E. (1993). Adolescent idiopathic scoliosis—Early menarche, normal growth. *Spine*, *18*(5), 529-535. https://doi.org/10.1097/00007632-199304000-00003.

Hasegawa, K., & Dubousset, J. F. (2022). Cone of Economy with the Chain of Balance—Historical Perspective and Proof of Concept. *Spine Surgery and Related Research*, *6*(4), 337-349. https://doi.org/10.22603/ssrr.2022-0038.

Janssen, M. M. A., de Wilde, R. F., Kouwenhoven, J.-W. M., & Castelein, R. M. (2011). Experimental animal models in scoliosis research: A review of the literature. *The Spine Journal: Official Journal of the North American Spine Society*, *11*(4), 347-358. https://doi.org/10.1016/j.spinee.2011.03.010.

Janssen, M. M. A., Kouwenhoven, J.-W. M., Schlösser, T. P. C., Viergever, M. A., Bartels, L. W., Castelein, R. M., & Vincken, K. L. (2011). Analysis of preexistent vertebral rotation in the normal infantile, juvenile, and adolescent spine. *Spine*, *36*(7), E486-491. https://doi.org/10.1097/BRS.0b013e3181f468cc.

Jarvis, J. G., Ashman, R. B., Johnston, C. E., & Herring, J. A. (1988). The posterior tether in scoliosis. *Clinical Orthopaedics and Related Research*, *227*, 126-134.

Kouwenhoven, J.-W. M., & Castelein, R. M. (2008). The Pathogenesis of Adolescent Idiopathic Scoliosis: Review of the Literature. *Spine*, *33*(26), 2898-2908. https://doi.org/10.1097/BRS.0b013e3181891751.

Kouwenhoven, J.-W. M., Smit, T. H., van der Veen, A. J., Kingma, I., van Dieën, J. H., & Castelein, R. M. (2007). Effects of dorsal versus ventral shear loads on the rotational stability of the thoracic spine: A biomechanical porcine and human cadaveric study. *Spine*, *32*(23), 2545-2550. https://doi.org/10.1097/BRS.0b013e318158cd86.

Mehlman, C. T., Araghi, A., & Roy, D. R. (1997). Hyphenated history: The Hueter-Volkmann law. *American Journal of Orthopedics (Belle Mead, N.J.)*, *26*(11), 798-800.

Meir, A. R., Fairbank, J. C., Jones, D. A., McNally, D. S., & Urban, J. P. (2007). High pressures and asymmetrical stresses in the scoliotic disc in the absence of muscle loading. *Scoliosis*, *2*(1), 4. https://doi.org/10.1186/1748-7161-2-4.

Millner, P. A., & Dickson, R. A. (1996). Idiopathic scoliosis: Biomechanics and biology. *European Spine Journal*, *5*(6), 362-373. https://doi.org/10.1007/BF00301963.

Nissinen, M., Heliövaara, M., Seitsamo, J., & Poussa, M. (1993). Trunk asymmetry, posture, growth, and risk of scoliosis. A three-year follow-up of Finnish prepubertal school children. *Spine*, *18*(1), 8-13. https://doi.org/10.1097/00007632-199301000-00002.

Normelli, H., Sevastik, J., & Akrivos, J. (1985). The length and ash weight of the ribs of normal and scoliotic persons. *Spine*, *10*(6), 590-592. https://doi.org/10.1097/00007632-198507000-00015.

Perdriolle, R., & Vidal, J. (1987). Morphology of scoliosis: Three-dimensional evolution. *Orthopedics*, *10*(6), 909-915. https://doi.org/10.3928/0147-7447-19870601-10.

Porter, R. W. (2001). The pathogenesis of idiopathic scoliosis: Uncoupled neuro-osseous growth? *European Spine Journal: Official Publication of the European Spine Society, the European Spinal Deformity Society, and the European Section of the Cervical Spine Research Society*, *10*(6), 473-481. https://doi.org/10.1007/s005860100311.

Roaf, R. (1960). Vertebral growth and its mechanical control. *The Journal of Bone and Joint Surgery. British Volume*, *42-B*, 40-59. https://doi.org/10.1302/0301-620X.42B1.40.

Roth, M. (1981). Idiopathic scoliosis from the point of view of the neuroradiologist. *Neuroradiology*, *21*(3), 133-138. https://doi.org/10.1007/BF00339521.

Schlösser, T. P. C., Janssen, M. M. A., Vrtovec, T., Pernuš, F., Oner, F. C., Viergever, M. A., Vincken, K. L., & Castelein, R. M. (2014). Evolution of the ischio-iliac lordosis during natural growth and its relation with the pelvic incidence. *European Spine Journal: Official Publication of the European Spine Society, the European Spinal Deformity Society, and the European Section of the Cervical Spine Research Society*, *23*(7), 1433-1441. https://doi.org/10.1007/s00586-014-3358-z.

Siu King Cheung, C., Tak Keung Lee, W., Kit Tse, Y., Ping Tang, S., Man Lee, K., Guo, X., Qin, L., & Chun Yiu Cheng, J. (2003). Abnormal peri-pubertal anthropometric measurements and growth pattern in adolescent idiopathic scoliosis: A study of 598 patients. *Spine*, *28*(18), 2152-2157. https://doi.org/10.1097/01.BRS.0000084265.15201.D5.

Skalli, W., & Vergari, C. (2018). Biomechanics of Adolescent Idiopathic Scoliosis. Içinde M. Machida, S. L. Weinstein, & J. Dubousset (Ed.), *Pathogenesis of Idiopathic Scoliosis* (ss. 75-97). Springer Japan. https://doi.org/10.1007/978-4-431-56541-3_4.

Stokes, I. A. (1997). Analysis of symmetry of vertebral body loading consequent to lateral spinal curvature. *Spine*, *22*(21), 2495-2503. https://doi.org/10.1097/00007632-199711010-00006.

Stokes, I. A., Burwell, R. G., & Dangerfield, P. H. (2006). Biomechanical spinal growth modulation and progressive adolescent scoliosis – a test of the "vicious cycle"

pathogenetic hypothesis: Summary of an electronic focus group debate of the IBSE. *Scoliosis*, *1*, 16. https://doi.org/10.1186/1748-7161-1-16.
Stokes, I. A. F. (2007). Analysis and simulation of progressive adolescent scoliosis by biomechanical growth modulation. *European Spine Journal*, *16*(10), 1621-1628. https://doi.org/10.1007/s00586-007-0442-7.
Stokes, I. A., Spence, H., Aronsson, D. D., & Kilmer, N. (1996). Mechanical modulation of vertebral body growth. Implications for scoliosis progression. *Spine*, *21*(10), 1162-1167. https://doi.org/10.1097/00007632-199605150-00007.
Veldhuizen, A. G., Wever, D. J., & Webb, P. J. (2000). The aetiology of idiopathic scoliosis: Biomechanical and neuromuscular factors. *European Spine Journal*, *9*(3), 178-184. https://doi.org/10.1007/s005860000142.
Villemure, I., & Stokes, I. A. F. (2009). Growth plate mechanics and mechanobiology. A survey of present understanding. *Journal of Biomechanics*, *42*(12), 1793-1803. https://doi.org/10.1016/j.jbiomech.2009.05.021.
Vital, J. M., & Senegas, J. (1986). Anatomical bases of the study of the constraints to which the cervical spine is subject in the sagittal plane A study of the center of gravity of the head. *Surgical and Radiologic Anatomy*, *8*(3), 169-173. https://doi.org/10.1007/BF02427845.
Wong, C. (2015). Mechanism of right thoracic adolescent idiopathic scoliosis at risk for progression; a unifying pathway of development by normal growth and imbalance. *Scoliosis*, *10*, 2. https://doi.org/10.1186/s13013-015-0030-2.
Ylikoski, M. (1993). Spinal growth and progression of adolescent idiopathic scoliosis. *European Spine Journal*, *1*(4), 236-239. https://doi.org/10.1007/BF00298366.

# Chapter 12

# The Effects of Early-Onset Scoliosis on Morbidity and Mortality of Untreated Patients

**Orkun Halaç**[1]
**and Ümit Aygün**[2,*]
[1]Department of Orthopedics and Traumatology, Ağrı Training and Research Hospital, Ağrı, Turkiye
[2] Department of Orthopedics and Traumatology, Ağrı İbrahim Çeçen University, Faculty of Medicine, Ağrı, Turkiye

## Abstract

Any spinal deformity that manifests before the age of 10 is referred to as early-onset scoliosis (EOS), regardless of the cause. The relationship between the lungs, spine, and thorax must be taken into consideration when evaluating deformity. Early-onset curves have higher progression risks, cardiorespiratory issues, and higher morbidity and mortality rates. Thoracic insufficiency syndrome, in which a deformed thorax is unable to sustain normal respiratory function or lung growth, could result from progressing deformity. The management and treatment of EOS should use a holistic strategy that takes into account the patient's quality of life and psychological wellbeing. For children, severe physical malformations can have significant short-term and long-term psychological repercussions, including poor self-esteem, social isolation, physical limitations, and anxiety or depression. The initial hopes for the correction of scoliotic deformity, promotion of thoracic growth, and enhancement of pulmonary function have not been met with growth-friendly surgical procedures.

---

* Corresponding Author's Email: aygun.umit55@gmail.com.

In: Early Onset Scoliosis
Editor: Ahmed Majid Heydar
ISBN: 979-8-89113-600-7

**Keywords:** early-onset scoliosis, untreated patients, morbidity, mortality, cardiopulmonary effect, psychological effect

## Introduction

Pathologies of the developing spine that present and proceed in a variety of ways are referred to as early-onset scoliosis (EOS). It has always been challenging to adopt a thorough definition of EOS that fosters consensus in diagnosis and management due to the challenging nature of the condition. Ponseti and Friedman coined the term EOS in 1950, to describe idiopathic scoliosis in children under the age of 10 (Ponseti & Friedman, 1950). They discovered that younger EOS patients had a poorer prognosis when compared to older people. Subsequently, in 1954, idiopathic scoliosis was classified into three age groups. These were infantile (3 years), juvenile (4-9 years), and adolescent (10 years to maturity) (James et al., 1959). Dickson, however, opposed the categorisation of juvenile idiopathic scoliosis in 1985 because patients might fall under the infantile category (Dickson, 1985). Years later, Dickson advocated categorising idiopathic scoliosis into early-onset (0–5 years) and late-onset (>5 years) cases (Dickson, 1994). Compared to treatment strategies for children over 10, those for children between 5 and 10 more closely resemble those used for children under 5, despite the adoption of this definition in recent research (El-Hawary & Akbarnia, 2015). Therefore, regardless of the origin, the Children Spine Study Group (CSSG) and the Growing Spine Study Group (GSSG) defined EOS as any spinal deformity present before the age of 10 (El-Hawary & Akbarnia, 2015; Williams et al., 2014). The lack of treatment for progressive EOS typically results in severe adult idiopathic scoliosis, a condition that lowers quality of life, puts general health at risk, and can eventually cause catastrophic cardiac-pulmonary consequences and early mortality.

This study describes the effects of EOS on morbidity and mortality in untreated patients. We outline our evidence based on empirical research regarding health-related issues, and the development of EOS.

## Natural Course and Systemic Effects

In individuals with EOS, it is generally recognised that the earlier the onset, the worse the eventual curvature, and the prognosis (James, 1954; Scott &

Morgan, 1955). Progressive curves typically result in substantial deformity, degeneration of the cardiovascular system, and reduced life expectancy (James et al., 1959; Pehrsson et al., 1992). Scott et al. discovered in 1955 that the predicted rate of EOS advancement is 5° per year, therefore, at the age of approximately 14, a youngster with a starting curve of 30° should have a major curve of about 100° (Scott & Morgan, 1955). If the deformity is not addressed once it reaches 70°, it may increase to more than 100°, which will impair its prognosis (James et al., 1959). In contrast to adolescent scoliosis, it was discovered that patients with EOS were more likely to experience severe scoliosis and greater morbidity and death (Pehrsson et al., 1992). Structural modifications that constrict the thoracic cavity and cause respiratory failure, cardiovascular problems, and restrictive lung disease cause increased mortality (Scott & Morgan, 1955; Branthwaite, 1986; Pehrsson et al., 1992; Swank et al., 1982). Consequently, to understand the detrimental effects of EOS on cardiopulmonary function, it should be evaluated in light of the interactions between lung, spine, and thorax development.

## Pulmonary Effect

As EOS progresses, lung development becomes a key factor. Alveoli experience their fastest growth up to 8 years old when it happens exponentially (Thurlbeck, 1975; Dunnill, 1962). This discovery assisted in changing the cut-off for EOS from 5 to 10 years of age. Early in childhood, restricted development of the thorax reduces volume, which has a negative impact on lung size in adulthood (Campbell et al., 2003). Patients with noticeable scoliosis during this crucial stage of lung development have been found to have lung hypoplasia, where there are few alveoli and arteries, which frequently include emphysematous abnormalities (Davies & Reid, 1971) (Figure 1).

Thoracic cage shape, volume, standing and sitting height, circumference, and eventually lung development are all influenced by synchronised spinal growth (Canavese & Dimeglio, 2013). The sitting height measurement provides a distorted picture of spinal development and generally refers to the height of the trunk. The acceleration and deceleration events follow a pre-set pattern. For up to 5 years of age, sitting height increases from 35 to 62 cm, or about 66% of the total sitting height (Dimeglio, 2001; Canavese & Dimeglio, 2013; Dimeglio, 1992). Sitting height increases by approximately 12 cm between the ages of 5 and 10 and an additional 12 cm throughout puberty

(Canavese & Dimeglio, 2013). The loss of sitting height in children with significant spinal abnormalities is correlated with the degree of deformity (Canavese & Dimeglio, 2013). The relationship between thoracic height and pulmonary function has been reported. The forced vital capacity (FVC) decreases with the length of the thoracic spine, increasing the risk of restrictive pulmonary illness (Karol et al., 2008). It was also reported that the height of the thoracic at skeletal maturity should be larger than 22 cm in order to prevent severe restrictive lung disease (FVC <50%) (Karol et al., 2008; Dimeglio & Canavese, 2012). Since humans lack the thoracic height necessary to prevent this respiratory disturbance at 5 years old, this became another justification to set the threshold for EOS at less than 10 years of age instead of 5 years. It is important to realise that the growth of the thoracic cage is altered as the spinal abnormality worsens. The rib cage contributes to the width and depth of the thoracic volume, whereas the thoracic spine provides the vertical component (Campbell & Smith, 2007). At birth, the volume of the thoracic cage is approximately 6% of full size, increases to 30% at age 5, and increases to 50% at age 10 (Charles et al., 2008; Canavese & Dimeglio, 2013).

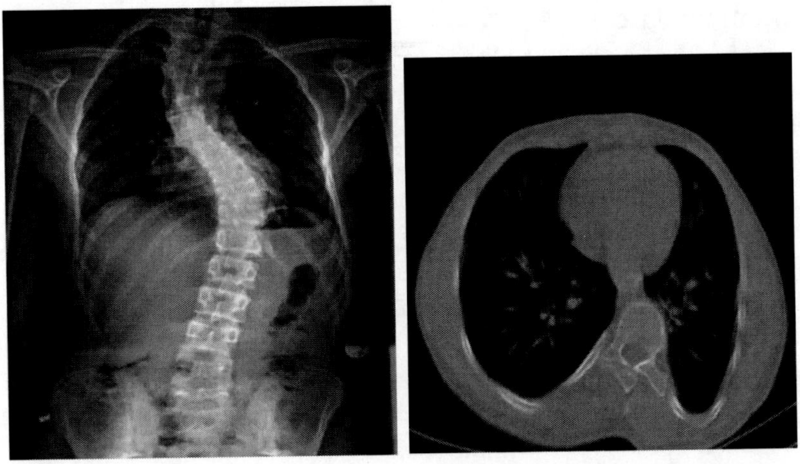

**Figure 1.** X-ray and axial section thorax computed tomography images reflecting the cardiopulmonary field of an untreated EOS patient with thoracic scoliosis.

## Thoracic Insufficiency Syndrome and Cardiac Effect

Early in life, it is understood that the spine and thorax undergo significant growth and development in a coordinated pattern. Therefore, during the crucial developmental phase, EOS causes structural changes in several interconnected growth processes. According to Campbell et al., a small, stiff, deformed thorax, which is unable to supply volume for lung expansion and hence performed poorly, characterises patients with EOS. This symptom was referred to as thoracic insufficiency syndrome (TIS), which is characterised by the incapacity of the thorax to support normal breathing or lung development (Campbell et al., 2003). This leads to a scoliotic heart, characterised as right ventricular hypertrophy connected with increased pulmonary vascular resistance; whether or not congestive heart failure is present, a deformed stiff chest cage causes lung, and respiratory diseases (Swank et al., 1982). It eventually interferes with heart function and lung development as the spinal deformity in EOS continues, resulting in a potentially fatal cor pulmonale and TIS (Canavese & Dimeglio, 2013).

It was reported that the prognosis of early-onset idiopathic scoliosis was poorer than that of the late-onset adolescent form in untreated idiopathic scoliosis patients (Pehrsson et al., 1992; Nilsonne & Lundgren, 1968). In comparison to the general population, both studies showed significantly higher rates of mortality from cardiovascular or respiratory disorders, with an increased risk of death after the age of 40. Patients with infantile and juvenile scoliosis had higher mortality rates than patients with adolescent scoliosis, but this does not mean that the adolescent form has never had cardiopulmonary failure leading to death (Asher & Burton, 2006). The severity of the curve is associated with mortality from untreated scoliosis. It was shown that only patients with a curve greater than 110°anda predicted vital capacity (VC) of less than 45% experienced respiratory failure (Pehrsson et al., 1991).In a 4-year study, without clinically significant cardiorespiratory embarrassment, it was discovered that 10 patients with kyphoscoliotic curves greater than 100° had survived into their seventh decade, although they concluded that a long and active life is incompatible with severe deformity (Rom & Miller, 1978). Untreated idiopathic scoliosis that develops beyond skeletal maturity presents a challenging interdisciplinary approach to treating the condition because of the diminished physiological reserve of the patient caused by age, chronic pain, and cardiopulmonary insufficiency. A surgeon's personal experience of a difficult procedure, knowledge of conflicting evidence of complications, and knowledge of the short to long-term outcomes of these comparatively uncommon spine surgeries are frequently used to determine the best course of surgical therapy.

## Morbidity and Mortality

As mentioned previously, during the first 5 years of life, the spine, chest wall, and respiratory system develop rapidly (Dimeglio, 1992). A change in the development of one of these parts may negatively impact the others. Cardiopulmonary impairment is more likely to occur with scoliosis that develops and manifests during this time (Muirhead & Conner, 1985). Ventilation abnormalities originate from infantile scoliosis altering the normal development of the alveoli and pulmonary arteries. The age at which scoliosis first appears is directly correlated with the severity of pulmonary involvement. The severity of disability increases with the earlier onset and development. Typically, restrictive lung disease with increased residual volume (RV) and decreased total lung capacity (TLC), VC represents pulmonary dysfunction. The restrictive pattern of the disease is influenced by the loss of compliance in both the lungs and the chest wall. Pulmonary hypertension and cor pulmonale are typically side effects of restrictive lung disease persistence. Given that gas exchange is usually normal, hypoxemia is associated with decreased tidal volume. As these individuals have a significant pulmonary reserve, respiratory failure rarely occurs in the early stages. Although this illness pattern has been repeatedly documented in the literature, children with diagnoses made in later childhood are far less likely to have respiratory failure (Kafer, 1976; Davies & Reid, 1971). Pehrsson et al. studied mortality and reasons for death among 115 untreated scoliosis patients in Sweden in 1992 and found that the fourth to fifth decade of life is when the scoliosis-related elevated risk of cardiovascular disease emerges. The mortality rate by age 40 was twice as high in people with idiopathic EOS as in the general group (Pehrsson et al., 1992).

The most obvious signs of the severity of EOS-related pulmonary problems include a complete history of the frequency and duration of hospital stays and intubations for respiratory compromise or pneumonia. It also serves as a loose indicator of whether their respiratory condition has improved gradually over time or remained stable. For instance, bilevel positive airway pressure (BiPAP) or continuous positive airway pressure (CPAP),if the patient requires non-invasive positive pressure ventilation (NPVV), the surgeon can administer it. In patients with severe EOS, nocturnal hypoxemia is frequently observed and is frequently treated with NPPV (Katz et al., 2010; Piesiak et al., 2015; Simonds & Elliott, 1995; Shneerson & Simonds, 2002). Patients with EOS can show signs of exercise intolerance, therefore it is important to determine if their hobbies or sports have changed. Previously active EOS patients can switch from vigorous exercises to more sedentary activities due to increased respiratory work. Patients should report if they are experiencing increased difficulty maintaining their normal pace during recess or exercise, such that they should change their workout to be appropriately lighter by avoiding hills and stairs, for example (Redding, 2014). The eating and sleeping habits of an EOS patient can also reveal any potential respiratory problems. Snoring in the past, agitation, fatigue, or restless sleep can be indicators of nocturnal hypoventilation (MacKintosh et al., 2020). As larger meals may exacerbate a restrictive chestwall condition and impede an already compromised diaphragmatic excursion, patients with EOS should eat smaller, more frequent meals (Redding, 2014). As a result, failure to thrive can be observed in patients with EOS. This could be because patients are unable to maintain the higher caloric intake that is frequently required in severe EOS, whereby the chest wall is constricted, making breathing difficult.

Patients with untreated scoliosis are more likely than the general population to experience both acute and chronic back discomfort, although symptoms that seldom result in impairment. Back discomfort in an adult with scoliosis is often asymmetrical, rarely severe, frequently extra vertebral, and cured with rest. Rarely is a long-term pain management regimen required, with the exception of patients with thoracolumbar curves, where a vertebral translatory shift has been indicated as the explanation. However, there is no relationship between back pain and the kind and degree of the curve, although there are reports of a rise in the frequency and intensity of pain with greater than 45° curves (Kostuik & Bentivoglio, 1981). Double curves appear to have the lowest probability of causing more discomfort. The convexity of the curve is where back pain is most frequently reported. Moreover, the onset of back discomfort in female patients may coincide with their first pregnancy. Another neurologic damage is uncommon; however, there may be lumbar radiculopathy and it appears to be restricted to the concave side of the compensatory curves (Beauchamp et al., 2019; Kostuik & Bentivoglio, 1981).

## Psychological Effect

EOS can also cause physical deformities in early childhood (such as trunkshift, shoulder imbalance, or pelvic obliquity) that can last throughout adolescence and adulthood and can get progressively worse. For the child and caregiver, having severe physical malformations may have significant short-term and long-term psychological repercussions, including poor self-esteem, social isolation, physical limitations, and anxiety or depression (Vitale et al., 2008a; Vitale et al., 2008b). The psychological impact of those factors is understandable when we take into account the additional medical appointments, hospital stays, comorbidities, and repeated surgical procedures (Marks et al., 2003). It has been reported that people with EOS have higher rates of sadness and anxiety, and greater difficulty in performing basic daily functions (Horton et al., 2005). Additionally, those with TIS have reported a lower quality of life than people with chronic illnesses such as malignancy or cardiac disease (Kaneko et al., 2016). Therefore, it is crucial to take radiographic measurements, scoliometer readings to determine trunk form, and surveys to determine the quality of life in terms of health.

Recurrent surgery in children has been linked to considerable psychiatric dysfunction (Marks et al., 2009). Patients with EOS frequently undergo repetitive surgeries because of the nature of the disease and current therapeutic approaches to treating EOS (such as growth-friendly procedures). This situation exposes patients to the negative effects of anaesthesia, hospitalisations, lengthening procedures, surgical complications, and follow-ups that together produce chronic stress (Redding et al., 2008; Hedequist & Emans, 2003; Marks et al., 2009; Adam et al., 2007). It was found that 58% of people who had multiple surgeries experienced psychological dysfunction, with positive correlations with anxiety, depression, and anger management, and this study was one of the first to examine the psychological effects of growth-friendly surgery in patients with EOS (Marks et al., 2009). They also discovered a connection between violence, breach of the law, and conduct issues in patients with EOS. More importantly than having several procedures, patients at risk of acquiring these lifelong psychological problems had an earlier surgical intervention (Matsumoto et al., 2014). This reinforces the idea that postponing surgery is advantageous in reducing such difficulties by allowing the body to mature and lessening the detrimental psychological effects (Brenner et al., 2001). However, relying on the healthcare system, frequent visits to the hospital, and disturbance of daily routines all contribute to the associated stress and psychological dysfunction (Adam et al., 2007). These data lead us to the conclusion that EOS is more than an orthopaedic problem with cardiopulmonary consequences. To achieve the best results in treatment, a multidisciplinary strategy that takes into account the psychological consequences and demands of these patients is necessary. Prioritising access to mental health services is essential to a comprehensive strategy for patient care, therapeutic success, and quality of life.

## Health-Related Quality of Life

The control of spine and thoracic cage deformity, reduction of cardiovascular dysfunction, psychological impact, and health-related quality of life metrics are the current focus of EOS treatment (Matsumoto et al., 2014; Campbell et al., 2003; Anari et al., 2020; Matsumoto et al., 2018). Understanding the natural history, development, and long-term effects of EOS has progressed. Similarly, during the past few decades, technological advancements have improved the number of therapy options available to patients with EOS (Skaggs et al., 2014; Beauchamp et al., 2019). Despite advancements, treating EOS remains difficult, as seen by the lack of agreement among experts (Hughes et al., 2020). The rapid proliferation of therapy alternatives has overtaken the body of research, which has increased management uncertainty (Park et al., 2016). In addition to the rapid proliferation of treatments, there are other challenges to obtaining high-level data, such as the small and varied patient population, the requirement for long duration of follow-ups, and the challenges in evaluating pulmonary outcomes in this population (Park et al., 2016; Yang et al., 2016). Although there is proof that treatments work to correct curvature and promote spine growth, questions remain regarding how these methods affect pulmonary function (Glotzbecker et al., 2014; Campbell et al., 2003). Traditional radiographic investigations have been found to not accurately indicate outcomes in EOS respiratory function (Yang et al., 2016; Glotzbecker et al., 2014). The improvement of the evaluation of the spine-thorax pulmonary link may result from advancements in imaging methods that give dynamic measurements in three dimensions in addition to alternative methods to measure pulmonary outcomes in treated children (Yang et al., 2016; Glotzbecker et al., 2014; Park et al., 2016). A greater understanding of how to prevent the final manifestation of TIS, which causes individuals with progressive scoliosis to have cardiac compromise, will be possible due to advancements in these areas (Campbell et al., 2003).

Future EOS management can be viewed with optimism if efforts are made to address these issues. For EOS research, the need for a consistent and effective methodology has been acknowledged. To strengthen the consistency and dependability of research, multicentre study groups such as the CSSG, GSSG, and Pediatric Spine Study Group have been established (Park et al., 2016; Yang et al., 2016). Finally, instruments such as the 24-item Early-Onset Scoliosis Questionnaire created by Matsumoto et al. will offer a high-quality and consistent assessment of the influence of each treatment strategy based on the dimensions of health-related quality of life and its psychological impact (Matsumoto et al., 2018).

## Conclusion

EOS refers to a variety of spinal deformities that manifest in patients 10 years of age or younger, ranging from mild idiopathic scoliosis to severe congenital scoliosis that can be fatal and cause fused ribs, as well as syndromic scoliosis that causes TIS. Similar to how the severity, extent, and evolution of the spine and thoracic deformities vary, so does the effect on the patient's breathing ability. Even though early and late-onset idiopathic scoliosis can be managed with exercises, bracing, or surgery, if left untreated, it could pose a major health risk. The likelihood of missing instances and the emergence of adult idiopathic scoliosis is low in contemporary healthcare systems with effective screening programs for school-age children and adolescents. School screening is an essential tool for the study of scoliosis etiology and an instrument for early detection and a reduction in the number of patients who will ultimately require operational treatment.

## References

Adam, C. J., Cargill, S. C., &Askin, G. N. (2007). Computed tomographic-based volumetric reconstruction of the pulmonary system in scoliosis. *J Pediatr Orthop*, 27(6), 677–681. https://doi.org/10.1097/BPO.0b013e318425ee.

Anari, J. B., Flynn, J. M., Campbell, R. M., & Cahill, P. J. (2020). Evaluation and treatment of early-onset scoliosis: A team approach. *JBJS Reviews,* 8(10), e20.00040. https://doi.org/10.2106/JBJS.RVW.20.00040.

Asher, M. A., & Burton, D. C. (2006). Adolescent idiopathic scoliosis: natural history and long term treatment effects. *Scoliosis,* 1(1), 2. https://doi.org/10.1186/1748-7161-1-2.

Beauchamp, E. C., Anderson, R. C. E., & Vitale, M. G. (2019). Modern surgical management of early onset and adolescent idiopathic scoliosis. *Neurosurgery*, 84(2), 291–304. https://doi.org/10.1093/neuros/nyy267.

Branthwaite, M. A. (1986). Cardiorespiratory consequences of unfused idiopathic scoliosis. *Br J Dis Chest,* 80 (4), 360–369. https://doi.org/10.1016/0007-0971(86)90089-6.

Brenner, D., Elliston, C., Hall, E., & Berdon, W. (2001). Estimated risks of radiation-induced fatal cancer from pediatric CT.*AJR Am J Roentgenol*, 176(2), 289–296. https://doi.org/10.2214/ajr.176.2.1760289.

Campbell, R. M., Jr, Smith, M. D., Mayes, T. C., Mangos, J. A., Willey-Courand, D. B., Kose, N., Pinero, R. F., Alder, M. E., Duong, H. L., & Surber, J. L. (2003). The characteristics of thoracic insufficiency syndrome associated with fused ribs and congenital scoliosis. *J Bone Joint Surg Am,* 85(3), 399–408. https://doi.org/10.2106/00004623-200303000-00001.

Campbell, R. M., Jr, & Smith, M. D. (2007). Thoracic insufficiency syndrome and exotic scoliosis. *J Bone Joint Surg Am*, 89(Supplement 1), 108–122.https://doi.org/10.2106/JBJS.F.00270.

Canavese, F., & Dimeglio, A. (2013). Normal and abnormal spine and thoracic cage development. *World J Orthop,* 4 (4), 167–174.https://doi.org/10.5312/wjo.v4.i4.167.

Charles, Y. P., Diméglio, A., Marcoul, M., Bourgin, J. F., Marcoul, A., & Bozonnat, M. C. (2008). Influence of idiopathic scoliosis on three-dimensional thoracic growth. *Spine (Phila Pa 1976),* 33 (11), 1209–1218. https://doi.org/10.1097/BRS.0b013e3181715272.

Davies, G., & Reid, L. (1971). Effect of scoliosis on growth of alveoli and pulmonary arteries and on right ventricle. *Arch Dis Child,* 46 (249), 623–632. https://doi.org/10.1136/adc.46.249.623.

Dickson, R. A. (1994). Early-onset idiopathic scoliosis. In S.Weinstein (Ed.), *The Pediatric Spine: Principles and Practice*(pp: 421- 429). New York: Raven Press.

Dickson, R. A. (1985). Conservative treatment for idiopathic scoliosis. *J Bone Joint Surg Br,* 67(2), 176–181. https://doi.org/10.1302/0301-620X.67B2.3872301.

Dimeglio, A., & Canavese, F. (2012). The growing spine: how spinal deformities influence normal spine and thoracic cage growth. *Eur Spine J*, 21(1), 64–70.https://doi.org/10.1007/s00586-011-1983-3.

Dimeglio, A. (1992). Growth of the spine Before age 5 years. *Journal of Pediatric Orthopaedics B,* 1(2), 102–107. https://doi.org/10.1097/01202412-199201020-00003.

Dimeglio, A. (2001). Growth in pediatric orthopaedics. *J Pediatr Orthop*, 21(4), 549–555. https://doi.org/10.1097/01241398-200107000-00026.

Dunnill, M. S. (1962). Postnatal growth of the lung. *Thorax,* 17, 329–333. https://doi.org/10.1136/thx.17.4.329.

El-Hawary, R., & Akbarnia, B. A. (2015). Early onset scoliosis - time for consensus. *Spine Deform*, 3(2), 105–106. https://doi.org/10.1016/j.jspd.2015.01.003.

Glotzbecker, M., Johnston, C., Miller, P., Smith, J., Perez-Grueso, F. S., Woon, R., Flynn, J., Gold, M., Garg, S., Redding, G., Flynn, J., Garg, S., Redding, G., Cahill, P., & Emans, J. (2014). Is there a relationship Between thoracic dimensions and pulmonary function in early-onset scoliosis? *Spine (Phila Pa 1976),* 39(19), 1590–1595. https://doi.org/10.1097/BRS.0000000000000449.

Hedequist, D. J., & Emans, J. B. (2003). The correlation of preoperative three dimensional computed tomography reconstructions with operative findings in congenital scoliosis. *Spine (Phila. Pa. 1976),* 28(22), 2531–2534. https://doi.org/10.1097/01.BRS.0000092382.80487.F0.

Horton, W. C., Brown, C. W., Bridwell, K. H., Glassman, S. D., Il Suk, S., & Cha, C. W. (2005). Is there an optimal patient stance for obtaining a lateral 36″ radiograph?: a critical comparison of three techniques. *Spine (Phila. Pa. 1976),* 30 (4), 427–433. https://doi.org/10.1097/01.brs.0000153698.94091.f8.

Hughes, M. S., Swarup, I., Makarewich, C. A., Williams, B. A., Talwar, D., Cahill, P. J., Flynn, J. M., & Anari, J. B. (2020). Expert consensus for early onset scoliosis surgery.

*J Pediatr Orthop,* 40(7), e621–e628. https://doi.org/10.1097/BPO.0000000000001473.

James, J. I. (1954). Idiopathic Scoliosis; the prognosis, diagnosis, and operative indications related to curve patterns and the age at onset. *J Bone Joint Surg Br*, 36-B(1), 36–49. https://doi.org/10.1302/0301-620X.36B1.36.

James, J. I., Lloyd-Roberts, G. C., & Pilcher, M. F. (1959). Infantile structural scoliosis. *J Bone Joint Surg Br*, 41-B, 719–735. https://doi.org/10.1302/0301-620X.41B4.719.

Kafer, E. R. (1976). Idiopathic scoliosis. Gas exchange and the age dependence of arterial blood. *J Clin Invest*, 58(4), 825-833. https://doi.org/10.1172/JCI108535.

Kaneko, K., Aota, Y., Sekiya, T., Yamada, K., & Saito, T. (2016). Validation study of arm positions for evaluation of global spinal balance in EOS imaging. *Eur J Orthop Surg Traumatol,* 26(7), 725–733. https://doi.org/10.1007/s00590-016-1813-8.

Karol, L. A., Johnston, C., Mladenov, K., Schochet, P., Walters, P., & Browne, R. H. (2008). Pulmonary function following early thoracic fusion in non-neuromuscular scoliosis. *J Bone Joint Surg Am*, 90(6), 1272–1281.https://doi.org/10.2106/JBJS.G.00184.

Katz, S. L., Gaboury, I., Keilty, K., Banwell, B., Vajsar, J., Anderson, P., Ni, A., & Maclusky, I. (2010). Nocturnal hypoventilation: predictors and outcomes in childhood progressive neuromuscular disease. *Arch Dis Child,* 95(12), 998–1003. https://doi.org/10.1136/adc.2010.182709.

Kostuik & Bentivoglio, 1981, as cited in Hu. (2006). *Adult scoliosis*. In: H. N. Herkowitz, S. R. Garfin, F. J. Eismont, G. R. Bell, R.A. Balderston, (Eds.) *Rothman-Simeone the Spine*, (pp. 1046-1057). Philadelphia, Pennsylvania, USA: Saunders Elsevier.

MacKintosh, E. W., Ho, M., White, K. K., Krengel, W. 3rd., Bompadre, V., Chen, M. L., & Redding, G.J. (2020). Referral indications and prevalence of sleep abnormalities in children with early onset scoliosis. *Spine Deform,* 8(3), 523–530. https://doi.org/10.1007/s43390-020-00080-x.

Marks, M. C., Stanford, C. F., Mahar, A. T., & Newton, P. O. (2003). Standing lateral radiographic positioning does not represent customary standing balance. *Spine (Phila.Pa.1976),* 28(11), 1176–1182. https://doi.org/10.1097/01.BRS.0000067271.00258.51.

Marks, M., Stanford, C., & Newton, P. (2009). Which lateral radiographic positioning technique provides the most reliable and functional representation of a patient's sagittal balance? *Spine (Phila Pa. 1976),* 34(9), 949–954. https://doi.org/10.1097/BRS.0b013e318199650a.

Matsumoto, H., Williams, B. A., Corona, J., Comer, J. S., Fisher, P. W., Neria, Y., Roye, B. D., Roye, D. P., & Vitale, M. G. (2014). Psychosocial effects of repetitive surgeries in children with early-onset scoliosis: are we putting them at risk? *J Pediatr Orthop,* 34(2), 172–178. https://doi.org/10.1097/BPO.0b013e3182a11d73.

Matsumoto, H., Williams, B., Park, H. Y., Yoshimachi, J. Y., Roye, B. D., Roye, D. P., Jr, Akbarnia, B. A., Emans, J., Skaggs, D., Smith, J. T., & Vitale, M. G. (2018). The final 24-item early onset scoliosis questionnaires (EOSQ-24): validity, reliability and responsiveness. *J Pediatr Orthop,* 38(3), 144–151. https://doi.org/10.1097/BPO.0000000000000799.

Muirhead, A., & Conner, A. N. (1985). The assessment of lung function in children with scoliosis. *J Bone Joint Surg Br,* 67(5), 699-702. https://doi.org/10.1302/0301-620X.67B5.4055863.

Nilsonne, U., & Lundgren, K. D. (1968). Long-term prognosis in idiopathic scoliosis. *Acta Orthop Scand,* 39(4), 456-465. https://doi.org/10.3109/17453676808989663.

Park, H. Y., Wright, J. G., & Vitale, M. G. (2016). Outcomes in children with early-onset scoliosis. In B. A. Akbarnia, M. Yazici& G. H. Thompson (Eds.), *The Growing Spine: Management of Spinal Disorders in Young Children* (pp. 909–917). Berlin, Heidelberg: Springer Berlin Heidelberg.

Pehrsson, K., Larsson, S., Oden, A., & Nachemson, A. (1992). Long-term follow-up of patients with untreated scoliosis. A study of mortality, causes of death, and symptoms. *Spine (Phila Pa 1976),* 17(9), 1091–1096. https://doi.org/10.1097/00007632-199209000-00014.

Pehrsson, K., Bake, B., Larsson, S., & Nachemson, A. (1991). Lung function in adult idiopathic scoliosis: a 20 year follow up. *Thorax*, 46(7), 474-478. https://doi.org/10.1136/thx.46.7.474.

Piesiak, P., Brzecka, A., Kosacka, M., & Jankowska, R. (2015). Efficacy of noninvasive volume targeted ventilation in patients with chronic respiratory failure due to kyphoscoliosis. *Adv Exp Med Biol,* 838, 53–58. https://doi.org/10.1007/5584_2014_68.

Ponseti, I. V., & Friedman, B. (1950). Prognosis in idiopathic scoliosis. *J Bone Joint Surg Am,* 32A(2), 381–395.

Redding, G. J. (2014). Early onset scoliosis: a pulmonary perspective. *Spine Deform,* 2(6), 425–429. https://doi.org/10.1016/j.jspd.2014.04.010.

Redding, G., Song, K., Inscore, S., Effmann, E., & Campbell, R. (2008). Lung function asymmetry in children with congenital and infantile scoliosis. *Spine J*, 8(4), 639–644. https://doi.org/10.1016/j.spinee.2007.04.020.

Rom, W. N., & Miller, A. (1978). Unexpected longevity in patients with severe kyphoscoliosis. *Thorax*, 33(1), 106-110. https://doi.org/10.1136/thx.33.1.106.

Scott, J. C., & Morgan, T. H. (1955). The natural history and prognosis of infantile idiopathic scoliosis. *J Bone Joint Surg Br*, 37-B(3), 400–413. https://doi.org/10.1302/0301-620X.37B3.400.

Shneerson, J. M., & Simonds, A. K. (2002). Noninvasive ventilation for chest wall and neuromuscular disorders. *Eur Respir J,* 20(2), 480–487. https://doi.org/10.1183/09031936.02.00404002.

Simonds, A. K., & Elliott, M. W. (1995). Outcome of domiciliary nasal intermit tent positive pressure ventilation in restrictive and obstructive disorders. *Thorax,* 50(6), 604–609. https://doi.org/10.1136/thx.50.6.604.

Skaggs, D. L., Akbarnia, B. A., Flynn, J. M., Myung, K. S., Sponseller, P. D., & Vitale, M. G. (2014). Chest Wall and Spine Deformity Study Group; Growing Spine Study Group; Pediatric Orthopaedic Society of North America; Scoliosis Research Society Growing Spine Study Committee. A classification of growth friendly spine implants. *J Pediatr Orthop,* 34(3), 260–274. https://doi.org/10.1097/BPO.0000000000000073.

Swank, S. M., Winter, R. B., & Moe, J. H. (1982). Scoliosis and cor pulmonale. *Spine (Phila Pa 1976),* 7(4), 343–354. https://doi.org/10.1097/00007632-198207000-00004.

Thurlbeck, W. M. (1975). Lung growth and alveolar multiplication. *Pathobiol Annu*, 5, 1–34.

Vitale, M. G., Matsumoto, H., Bye, M. R., Gomez, J. A., Booker, W. A., Hyman, J. E., & Roye, D. P. (2008a). A retrospective cohort study of pulmonary function, radiographic measures, and quality of life in children with congenital scoliosis. *Spine (Phila. Pa. 1976),* 33(11), 1242–1249. https://doi.org/10.1097/BRS.0b013e3181714536.

Vitale, M. G., Matsumoto, H., Roye, D. P., Gomez, J. A., Betz, R. R., Emans, J. B., Skaggs, D. L., Smith, J. T., Song, K. M., & Campbell, R. M. (2008b). Health related quality of life in children with thoracic insuffciency syn drome. *J Pediatr Orthop*, 28(2), 239–243. https://doi.org/10.1097/BPO.0b013e31816521bb.

Williams, B. A., Matsumoto, H., McCalla, D. J., Akbarnia, B. A., Blakemore, L. C., Betz, R. R., Flynn, J. M., Johnston, C. E., McCarthy, R. E., Roye, D. P., Skaggs, D. L., Smith, J. T., Snyder, B. D., Sponseller, P. D., Sturm, P. F., Thompson, G. H., Yazici, M., & Vitale, M. G. (2014). Development and initial validation of the classification of early-onset scoliosis (C-EOS). *J Bone Joint Surg Am*, 96(16), 1359–1367. https://doi.org/10.2106/JBJS.M.00253.

Yang, S., Andras, L. M., Redding, G. J., & Skaggs, D. L. (2016) Early-onset scoliosis: a review of history, current treatment, and future directions. *Pediatrics,* 137(1), 1-12. https://doi.org/10.1542/peds.2015-0709.

## Chapter 13

# Consequences of Early Spinal Fusion of EOS

**Recep Dinçer*, MD**
Department of Orthopedics and Traumatology, Suleyman Demirel University, Isparta, Turkiye

## Abstract

Early-onset scoliosis (EOS) is the complex deformity of the spine that occurs in children under ten years of age and an abnormal curvature of the spine greater than ten degrees. One of the treatment options for early-onset scoliosis is early spinal fusion. In EOS with severe spinal scoliosis or kyphosis, multilevel posterior spinal fusion (PSF) is not the standard surgical treatment. Nevertheless, fusion may be considered and severe cases, such as congenital deformities or syndromic entities based on the prognosis of the disease. EOS produces restrictive lung disease by constraining and deforming the intrathoracic space, increasing the rigidity of the chest wall, and impairing respiratory muscle function. Children who have undergone spinal fusion may experience reduced lung function due to the decreased ability of the chest wall to expand during breathing. Spinal fusion involves fusing the vertebrae together, which reduces the flexibility of the spine. This can severely limit the ability of the child to grow taller as the spine cannot elongate anymore. This is particularly problematic for younger children who have not yet reached their full potential in height. Children who undergo spinal fusion may require additional surgeries to correct for complications that arise from the initial procedure.

**Keywords:** early spinal fusion, consequences of early fusion, early-onset fusion

---

* Corresponding Author's Email: recebed@gmail.com.

In: Early Onset Scoliosis
Editor: Ahmed Majid Heydar
ISBN: 979-8-89113-600-7

## Introduction

Early-onset scoliosis (EOS) is a sophisticated deformity that occurs in children under ten years of age of the spine. It is characterized by an abnormal curvature of the spine greater than 10°. Surgery is one of the treatment options for EOS, and it has always been a challenge for spine surgeons. Early spinal fusion was used as the final surgical treatment. This involves immobilizing the spine by fusing the affected vertebrae together. Multilevel posterior spinal fusion (PSF) is no longer the standard surgical treatment option for EOS. However, fusion remains the main surgical treatment option, mostly in congenital disorders and in special syndromic conditions.

The goal of EOS treatment is to control spinal deformity without interference of spinal growth, but early definitive fusion before the age of 10 years may not prevent the progression of the deformity. This may lead to another deformity, the thoracic insufficiency syndrome, and the crankshaft phenomenon described by Dubousset et al. (1989) (Dubousset et al., 1989; Campbell, 2007). Therefore, early combined anterior/posterior fusion was considered the definitive treatment for late EOS children with severe spinal deformity, to arrest anterior vertebral growth in EOS and prevent the complications mentioned above.

EOS may lead to chronic respiratory diseases due to the progression of deformities in the thoracic region (Branthwaite, 1986). In this age group, the treatment of respiratory problems begins before the spine treatment and continues after the final surgical treatment. In EOS, intrathoracic volume and lung compliance decrease due to increased stiffness of the chest wall (Redding, 2014). For the lung to show its normal function, there must be sufficient thoracic cavity volume and a functional diaphragm. In children with EOS, severe thoracic deformity and decreased lung and diaphragm functions endanger respiratory functions. While early spinal fusion has been shown to be effective in correcting spinal deformities, it comes with a number of consequences. We will list the consequences of the early fusion from positive to negative results.

### Scoliosis Improvement

Early fusion in early-onset scoliosis (EOS) improves abnormal curves in the spine and facilitates the achievement of a more robust spinal architecture. In children with progressive early-onset idiopathic scoliosis, posterior spinal fusion was recommended at the age of 10 to control the more rapid deterioration, which usually occurs during the pre-adolescent growth spurt and cannot be adequately controlled with a brace (James, 1975). This approach has the potential to prevent more serious complications that may arise at later ages. Surgical intervention can stop the progression of scoliosis and reduce spine deformity by ensuring that the spine is aligned and improved more accurately.

## Quality of Life

The physical and psychosocial effects of scoliosis may adversely affect the quality of life. After early fusion, the deformity in the spine improves and the secondary pains due to the deformity regress. Respiratory functional capacity increases due to increased thoracic volume, which improves the quality of life of patients (Götze, 2002). However, children who undergo spinal fusion may experience a reduced quality of life compared to their peers. The procedure can be physically challenging, and children may have to wear a brace for a prolonged period of time. This can lead to limitations in their physical activities and social interactions. Additionally, the procedure may be emotionally taxing for the child and their caregivers. Studies have shown that children who undergo spinal fusion have lower health-related quality of life scores compared to non-fused children (Cahill, 2012). If early definitive fusion is recommended, reoperation rates must be examined in publications reporting early fusion results. Long-term results of in situ fusion in 43 patients with congenital scoliosis were published by Goldberg et al. Sixteen of them (37.2%), who were at least 15 years old at the last follow-up, underwent reoperation due to "adding on" and/or progression of their deformity following in situ fusion (Goldberg, 2002). Reoperation is not uncommon in young children after what was intended to be a definitive circumferential fusion. Although early definitive fusion continues to have a role in isolated spinal deformities, particularly in the lumbar spinal column, the effect of fusion before the age of 5 on the growth of the chest cage is life-changing for many children (Mehta, 2005).

## Respiratory Compromises-Thoracic Insufficiency Syndrome

As in EOS, respiratory failure may occur in early spinal fusion. Although lung volume continues to increase until mid-adolescence, alveolar proliferation is complete at eight years of age. Therefore, surgery is recommended in the first 8 years of life to restore the balance between alveolar and respiratory volume in pulmonary development (Karol, 2011). Primary abnormalities in rib cage, such as absent or fused ribs in forward curves in syndromic or neuromuscular EOS, add further thoracic disability. Because of the potential spine and thoracic growth inhibition or additional comorbidities resulting from early fusion for spinal deformity, this may not be practical for the treatment of curves (e.g., the patient may be too small for standard spinal implants, or the lung function may be so poor that the patient cannot survive surgery) (Campbell, 2007). Early fusion can correct respiratory functions and reduce the risk of respiratory failure by ensuring correct alignment of the spine. The spine is an important component of the chest wall, and any impairment of spinal mobility can impact the function of the lungs. Children who have undergone spinal fusion may experience reduced lung function due to the decreased ability of the chest wall to expand during breathing. Therefore, the inability of the rib cage to support normal breathing or lung growth is called thoracic insufficiency syndrome. Describes a generalized disease that affects the biomechanical ability of the lungs to accompany the enlargement of the thorax to serve as respiratory motors (Campbell, 2003). Studies have shown that children with early-onset scoliosis that undergo spinal fusion have a higher risk of developing respiratory complications compared to those who do not undergo spinal fusion (Emans et al., 2005). Karol et al. (2008) detected signs of severe restrictive lung disease on pulmonary function tests in 43% of patients, concluding that early anterior and posterior spinal fusion does not provide satisfactory pulmonary function in children younger than six years of age. The age of children with <50% forced vital capacity, representing severe restrictive pulmonary function, ranged from four months to 5.8 years. If patients with early definitive fusions initially have decreased pulmonary reserve, the expected loss of volume in adulthood has serious health implications (Karol et al., 2008).

## Lack of Growth Potential

One of the most significant consequences of early spinal fusion is that it can limit the growth potential of children. Spinal fusion involves fusing the vertebrae together, which reduces the flexibility of the spine. Bowen et al. found that thoracic growth, measured as height of T1-T12, in patients who underwent fusion before the age of 5 due to congenital scoliosis, remained

0.49 cm shorter than in non-fusional patients with congenital scoliosis (Bowen, 2008). Karol et al. found that 57% of patients who underwent definitive fusion before the age of 8 had a thoracic height less than the average thoracic height of a 5-year-old child (Karol, 2008). This can severely limit the ability of the child to grow taller as the spine cannot elongate anymore. This is particularly problematic for younger children who have not yet reached their full potential in height.

## Increased Risk of Complications

Early spinal fusion is a complex procedure that carries a high risk of complications. Complications can range from minor to life-threatening and can include infection, bleeding, nerve damage, and spinal instability. Children who undergo spinal fusion may require additional surgeries to correct complications that arise from the initial procedure. Studies have shown that the risk of complications increases with longer fusion constructs and the use of more aggressive instrumentation (Karol et al., 2011). Goldberg et al. (2002) stated that in 43 patients with congenital scoliosis to whom they applied in situ fusion, 16 (37.2%) of 43 patients required re-operation as a result of 'adding-on' and/or progression (Goldberg et al., 2002). Dubousset reported that the scoliotic deformity progressed after definitive posterior spine fusion (PSF) in patients with paralytic scoliosis and named it the 'Crancshaft phenomenon'. He noted that the deformity increased as the patient got older, was evident only in young patients, and was not associated with pseudoarthrosis within the fusion mass (Dubousset, 1973). Dubousset et al. demonstrated that the progression of deformity is inevitable in skeletally immature patients who undergo only posterior fusion for idiopathic or paralytic scoliosis. In addition, they showed a correlation between the immature skeleton and the degree of deformity during fusion (Dubousset, 1989). Curvature progression may occur despite attempts to achieve circumferential fusion of the spine in young children. Whether this is the result of pseudarthrosis due to the difficulty of achieving fusion in younger children, the addition of deformity at the cephalic or caudal ends of the initial fusion, or the evolution of the deformity as a result of the continued growth of the neurocentral synchondroses has not been determined (Zhang & Sucato, 2008).

### Increased Healthcare Costs

Early spinal fusion is an expensive procedure that requires a prolonged hospital stay and follow-up care. Postoperative follow-up and rehabilitation are crucial to optimize surgical outcomes and ensure long-term success. Children who undergo spinal fusion may require multiple surgeries to correct complications. This can lead to higher healthcare costs, which can be a burden for families. Additionally, the reduced quality of life and increased healthcare needs associated with spinal fusion can impact the ability of the child to participate in school and other activities, which can further impact their future economic potential.

## Conclusion

Early spinal fusion is an effective treatment option for early-onset scoliosis; however, it comes with a number of consequences. These include reduced growth potential, respiratory compromise, increased risk of complications, reduced quality of life, and increased healthcare costs. It is important for clinicians to weigh the benefits and risks of spinal fusion and consider alternative treatments when appropriate. Parents and caregivers should also be informed about the potential consequences of spinal fusion so they can make accurate decisions about their child's treatment.

## References

Bowen, R. E., Scaduto, A. A., & Banuelos, S. (2008). Does early thoracic fusion exacerbate preexisting restrictive lung disease in congenital scoliosis patients? *Journal of Pediatric Orthopedics, 28*(5), 506-511. https://doi.org/10.1097/BPO.0b013e31817b931c.

Branthwaite, M. A. (1986). Cardiorespiratory consequences of unfused idiopathic scoliosis. *British Journal of Diseases of the Chest, 80*, 360-369. https://doi.org/10.1016/0007-0971(86)90089-6.

Cahill, P. J., & Samdani, A. F. (2012). Early-onset scoliosis. *Orthopedics, 35*(12), 1001-1003. https://doi.org/10.3928/01477447-20121120-02.

Campbell, R. M. Jr., & Smith, M. D. (2007). Thoracic insufficiency syndrome and exotic scoliosis. *JBJS, 89*(Suppl 1), 108-122. https://doi.org/10.2106/JBJS.F.00270.

Campbell, R. M., Smith, M. D., Mayes, T. C., Mangos, J. A., Willey-Courand, D. B., Kose, N., Pinero, R. F., Alder, M. E., Duong, H. L., Surber, J. L. (2003). The characteristics of thoracic insufficiency syndrome associated with fused ribs and congenital scoliosis. *Journal of Bone and Joint Surgery Am, 85*, 399-408. http://doi.org/10.2106/00004623-200303000-00001.

Dubousset, J. (1973). Recidive d'une scoliose lombaire et d'un bassin oblique apres fusion precoce: Le phenomene due villebrequin in [Recurrence of lumbar scoliosis and oblique pelvis after precocious fusion: The phenomenon due to villebrequin in], *Proceedings Group Etude de la Scoliose*. Paris, France, CRF Massues, pp 62-66.

Dubousset, J., Herring, J. A., & Shufflebarger, H. (1989). The crankshaft phenomenon. *Journal of Pediatric Orthopedics, 9*(5), 541-550. https://doi.org/10.1097/01241398-198909010-00008.

Emans, J. B., Caubet, J. F., Ordonez, C. L., Lee, E. Y., & Ciarlo, M. (2005). The treatment of spine and chest wall deformities with fused ribs by expansion thoracostomy and insertion of vertical expandable prosthetic titanium rib: growth of thoracic spine and improvement of lung volumes. *Spine, 30*(17S), S58-S68. https://doi.org/10.1097/01.brs.0000175194.31986.2f.

Goldberg, C. J., Moore, D. P., Fogarty, E. E., & Dowling, F. E. (2002). Long-term results from in situ fusion for congenital vertebral deformity. *Spine, 27*(6), 619-628. https://doi.org/10.1097/00007632-200203150-00011.

Götze, C., Liljenqvist, U. R., Slomka, A., Götze, H. G., & Steinbeck, J. (2002). Quality of life and back pain: outcome 16.7 years after Harrington instrumentation. *Spine, 27*(13), 1456–1464. https://doi.org/10.1097/00007632-200207010-00016.

James, J. I. P. (1975). The management of infants with scoliosis. *The Journal of Bone and Joint Surgery. British Volume, 57*(4), 422-429. https://doi:10.1302/0301-620X.57B4.422.

Karol, L. A., Johnston, C., Mladenov, K., Schochet, P., Walters, P., & Browne, R. H. (2008). Pulmonary function following early thoracic fusion in non-neuromuscular scoliosis. *JBJS, 90*(6), 1272-1281. https://doi.org/10.2106/JBJS.G.00184.

Karol, L. A. (2011). Early definitive spinal fusion in young children: what we have learned. *Clinical Orthopaedics and Related Research®, 469*, 1323-1329. https://doi.org/10.1007/s11999-010-1622-z.

Mehta, M. H. (2005). Growth as a corrective force in the early treatment of progressive infantile scoliosis. *The Journal of Bone and Joint Surgery. British Volume, 87*(9), 1237-1247. https://doi.org/10.1302/0301-620X.87B9.16124.

Redding, G. J. (2014). Early onset scoliosis: a pulmonary perspective. *Spine Deformity, 2*, 425-429. https://doi.org/10.1016/j.jspd.2014.04.010.

Zhang, H., & Sucato, D. J. (2008). Unilateral Pedicle Screw Epiphysiodesis of the Neurocentral Synchondrosis: Production of Idiopathic-Like Scoliosis in an Immature Animal Model. *JBJS, 90*(11), 2460-2469. https://doi.org/10.2106/JBJS.G.01493.

## Chapter 14

# Prognosis of Both Surgical and Non-Surgical Treatments of EOS

**Kayra Barut[1], MD**
**and Hüseyin Sina Coşkun[2,*]**
[1]EMOT Plus Hospital, Department of Physical Medicine and Rehabilitation, İzmir, Turkiye
[2]Department of Orthopaedics and Traumatology, Ondokuz Mayıs University, Samsun, Turkiye

## Abstract

Early-onset scoliosis (EOS) is a form of scoliosis that occurs before the age of ten, regardless of the etiology. The severity of EOS ranges from mild to severe and can cause long-term health problems if not diagnosed and treated early. EOS affects fewer people than adolescent idiopathic scoliosis but requires specialized treatment. The conservative treatment methods can be listed as bracing and casting. The main goals of surgical treatment are to stop the progression of the curve and allow the thorax to grow normally. Thus, surgeries that allow spinal growth, which are also called "growth-friendly" surgeries, are first considered rather than spinal fusions. The prognosis of both conservative surgical treatments of EOS is determined by various factors, such as the patient's age, flexibility, and the magnitude of the curve. Congenital and neuromuscular scoliosis tends to progress more rapidly than idiopathic disorders. This chapter explores the prognosis of conservative and surgical treatment of EOS and the outcomes associated with different surgical approaches used to manage the condition.

* Corresponding Author's Email: sina.coskun@hotmail.com.

In: Early Onset Scoliosis
Editor: Ahmed Majid Heydar
ISBN: 979-8-89113-600-7

**Keywords:** early-onset scoliosis, prognosis, conservative treatment, growth-friendly surgery

## Introduction

Early-onset scoliosis (EOS) occurs before age ten, regardless of the etiology (Yang et al., 2016). Early-onset scoliosis treatment is challenging in many aspects. In early posterior spinal fusions, the spine is at risk of developing the crankshaft phenomenon. If surgical treatment is delayed, the control of the curves becomes difficult. Conservative treatments, especially congenital cases, can be more challenging than classical idiopathic scoliosis. Treatment in early-onset scoliosis aims to correct the deformity and protect this condition while at the same time not harming the physiological development of the spine. In the same way, considering its intertwined development with the spine, the development of the thorax and the development of the pulmonary structures are critical in this treatment.

Although there are many options to treat these challenging spinal deformities, treatments can be classified into two main groups: Surgical and conservative.

Bracing and casting are the main methods of conservative treatment. Today, there is no consensus on the role of physical therapy in the treatment of scoliosis. Scoliosis-specific exercises may be effective in improving measures of spinal deformity in people with AIS, but the evidence is of very low quality (Thompson et al., 2019).

"Growth-friendly" surgical procedures are the treatment of choice when surgery is needed in groups of patients with EOS. Spinal fusion is rarely performed in early-onset scoliosis cases, as it disturbs the anterior-posterior balance of the spine and may also cause the "Crankshaft phenomenon." Also, the compromises of the thorax and the pulmonary structures are well documented in the current literature on early spinal fusion cases (Karol et al., 2008; Vitale et al., 2008). The "tweener" term has been described in the literature to better understand the treatment options and the prognosis of older patients with EOS. The authors questioned whether these groups of patients may benefit from spinal fusion or growth-friendly surgeries, but this new term needs further clarification to be better understood (Quan et al., 2023).

## Conservative Treatment and Prognosis of EOS

The aim of conservative treatment in the group of patients with EOS is to prevent the progression of the curve and reduce the number of surgical interventions.

Cobb angle greater than 25° in EOS is a poor prognostic factor indicating a high risk of progression of the curve. However, rather than evaluating the Cobb angle alone, it would be more accurate to evaluate it with other poor prognostic factors, such as the costovertebral angle ratio and the degree of axial rotation (Mehta, 1972; Perdriolle & Vidal, 1985). Curvatures may be more progressive in EOS compared to adolescent idiopathic scoliosis (AIS), and respiratory problems may be seen at higher rates in the thoracic curves.

However, despite all these risks, no complete treatment protocol has been established for this type of curve. The importance of conservative treatment has increased recently because early surgical interventions can cause short stature, affected rib cage development, and the crankshaft phenomenons.

In cases where the curve is greater than 25°, bracing is the primary treatment method to prevent curve progression in conservative treatment (Negrini et al., 2015). In 2011, the importance of bracing and casting treatment in conservative treatment was mentioned by the Pediatric Orthopedic Society of North America (POSNA) (Fletcher et al., 2011). Recently, it has been clearly shown by the BRAIST study that the use of corsets in AIS under appropriate conditions reduces the need for surgery by preventing the progression of the curvature (Weinstein et al., 2013).

In a 43-year retrospective study by Harshavardhana and Lonstein, 125 children with juvenile idiopathic scoliosis (JIS) were included. In the study, Milwaukee (STLSO) and Boston (TLSO) braces were used for at least 20 hours a day, and it was shown that the frequency of surgery was reduced, and the timing of surgery was delayed with the use of braces (Harshavardhana & Lonstein, 2018).

In another retrospective study conducted in 2014, 88 patients with juvenile idiopathic scoliosis were included. 28% of the patients had a stable or reduced Cobb angle, 72% had progressed in their curve, and 50% had been operated on. The patients were followed up with TLSO, Milwaukee, and Charleston night brace. It was determined that most patients who underwent surgery had curves with Cobb degrees of 30° and above. In addition, it has been stated that Lenke VI type curves give the best result to the brace (Khoshbin et al., 2015).

In the study where Kahanovitz evaluated 15 JIS patients, it was emphasized that part-time bracing gave good results when the Cobb angle was less than 35°, and the Mehta angle was less than 20° (Kahanovitz et al., 1982). In another study by Jarvis, 37 JIS type curves were evaluated, and part-time brace use was reported to be 51% successful (Jarvis et al., 2008). In a 30-year retrospective study, it was stated that brace treatment in JIS successfully stopped the progression of the curve and prevented spinal fusion surgery. It was emphasized that 36% of the evaluated patients were unsuccessful despite brace treatment (Babaee et al., 2020).

In our daily routine clinical practice, we use TLSO and Rigo-Chenau braces for EOS patients with a Cobb angle between 25-45. An example of a case is given in Figure 1.

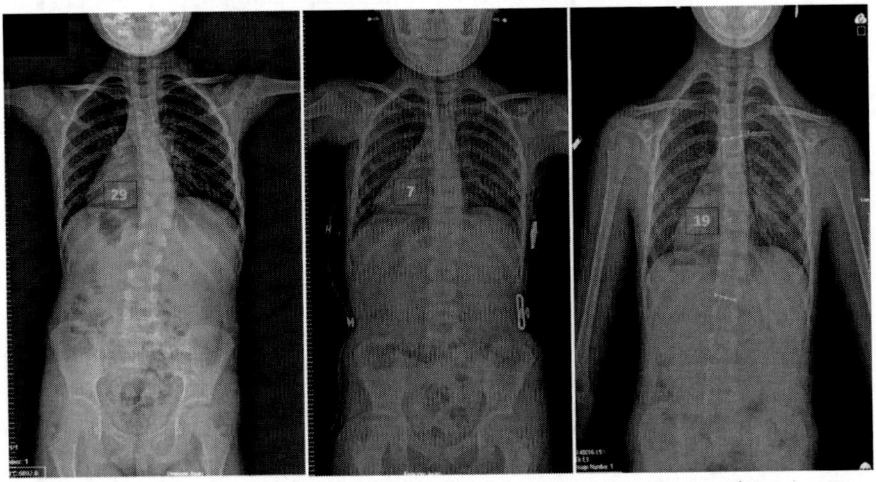


a) b) c)

**Figure 1.** a) A seven-year-old female diagnosed with juvenile idiopathic scoliosis. The Cobb angle between T5-T12 measured 29°. b) Modified TLSO brace treatment has been started. In-brace correction at the third week follow-up showed a Cobb angle reduced from 29° to 7°. c) In the one-year follow-up, the brace was removed the night before the clinical control. A 6 cm growth in her height has been noted with a Cobb reduction of 10 degrees, with maintained coronal balance (from 29 to 19).

Another conservative treatment modality for EOS is casting. Serial casting is a time-gaining method for postponing surgical interventions in early-onset scoliosis, although it has some adverse effects that should be considered and discussed with the family beforehand (Senkoylu et al., 2020).

In the casting process for EOS, force is applied to the chest wall and axial skeleton in the direction of traction-derotation without or under general anesthesia. Frequently used casting methods are Risser Cast and elongation-derotation-flexion (EDF) plasters (Fedorak & D'Astous, 2018; Mahajan et al., 2020). If the serial casting method starts before age 2, it can make a near-total correction in idiopathic curves less than 60° (Sanders et al., 2009). In the study by Waldron et al., in which 20 patients with EOS were evaluated, it was stated that 65% did not need surgery with Risser casting (Waldron et al., 2013).

Serial casting of EDF can modulate spinal growth and can—at least in some cases—prevent the progression of spinal deformity. The serial casting technique of EDF has become an accepted treatment option for managing children with idiopathic and juvenile EOS (Canavese & Dimeglio, 2020).

In summary, the prognosis of conservative treatment depends on various factors, such as age, Cobb angle magnitude, Mehta angle, and curve flexibility. It must be kept in mind that the remaining growth potential plays an essential role in the progress of the curve. Congenital and neuromuscular cases curves tend to worsen during the child's growth. In every child with EOS, detailed imaging such as MRI must be carried out to enlighten if there is a secondary reason for scoliosis or any accompanying deformity.

## Surgical Prognosis of EOS

The prognosis of surgical treatment of EOS relies on various factors, such as the timing of surgery, surgical technique, implant selection, and postoperative care. The goal of surgical intervention in EOS is to prevent the progression of the curve, correct spinal alignment, and allow normal growth and development of the spine. Growth-friendly surgeries are often performed as a surgical technique rather than spinal fusions.

Skaggs et al. described treatment options for growing children (Skaggs et al., 2014). Up to their study, growth-friendly spinal implant systems are divided into three categories based on the forces of correction that the implants exert on the spine:

- Distraction-based
- Compression-based
- Guided growth.

Each type of system has potential benefits and shortcomings. There is not enough literature to show the superiority of the systems over each other.

Harrington widely used distraction-based systems in 1962 (Harrington, 1962). These systems provide the correction by mechanically applying a distractive force between the affected segments (Tello, 1994). These systems included the traditional growing rods (single and dual), vertical expandable titanium ribs (VEPTR), and magnetically controlled growing rods (MCGR).

Despite high rates of complication, growing rods (GR) treatment successfully controls the deformity while preserving the growth of the spine and thorax. One disadvantage of the traditional GR systems is multiple surgeries and the need for definitive fusion at the end of the procedure. Although preliminary results are promising, there are still significant challenges and unknowns for MCGR (Bekmez et al., 2017).

Scoliosis can be equally controlled after conversion from traditional growing rods to MCGR, but spinal growth from baseline is less in the conversion patients than in the primary group (Keskinen et al., 2016). The MCGR technique reduces the number of procedures compared to the classical GR systems. Up to another study in the literature, MCGR provides satisfactory correction for deformities and avoids repeated surgical procedures for lengthening. However, it has a substantial complication rate. Although less frequent than in GR, the law of diminishing returns also applies to MCGR (Lebon et al., 2017).

A meta-analysis revealed that patients with dual-growing rods had fewer complications than those with single-growing rods. However, neither deformity correction, spinal growth, nor other complications differed between single and dual-growing rods. Therefore, the authors stated that dual-growing rods do not provide substantial advantages over single-growing rods in treating EOS (Wang et al., 2023).

These distraction-based techniques help restore the coronal balance of the spine while allowing the spine to grow. Although these systems are widely used in groups of patients with EOS, there are several disadvantages of these systems. First, these are static systems. Second, these systems had difficulties in restoring sagittal plane deformities. Third, the need for multiple surgeries is another disadvantage. So, patients must be well informed about this long treatment process before surgery.

Compression-based systems included the staples and the anterior vertebral body tethering. In recent years, AVBT has increased popularity with its widespread use. The clinical results seem promising, but the indications of the technique are not consensus. Thoracoscopic procedures of VBT are technically demanding but preserve the lung functions better than the open technique in the long term. VBT is not widely used in the group of patients with EOS, so further studies are needed to clarify the prognosis of this promising system (Baker et al., 2021). These compression-based systems are discussed in detail in another chapter.

In the Shilla growth guidance technique (SGGT), the dual rods are fixed to the curve's apex by pedicle screws with limited fusion. The growth of the spine occurs in a proximal and distal direction through the sliding pedicle screws placed without disturbing the facet joints. Thirty-eight patients were retrospectively analyzed. If treated by conventional methods growing rod distraction, these patients would have had 49 scheduled lengthening procedures after their initial correction. At a 2-year follow-up, SGGT provides a satisfactory curve correction in children's deformity with an acceptable complication rate. (McCarthy et al., 2014). This surgical intervention is technically demanding, and special pedicle screws are required. Revision rates can be higher than those of other growth-sparing procedures.

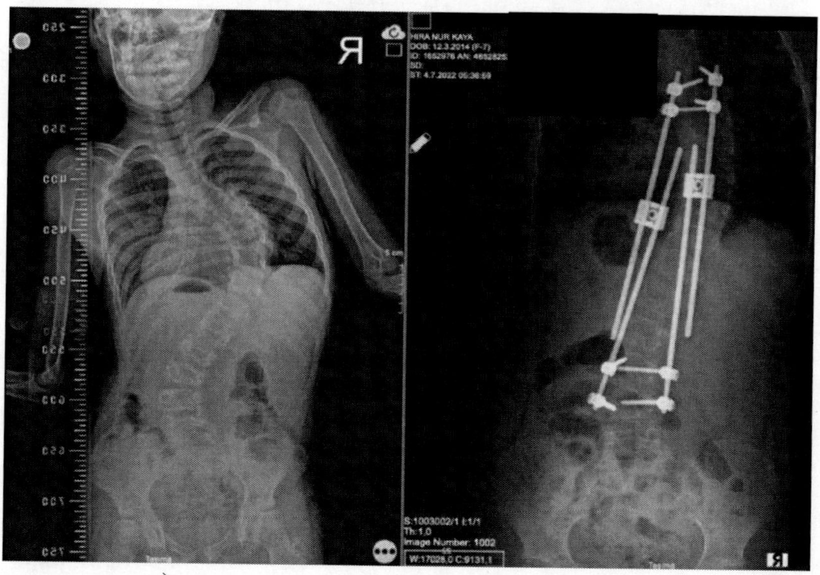

a) b)

**Figure 2.** a) A seven-year-old female presented with a very aggressive curve; Multiple genetic anomalies have been detected on her clinical examination. The Cobb angle T6-T12 was almost 90°. b) After the implantation of the growth guidance system, her coronal balance improved, and the Cobb angle between the same levels was reduced to 45°.

There are several growth guidance systems described in the literature. In Figure 2, a case example is given. Unlike the Shilla procedure, the cranial and the caudal end vertebrae were fused, and the construct was placed between them.

The conversion to definitive fusion is a debate. A current analysis evaluated the outcomes of graduates from growing rods who underwent final fusion or observation with implants in-situ. The meta-analysis showed a significantly higher revision rate in patients undergoing a definitive fusion procedure (Ahuja et al., 2023). The results this study can be a game changer in treating EOS with growing rods.

Spinal fusion in young children to treat early-onset scoliosis is not optimal because it limits growth and contributes to long-term lung compromise (Alkhalife et al., 2019). It can be considered in early-onset scoliosis (EOS) around triradiate cartilage closure (Simon et al., 2021). In severe cases, osteotomies such as vertebral column resections can be performed, but as an alternative, halo gravity traction must be considered before the surgical intervention.

One concern about the instrumentation in EOS patients is the development of the spinal canal. The disruption of the growth of the spinal canal is a question that every pediatric spine surgeon should be aware of. The current literature demonstrates that posterior instrumentation can be used safely in EOS regarding spinal canal development. In addition, pedicle screw instrumentation performed before the age of five years does not damage the growth of pedicles, the transverse plane of the vertebral body, or the spinal canal. It can safely treat deformities in this age group (Olgun et al., 2012). In another study conducted with 11 patients with congenital scoliosis with an average follow-up of 7.2 years, Hamzaoğlu et al. demonstrated that pedicle screw instrumentation has no adverse effect on the further spinal body, pedicle, and canal growth and does not result in iatrogenic spinal canal stenosis (Kahraman et al., 2016).

Despite all these encouraging articles, spinal canal development in patients with EOS must be a concern for the spine surgeon when surgical interventions are considered.

In summary, all surgical interventions in patients with EOS follow the same goals; minimizing and controlling the spinal deformity while maximizing the thoracic functions and the motion of the chest and spine. These goals are standard for the current treatment of EOS (El-Hawary & Akbarnia, 2015). Pediatric spine surgeons must be familiar with the prognoses of EOS patients and possible complications while treating them with conservative and surgical methods.

## Conclusion

EOS is a severe condition that requires early detection and intervention to prevent long-term complications. Indeed, the early start of the treatment is essential for a better prognosis. The first step of the treatment is always conservative. Bracing and casting are associated with a good long-term prognosis in the current literature. Sometimes, these treatments are used in severe curves for a time-buying strategy. Surgical interventions must be considered if these methods cannot control the progress of the curve. Unlike the adolescent group, spinal fusion is rarely considered in the EOS patient groups. Instead, growth-friendly surgery, which allows the thorax and spine to grow within the instrumentation, is the treatment of choice. There are several techniques, and the pediatric spine surgeon must choose the one they are familiar with.

## References

Ahuja, K., Ifthekar, S., Mittal, S., Bali, S. K., Yadav, G., Goyal, N., Sudhakar, P. V., & Kandwal, P. (2023). Is Final Fusion Necessary for Growing-Rod Graduates: A Systematic Review and Meta-Analysis. *Global Spine J, 13*(1), 209-218. https://doi.org/10.1177/21925682221090926.

Alkhalife, Y. I., Padhye, K. P., & El-Hawary, R. (2019). New Technologies in Pediatric Spine Surgery. *Orthop Clin North Am, 50*(1), 57-76. https://doi.org/10.1016/j.ocl.2018.08.014.

Babaee, T., Kamyab, M., Ganjavian, M. S., Rouhani, N., & Jarvis, J. (2020). The success rate of brace treatment for juvenile-onset idiopathic scoliosis up to skeletal maturity. *International Journal of Spine Surgery, 14*(5), 824-831.

Baker, C. E., Milbrandt, T. A., & Larson, A. N. (2021). Anterior vertebral body tethering for adolescent idiopathic scoliosis: early results and future directions. *Orthopedic Clinics, 52*(2), 137-147.

Bekmez, S., Dede, O., & Yazici, M. (2017). Advances in growing rod treatment for early onset scoliosis. *Curr Opin Pediatr, 29*(1), 87-93. https://doi.org/10.1097/mop.0000000000000432.

Canavese, F., & Dimeglio, A. (2020). Serial elongation derotation flexion casting in children with infantile and juvenile scoliosis. *Annals of Translational Medicine, 8*(2).

El-Hawary, R., & Akbarnia, B. A. (2015). Early Onset Scoliosis - Time for Consensus. *Spine deformity*, *3*(2), 105-106. https://doi.org/10.1016/j.jspd.2015.01.003.

Fedorak, G., & D'Astous, J. (2018). EDF casting for early-onset scoliosis. *Early Onset Scoliosis: A Clinical Casebook*, 17-34.

Fletcher, N. D., Larson, A. N., Richards, B. S., & Johnston, C. E. (2011). Current treatment preferences for early onset scoliosis: a survey of POSNA members. *Journal of pediatric orthopaedics*, *31*(3), 326-330.

Harrington, P. R. (1962). Treatment of scoliosis: correction and internal fixation by spine instrumentation. *JBJS*, *44*(4), 591-634.

Harshavardhana, N. S., & Lonstein, J. E. (2018). Results of bracing for juvenile idiopathic scoliosis. *Spine deformity*, *6*(3), 201-206.

Jarvis, J., Garbedian, S., & Swamy, G. (2008). Juvenile idiopathic scoliosis: the effectiveness of part-time bracing. *Spine*, *33*(10), 1074-1078.

Kahanovitz, N., Levine, D. B., & Lardone, J. (1982). The Part-time Milwaukee Brace Treatment of Juvenile Idiopathic Scoliosis: Long-term Follow-up. *Clinical Orthopaedics and Related Research (1976-2007)*, *167*, 145-151.

Kahraman, S., Karadereler, S., Cobanoglu, M., Yilar, S., Mutlu, A., Ulusoy, L. O., & Hamzaoglu, A. (2016). Does pedicle screw fixation under age 5 cause spinal canal narrowing? A CT study with minimum 5 years follow-up. *European Spine Journal*, *25*, 1665-1673.

Karol, L. A., Johnston, C., Mladenov, K., Schochet, P., Walters, P., & Browne, R. H. (2008). Pulmonary function following early thoracic fusion in non-neuromuscular scoliosis. *JBJS*, *90*(6), 1272-1281.

Keskinen, H., Helenius, I., Nnadi, C., Cheung, K., Ferguson, J., Mundis, G., Pawelek, J., & Akbarnia, B. A. (2016). Preliminary comparison of primary and conversion surgery with magnetically controlled growing rods in children with early onset scoliosis. *Eur Spine J*, *25*(10), 3294-3300. https://doi.org/10.1007/s00586-016-4597-y.

Khoshbin, A., Caspi, L., Law, P. W., Donaldson, S., Stephens, D., da Silva, T., Bradley, C. S., & Wright, J. G. (2015). Outcomes of bracing in juvenile idiopathic scoliosis until skeletal maturity or surgery. *Spine*, *40*(1), 50-55.

Lebon, J., Batailler, C., Wargny, M., Choufani, E., Violas, P., Fron, D., Kieffer, J., Accadbled, F., Cunin, V., & De Gauzy, J. S. (2017). Magnetically controlled growing rod in early onset scoliosis: a 30-case multicenter study. *Eur Spine J*, *26*(6), 1567-1576. https://doi.org/10.1007/s00586-016-4929-y.

Mahajan, R., Kishan, S., Mallepally, A. R., Shafer, C., Marathe, N., & Chhabra, H. S. (2020). Evolution of casting techniques in early-onset and congenital scoliosis. *Journal of Clinical Orthopaedics and Trauma*, *11*(5), 810-815.

McCarthy, R. E., Luhmann, S., Lenke, L., & McCullough, F. L. (2014). The Shilla growth guidance technique for early-onset spinal deformities at 2-year follow-up: a preliminary report. *J Pediatr Orthop*, *34*(1), 1-7. https://doi.org/10.1097/BPO.0b013e31829f92dc.

Mehta, M. (1972). The rib-vertebra angle in the early diagnosis between resolving and progressive infantile scoliosis. *The Journal of bone and joint surgery. British volume*, *54*(2), 230-243.

Negrini, S., Minozzi, S., Bettany-Saltikov, J., Chockalingam, N., Grivas, T. B., Kotwicki, T., Maruyama, T., Romano, M., & Zaina, F. (2015). Braces for idiopathic scoliosis in adolescents. *Cochrane Database of Systematic Reviews,* (6), CD006850.

Olgun, Z. D., Demirkiran, G., Ayvaz, M., Karadeniz, E., & Yazici, M. (2012). The effect of pedicle screw insertion at a young age on pedicle and canal development. *Spine, 37*(20), 1778-1784.

Perdriolle, R., & Vidal, J. (1985). Thoracic idiopathic scoliosis curve evolution and prognosis. *Spine, 10*(9), 785-791.

Quan, T., Matsumoto, H., Bonsignore-Opp, L., Ramo, B., Murphy, R. F., Brooks, J. T., Welborn MC, Emans JB, Anari JB, Johnston CE, Akbarnia BA, McCarthy R, Flynn J, Sawyer JR, Vitale MG, Roye BD, & Pediatric Spine Study Group (2023). Definition of Tweener: Consensus Among Experts in Treating Early-onset Scoliosis. *Journal of Pediatric Orthopaedics, 43*(3):e215-e222.

Sanders, J. O., D'Astous, J., Fitzgerald, M., Khoury, J. G., Kishan, S., & Sturm, P. F. (2009). Derotational casting for progressive infantile scoliosis. *Journal of pediatric orthopaedics, 29*(6), 581-587.

Senkoylu, A., Riise, R. B., Acaroglu, E., & Helenius, I. (2020). Diverse approaches to scoliosis in young children. *EFORT Open Reviews, 5*(10), 753-762. https://doi.org/10.1302/2058-5241.5.190087.

Simon, A. L., Angelliaume, A., Happiette, A., Huneidi, M., Julien-Marsollier, F., & Ilharreborde, B. (2021). Halo-gravity traction followed by definitive fusion in severe early onset scoliosis: results of a trunk analysis based on biplanar 3D reconstructions. *Eur Spine J, 30*(12), 3540-3549. https://doi.org/10.1007/s00586-021-06986-y.

Skaggs, D. L., Akbarnia, B. A., Flynn, J. M., Myung, K. S., Sponseller, P. D., & Vitale, M. G. (2014). A classification of growth friendly spine implants. *Journal of pediatric orthopaedics, 34*(3), 260-274.

Tello, C. A. (1994). Harrington instrumentation without arthrodesis and consecutive distraction program for young children with severe spinal deformities: experience and technical details. *Orthopedic Clinics of North America, 25*(2), 333-351.

Thompson, J. Y., Williamson, E. M., Williams, M. A., Heine, P. J., Lamb, S. E., & Group, A. C. S. (2019). Effectiveness of scoliosis-specific exercises for adolescent idiopathic scoliosis compared with other non-surgical interventions: a systematic review and meta-analysis. *Physiotherapy, 105*(2), 214-234. https://doi.org/10.1016/j.physio.2018.10.004.

Vitale, M. G., Matsumoto, H., Bye, M. R., Gomez, J. A., Booker, W. A., Hyman, J. E., & Roye Jr, D. P. (2008). A retrospective cohort study of pulmonary function, radiographic measures, and quality of life in children with congenital scoliosis: an evaluation of patient outcomes after early spinal fusion. *Spine, 33*(11), 1242-1249.

Waldron, S. R., Poe-Kochert, C., Son-Hing, J. P., & Thompson, G. H. (2013). Early onset scoliosis: the value of serial risser casts. *J Pediatr Orthop, 33*(8), 775-780. https://doi.org/10.1097/bpo.0000000000000072.

Wang, T., Fan, N., Zang, L., Yuan, S., Du, P., Si, F., Wang, A., Li, J., Kong, X., & Zhu, W. (2023). Comparative efficacy and complications of single and dual growing rods for early-onset scoliosis: an updated meta-analysis. *Eur Spine J, 32*(1), 167-180. https://doi.org/10.1007/s00586-022-07488-1.

Weinstein, S. L., Dolan, L. A., Wright, J. G., & Dobbs, M. B. (2013). Effects of bracing in adolescents with idiopathic scoliosis. *New England Journal of Medicine*, *369*(16), 1512-1521.

Yang, S., Andras, L. M., Redding, G. J., & Skaggs, D. L. (2016). Early-Onset Scoliosis: A Review of History, Current Treatment, and Future Directions. *Pediatrics*, *137*(1). https://doi.org/10.1542/peds.2015-0709.

# Chapter 15

# Non-Surgical Treatment of EOS

**Ahmet Çağrı Uyar*, MD**
Department of Orthopedics and Traumatology, University of Health Sciences,
Kocaeli Derince Training and Research Hospital, Kocaeli, Turkiye

## Abstract

Early-onset scoliosis (EOS) is defined as a spinal curvature above 10° in the coronal plane that occurs in children aged under ten. Together with spinal deformity, thoracic deformity may reduce chest volume and cause abnormal respiratory patterns and cardiopulmonary diseases. In EOS, conservative methods applied to terminate the progression of the curvature and correct the curvature while preserving the pulmonary and cardiac functions and controlling the growth of the spine and thorax include observation, physical therapy, serial casting, and bracing. Bracing and plaster treatments and physiotherapy practices contribute to the arrest and regression of the curvature when started at early ages and are effective in delaying the time of surgical intervention in older ages and high-degree curvatures. Conservative treatment methods reduce the need for surgical treatment in EOS.

**Keywords:** scoliosis, brace, casting, physiotherapy

## Introduction

Early-onset scoliosis (EOS) is defined as a spinal curvature above 10° in the coronal plane that occurs in children under the age of five. Some studies have

* Corresponding Author's Email: ahmetcagriuyar@gmail.com.

In: Early Onset Scoliosis
Editor: Ahmed Majid Heydar
ISBN: 979-8-89113-600-7

described EOS for children aged under ten (El-Hawary & Akbarnia, 2015; Thorsness et al., 2015; Yang et al., 2016). Together with spinal deformity, thoracic deformity may reduce chest volume and cause abnormal respiratory patterns and cardiopulmonary diseases. The etiology of EOS may be idiopathic, secondary to neuromuscular diseases, or associated with systemic syndromes or structural congenital deformities (Yang et al., 2016). Although the etiology of idiopathic EOS is associated with genetic factors, melatonin disorders, neurologic mechanisms, thrombocyte anomalies, and biomechanical factors, the true etiology is unknown; therefore, it is defined as a multifactorial disease (El-Hawary & Akbarnia, 2015; Lowe et al., 2000). The main goal of the treatment of EOS is to terminate the progression of the curvature and correct the curvature, protect the pulmonary and cardiac functions, and provide the growth of the spine and thorax in a controlled manner. The methods used in the conservative treatment of EOS include observation, physical therapy, serial casting, and bracing.

## Observation

Observation is not a treatment method in EOS, but it plays an important role in the planning of conservative and surgical treatment. It was observed that 5% of patients with curvature above 10° progressed to 30° (Bilgiç & Erşen, 2017; Deurloo & Verkerk, 2015). When growth was complete, patients with a curvature above 30 degrees were found to be more at risk of progressing the curvature in adulthood (Burger et al., 2019). The clinical follow-up of the patients is planned according to the potential of curvature progression and the patient is kept under observation. Curvatures below 25° are usually monitored at 6-12-month intervals (Burger et al., 2019).

### Physiotherapy

In adulthood, a curvature of 30° or above in EOS negatively affects thorax deformity, respiratory capacity, and quality of life (Romano et al., 2012). Scoliosis-specific exercises are among the main treatment options for preventing curvature progression (Lonstein, 2006; Romano et al., 2012). Various scoliosis-specific exercise programs have been prepared that offer patients a more effective treatment option. The common goal of these programs is to stop the progression of the curvature, prevent respiratory problems, reduce torso rotation, reduce the need for surgical treatment, and increase the quality of life (Berdishevsky et al., 2016). Scoliosis-specific exercises consist of personalized exercises that are taught to patients in the scoliosis treatment center and include a series of specific physical movements aimed at reducing the deformity. Exercises lead to mechanical changes in the muscles and other soft tissues of the spine. It is also believed that these exercises change motor control of the spine by triggering neurological changes (Hawes, 2003). Exercise programs also include patient training, sitting and standing training, and regulation of activities of daily living. The main scoliosis-specific exercise schools are located in Lyon (France), Schroth (Germany), SEAS (Italy), Barcelona (Spain), Dobomed (Poland), SideShift (England), and FITTS (Poland) (Berdishevsky et al., 2016).

Among these exercise programs, the most common is the Schroth method, which is still frequently used today. The method developed by Katharina Schroth in 1920 aims to achieve and maintain normal postural alignment through sensorimotor, respiratory, and postural exercises (Kuru et al., 2016; Schreiber et al., 2016). Studies have reported a reduction in Cobb angle, an improvement in torso rotation, and an increase in quality of life through Schroth exercises (Berdishevsky et al., 2016; Schreiber et al., 2016). Similar results can be achieved with other scoliosis-specific exercise techniques.

Alternative physiotherapy techniques such as yoga and pilates are also being applied to the treatment of EOS with increasing frequency. However, scientific data on these techniques are quite insufficient (Kim, 2014).

## Serial Casting

Cotrel and Morel described the elongation-derotation-flexion casting technique for the treatment of scoliosis in 1964 (Cotrel & Morel, 1964). Serial casting treatment contributes to the correction of the curvature in children under the age of two with infantile idiopathic scoliosis and mild to moderate curvatures (Mehta, 2005; Sanders et al., 2009). In different studies, it has been shown to slow the progression of the curvature and reduce the need for surgical treatment in older children and non-idiopathic scoliosis (Cao et al., 2017; Demirkiran et al., 2015; Fletcher et al., 2012; Gussous et al., 2015; Sanders et al., 2009). In the literature, there are not enough studies that examine the effect of serial casting treatment on the growth of the thoracic spine. Torso casting is also recommended in idiopathic EOS to delay surgical treatment in case of failure of bracing treatment. In cases where the degree and rigidity of the curvature increase, body casts can be used in children who cannot tolerate the use of braces. Thus, the difficulties in using braces in young children are eliminated (Dede & Sturm, 2016; Okkaoğlu et al., 2018). Plaster treatment has also been reported to reduce the curvature in addition to delaying surgical treatment (Mehta, 2005; Okkaoğlu et al., 2018). Although different torso casting techniques have been reported, their clinical follow-up is similar. Casting is performed under anesthesia every two to three months in children under the age of two. As age progresses, the frequency of casting decreases. The disadvantage of serial casting is that the patient receives anesthesia at frequent intervals. However, rapid correction can be achieved at young ages with rapid spinal growth (Dimeglio, 1992).

Serial casting is an effective treatment method to correct for curvature in idiopathic EOS. It is an effective method in terms of keeping the curvature under control and delaying the surgery in the period leading up to surgery in children aged two and over with a greater degree of rigid curvature and in patients with non-idiopathic EOS.

## Brace Treatment

There are not enough studies examining the use of brace treatment, which is used effectively in the treatment of adolescent idiopathic scoliosis, in the treatment of EOS (Weinstein et al., 2013). The use of braces in the treatment of EOS is used to maintain the spinal curvature under control during the growth of skeletal growth. It is also used as a complementary method after serial casting. Despite the lack of studies, it is the most commonly used method in the conservative treatment of EOS (Sauvagnac & Rigo, 2022; Thorsness et al., 2015). Bracing treatment aims to correct the scoliotic shape of the spine by applying pressure to certain points of the torso and controlling the progression of the curvature (Bilgiç et al., 2012). In many studies, it has been reported that bracing treatment is the most appropriate treatment option for curvatures of 25°-45° with potential progression (Bilgiç et al., 2012; Carr et al., 1980; Emans et al., 1986; Kuroki, 2018). The abdomen is generally wider in the younger age group. This may complicate the implementation of the brace. In young children, bracing requires an experienced orthotic specialist and a well-trained family for the use of braces (Thorsness et al., 2015). Various orthoses have been designed for the treatment of scoliosis. These include the Milwaukee brace (cervico-thoraco-lumbo-sacral orthosis), the Boston brace (thoraco-lumbo-sacral orthosis), the Charleston brace, the Providence brace, and the SpineCor brace.

The Milwaukee brace was used by Walter Blount in 1946 after surgical treatment of polio patients with neuromuscular scoliosis. Blount reported the results of Milwaukee applications in the treatment of adolescent idiopathic scoliosis in 1958 (Blount et al., 1958). The Milwaukee brace is used for 23 hours. It cannot be removed except for necessary cases such as showering and exercising. Milwaukee brace was the first type of brace used in the treatment of scoliosis. The device has a wide one-piece bar at the front and two thinner bars on the backside. Traction is provided between the pelvic part and the neck ring and corrective forces are applied to the apex points of the curvature through side supports (Figure 1). Thus, force is applied in two planes. Milwaukee brace is both cosmetically inappropriate and complicates patient compliance since its parts are uncomfortable (Lonstein & Winter, 1994; Noonan et al., 1996). Despite these disadvantages, it has been and is still widely used as an orthosis that can apply corrective force in both planes (Noonan et al., 1996; Sauvagnac & Rigo, 2022).

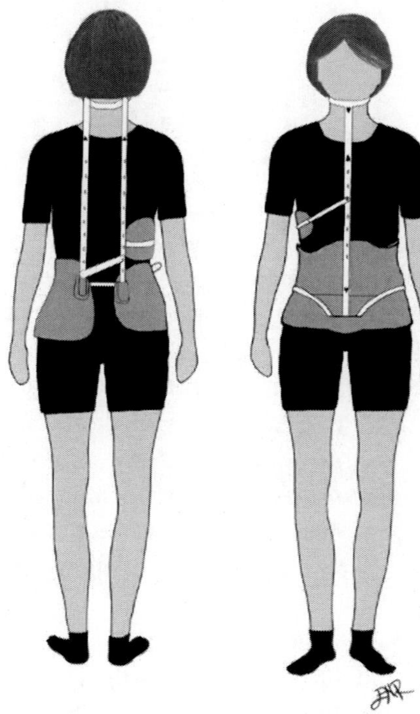

**Figure 1.** Milwaukee brace.

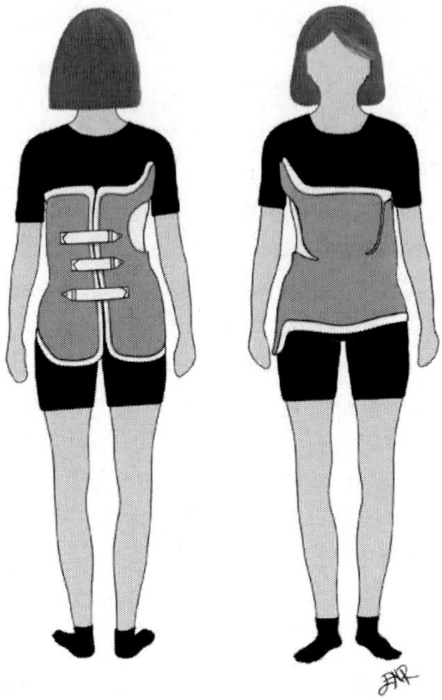

**Figure 2.** Boston brace.

Boston brace is a thoraco-lumbo-sacral orthosis developed at Boston Children's Hospital in 1972 (Figure 2). The Boston brace is similar to the Milwaukee brace in terms of active and passive forces points of application and usage characteristics. Due to its lower profile and more open design, it is easier to use compared to the Milwaukee brace. Patient compliance is better compared to the Milwaukee brace. The recommended duration of daily use for the Boston brace is 18-23 hours.

Night braces have been designed to increase patient compliance. The first designed night brace was the Charleston brace, which was developed by Frederick Reed Charleston in 1979. The Charleston brace is produced using mold obtained by applying plaster to the patient after lateral bending to ensure maximum correction of the curvature. Overcorrection is achieved with lateral bending forces. It is recommended to use it for eight to 10 hours (Bilgiç et al., 2012; Wiemann et al., 2014).

Another night brace is the Providence brace which was developed in 1992. Opposing forces are applied to the apexes of the curvature, pushing the apex towards the midline or further. D'Amato et al. reported excellent results in patients who used the Providence brace (Roland D'Amato et al., 2001). It has been reported that the Providence brace is more effective in curvatures below 35 degrees. In another study, the Providence brace was found to be more successful in the improvement of the curvature and reduction in the progression towards surgery in adolescent idiopathic scoliosis patients with a curvature of 25°-40° compared to the thoraco-lumbo-sacral orthosis (Janicki et al., 2007).

A non-rigid and dynamic brace system called SpineCor was described by Charles Rivard and Christine Coillard in 1998. The SpineCor brace consists of a thermoplastic pelvic floor, femoral and groin straps, a cotton vest on the back, and four adjustable correcting straps. The placement and tension of the band can be adjusted according to the curvature type. Strap tension and configuration are set up with computer support. The SpineCor brace was found to be more effective in low and moderate curvatures (Coillard et al., 2003). In their study, Coillard et al. reported improvement from the initial curvature in half of patients and worsening by less than 5° in 7% (Coillard et al., 2003). The advantage of this brace is that it is easy to use in terms of cosmetics and provides mobility compared to other braces.

The success of bracing treatment depends on many variables such as the type of curvature, the type of brace used, the application technique, the duration of use, and patient compliance. In a study conducted to examine the suitability of the use of braces, mechanical sensors were used, and it was found that the rate of use of braces with appropriate force and time was 60% (Rahman et al., 2015).

## Conclusion

While the EOS treatment aims to stop the progression of the curvature and correct the curvature, it is also very important to protect the pulmonary and cardiac functions and provide the growth of the spine and thorax in a controlled manner. The primary goal of conservative methods in the treatment of EOS is to arrest or reduce the increase in the rotation of the curvature in the growing spine and thorax. The risk of pulmonary restrictive lung diseases also increases with increased thoracic deformities. The progression of the curvature can be stopped, and improvement can be achieved, especially in children aged under 2, for whom conservative treatment is initiated in the early period. The regular physical examination of patients for the follow-up of the curvature and the continuity of the treatment is of great importance. Many different exercise procedures have been developed in physiotherapy. The clinical results of different exercise methods are similar. Bracing and serial casting are conservative treatment methods that require a high level of patient compliance. Good clinical results have been reported with both techniques. Different conservative treatment methods are applied in combination or complementarily. No consensus was reached regarding which treatment method should be applied to which patient. Conservative methods applied by determining patient-specific treatment reduce the need for surgical treatment in EOS.

## References

Berdishevsky, H., Lebel, V. A., Bettany-Saltikov, J., Rigo, M., Lebel, A., Hennes, A., Romano, M., Białek, M., M'hango, A., Betts, T., de Mauroy, J. C., & Durmala, J. (2016). Physiotherapy scoliosis-specific exercises - a comprehensive review of seven major schools. *Scoliosis and Spinal Disorders, 11*(1). https://doi.org/10.1186/s13013-016-0076-9.

Bilgiç, S., & Erşen, Ö. (2017). Adolesan İdiyopatik Skolyoz Konservatif Tedavisi [Conservative Treatment of Adolescent Idiopathic Scoliosis]. *Türkiye Klinikleri Ortopedi Travmatoloji - Özel Konular, 10*(2), 118–123. https://www.turkiyeklinikleri.com/article/tr-adolesan-idiyopatik-skolyoz-konservatif-tedavisi-79643.html.

Bilgiç, S., Erşen, Ö., & Şehirlioğlu, A. (2012). Adölesan İdiopatik skolyozda breys tedavisi [Brace treatment in adolescent idiopathic scoliosis]. *Journal of Clinical and Analytical Medicine, 3*(1), 112–116. https://doi.org/10.4328/jcam.231.

Blount, W. P., Schmidt, A. C., Keever, E. D., & Leonard, E. T. (1958). The Milwaukee Brace in the Operative Treatment of Scoliosis: JBJS. *The Journal of Bone & Joint Surgery, 40*(3), 511–525. https://journals.lww.com/jbjsjournal/Citation/1958/40030/The_Milwaukee_Brace_in_the_Operative_Treatment_of.3.aspx.

Burger, M., Coetzee, W., du Plessis, L. Z., Geldenhuys, L., Joubert, F., Myburgh, E., Rooyen, C. van, & Vermeulen, N. (2019). The effectiveness of Schroth exercises in adolescents with idiopathic scoliosis: A systematic review and meta-analysis. *The South African Journal of Physiotherapy, 75*(1). https://doi.org/10.4102/sajp.v75i1.904.

Cao, J., Zhang, X. J., Sun, N., Sun, L., Guo, D., Qi, X. Y., Bai, Y. S., & Sun, B. S. (2017). The therapeutic characteristics of serial casting on congenital scoliosis: a comparison with non-congenital cases from a single-center experience. *Journal of Orthopaedic Surgery and Research, 12*(1). https://doi.org/10.1186/s13018-017-0554-7.

Carr, W. A., Moe, J. H., Winter, R. B., & Lonstein, J. E. (1980). Treatment of idiopathic scoliosis in the Milwaukee brace: JBJS. *The Journal of Bone & Joint Surgery, 4*(62), 599–612. https://journals.lww.com/jbjsjournal/Abstract/1980/62040/Treatment_of_idiopathic_scoliosis_in_the_Milwaukee.15.aspx.

Coillard, C., Leroux, M. A., Zabjek, K. F., & Rivard, C. H. (2003). SpineCor--a non-rigid brace for the treatment of idiopathic scoliosis: post-treatment results. *European Spine*

*Journal: Official Publication of the European Spine Society, the European Spinal Deformity Society, and the European Section of the Cervical Spine Research Society, 12*(2), 141–148. https://doi.org/10.1007/s00586-002-0467-x.

Cotrel, Y., & Morel, G. (1964). The Elongation-Derotation-Flexion Technic in the Correction of Scoliosis. *Revue de Chirurgie Orthopedique et Reparatrice de L'appareil Moteur, 50*, 59–75. https://europepmc.org/article/med/14139818.

Dede, O., & Sturm, P. F. (2016). A brief history and review of modern casting techniques in early onset scoliosis. *Journal of Children's Orthopaedics, 10*(5), 405–411. https://doi.org/10.1007/s11832-016-0762-4/asset/images/large/10.1007_s11832-016-0762-4-fig2.jpeg.

Demirkiran, H. G., Bekmez, S., Celilov, R., Ayvaz, M., Dede, O., & Yazici, M. (2015). Serial derotational casting in congenital scoliosis as a time-buying strategy. *Journal of Pediatric Orthopedics, 35*(1), 43–49. https://doi.org/10.1097/bpo.0000000000000229.

Deurloo, J. A., & Verkerk, P. H. (2015). To screen or not to screen for adolescent idiopathic scoliosis? A review of the literature. *Public Health, 129*(9), 1267–1272. https://doi.org/10.1016/j.puhe.2015.07.021.

Dimeglio, A. (1992). Growth of the Spine Before Age 5 Years. *Journal of Pediatric Orthopaedics Part B, 1*(2), 102–107. https://doi.org/10.1097/01202412-199201020-00003.

El-Hawary, R., & Akbarnia, B. A. (2015). Early Onset Scoliosis - Time for Consensus. *Spine Deformity, 3*(2), 105–106. https://doi.org/10.1016/j.jspd.2015.01.003.

Emans, J. B., Kaelin, A., Bancel, P., Hall, J. E., & Miller, M. E. (1986). The Boston bracing system for idiopathic scoliosis. Follow-up results in 295 patients. *Spine, 11*(8), 792–801. https://doi.org/10.1097/00007632-198610000-00009.

Fletcher, N. D., McClung, A., Rathjen, K. E., Denning, J. R., Browne, R., & Johnston, C. E. (2012). Serial casting as a delay tactic in the treatment of moderate-to-severe early-onset scoliosis. *Journal of Pediatric Orthopaedics, 32*(7), 664–671. https://doi.org/10.1097/bpo.0b013e31824bdb55.

Gussous, Y. M., Tarima, S., Zhao, S., Khan, S., Caudill, A., Sturm, P., & Hammerberg, K. W. (2015). Serial Derotational Casting in Idiopathic and Non-Idiopathic Progressive Early-Onset Scoliosis. *Spine Deformity, 3*(3), 233–238. https://doi.org/10.1016/j.jspd.2014.10.001.

Hawes, M. C. (2003). The use of exercises in the treatment of scoliosis: an evidence-based critical review of the literature. *Pediatric Rehabilitation, 6*(3–4), 171–182. https://doi.org/10.1080/0963828032000159202.

Janicki, J. A., Poe-Kochert, C., Armstrong, D. G., & Thompson, G. H. (2007). A comparison of the thoracolumbosacral orthoses and providence orthosis in the treatment of adolescent idiopathic scoliosis: results using the new SRS inclusion and assessment criteria for bracing studies. *Journal of Pediatric Orthopedics, 27*(4), 369–374. https://doi.org/10.1097/01.bpb.0000271331.71857.9a.

Kim, H. S. (2014). Evidence-Based of Nonoperative Treatment in Adolescent Idiopathic Scoliosis. *Asian Spine Journal, 8*(5), 695. https://doi.org/10.4184/asj.2014.8.5.695.

Kuroki, H. (2018). Brace treatment for adolescent idiopathic scoliosis. *Journal of Clinical Medicine, 7*(6). https://doi.org/10.3390/jcm7060136.

Kuru, T., Yeldan, İ., Dereli, E. E., Özdinçler, A. R., Dikici, F., & Çolak, İ. (2016). The efficacy of three-dimensional Schroth exercises in adolescent idiopathic scoliosis: a randomised controlled clinical trial. *Clinical Rehabilitation, 30*(2), 181–190. https://doi.org/10.1177/0269215515575745.

Lonstein, J. E. (2006). Scoliosis: surgical versus nonsurgical treatment. *Clinical Orthopaedics and Related Research, 443*, 248–259. https://doi.org/10.1097/01.blo.0000198725.54891.73.

Lonstein, J. E., & Winter, R. B. (1994). The Milwaukee brace for the treatment of adolescent idiopathic scoliosis. A review of one thousand and twenty patients. *The Journal of Bone and Joint Surgery. American Volume, 76*(8), 1207–1221. https://doi.org/10.2106/00004623-199408000-00011.

Lowe, T. G., Edgar, M., Margulies, J. Y., Miller, N. H., Raso, V. J., Reinker, K. A., & Rivard, C. H. (2000). Etiology of idiopathic scoliosis: current trends in research. *The Journal of Bone and Joint Surgery. American Volume, 82*(8), 1157–1168. https://doi.org/10.2106/00004623-200008000-00014.

Mehta, M. H. (2005). Growth as a corrective force in the early treatment of progressive infantile scoliosis. *The Journal of Bone and Joint Surgery. British Volume, 87*(9), 1237–1247. https://doi.org/10.1302/0301-620x.87b9.16124.

Noonan, K. J., Weinstein, S. L., Jacobson, W. C., & Dolan, L. A. (1996). Use of the Milwaukee brace for progressive idiopathic scoliosis. *The Journal of Bone and Joint Surgery. American Volume, 78*(4), 557–567. https://doi.org/10.2106/00004623-199604000-00009.

Okkaoğlu, M. C., Demirkale, İ., & Altay, M. (2018). Gövde alçıları ve endikasyonları [Body casts and indications]. *TOTBİD Dergisi, 17*(3), 290–295. https://doi.org/10.14292/totbid.dergisi.2018.36.

Rahman, T., Sample, W., Yorgova, P., Neiss, G., Rogers, K., Gabos, P., Kritzer, D., & Bowen, J. R. (2015). Electronic monitoring of orthopedic brace compliance. *Journal of Children's Orthopaedics, 9*(5), 365–369. https://doi.org/10.1007/s11832-015-0679-3.

Roland D'Amato, C., Griggs, S., & McCoy, B. (2001). Nighttime bracing with the Providence brace in adolescent girls with idiopathic scoliosis. *Spine, 26*(18), 2006–2012. https://doi.org/10.1097/00007632-200109150-00014.

Romano, M., Minozzi, S., Bettany-Saltikov, J., Zaina, F., Chockalingam, N., Kotwicki, T., Maier-Hennes, A., & Negrini, S. (2012). Exercises for adolescent idiopathic scoliosis. *The Cochrane Database of Systematic Reviews, 2012*(8). https://doi.org/10.1002/14651858.cd007837.pub2.

Sanders, J. O., D'Astous, J., Fitzgerald, M., Khoury, J. G., Kishan, S., & Sturm, P. F. (2009). Derotational casting for progressive infantile scoliosis. *Journal of Pediatric Orthopaedics, 29*(6), 581–587. https://doi.org/10.1097/bpo.0b013e3181b2f8df.

Sauvagnac, R., & Rigo, M. (2022). Evolution of Early Onset Scoliosis under Treatment with a 3D-Brace Concept. *Journal of Clinical Medicine, 11*(5). https://doi.org/10.3390/jcm11051186.

Schreiber, S., Parent, E. C., Moez, E. K., Hedden, D. M., Hill, D. L., Moreau, M., Lou, E., Watkins, E. M., & Southon, S. C. (2016). Schroth Physiotherapeutic Scoliosis-Specific Exercises Added to the Standard of Care Lead to Better Cobb Angle Outcomes in

Adolescents with Idiopathic Scoliosis - an Assessor and Statistician Blinded Randomized Controlled Trial. *PloS One, 11*(12). https://doi.org/10.1371/journal.pone.0168746.

Thorsness, R. J., Faust, J. R., Behrend, C. J., & Sanders, J. O. (2015). Nonsurgical Management of Early-onset Scoliosis. *Journal of the American Academy of Orthopaedic Surgeons, 23*(9), 519–528. https://doi.org/10.5435/jaaos-d-14-00019.

Weinstein, S. L., Dolan, L. A., Wright, J. G., & Dobbs, M. B. (2013). Effects of bracing in adolescents with idiopathic scoliosis. *The New England Journal of Medicine, 369*(16), 1512–1521. https://doi.org/10.1056/nejmoa1307337.

Wiemann, J. M., Shah, S. A., & Price, C. T. (2014). Nighttime bracing versus observation for early adolescent idiopathic scoliosis. *Journal of Pediatric Orthopaedics, 34*(6), 603–606. https://doi.org/10.1097/bpo.0000000000000221.

Yang, S., Andras, L. M., Redding, G. J., & Skaggs, D. L. (2016). Early-onset scoliosis: A review of history, current treatment, and future directions. *Pediatrics, 137*(1). https://doi.org/10.1542/peds.2015-0709/52909.

## Chapter 16

# Physiotherapy in Idiopathic Early-Onset Scoliosis

**Burçin Akçay[1,*], PT, PhD**
**and Tuğba Kuru Çolak[2], PT, PhD**
[1]Department of Physiotherapy and Rehabilitation, Faculty of Health Sciences, Bandırma Onyedi Eylül University, Balıkesir, Turkiye
[2]Department of Physiotherapy and Rehabilitation, Faculty of Health Sciences, Marmara University, Istanbul, Turkiye

## Abstract

Scoliosis noticed in a child under the age of ten for any reason is defined as early-onset scoliosis. Conservative treatment of idiopathic early-onset scoliosis includes observation, physiotherapy, casting, and bracing treatment. Physiotherapy and rehabilitation play an important role in the treatment of early-onset scoliosis, as in other scoliosis treatments.

Despite the insufficiency of studies on physiotherapy in the literature, these conducted studies have shown that it is possible to stop progression and reduce curvature when treating EOS with physiotherapy.

Physiotherapy methods should be tried to delay or eliminate the indication for surgery, especially during this period, when lung and thorax development and spinal elongation continue. Physiotherapy methods are important for the development and support of both the musculoskeletal and cardiorespiratory systems.

**Keywords:** early-onset, exercise, physiotherapy, rehabilitation, scoliosis, spine

---

* Corresponding Author's Email: bakcay@bandirma.edu.tr.

In: Early Onset Scoliosis
Editor: Ahmed Majid Heydar
ISBN: 979-8-89113-600-7

## Introduction

Currently, scoliosis diagnosed before the age of 10 years for any reason, whether idiopathic or not, is defined as early-onset scoliosis (EOS) (Skaggs et al., 2015). According to the classification made by the Scoliosis Research Society (SRS), EOS is subdivided into idiopathic, congenital, thoracogenic, neuromuscular, and syndromic (Skaggs et al., 2015). Scoliosis below 3 years of age is considered in the infantile scoliosis group and will not be discussed in this chapter. Idiopathic EOS, which has received the most attention in the literature, will be the subject of this chapter.

Currently, conservative treatment of idiopathic early-onset scoliosis includes observation, physiotherapy, casting, and bracing treatment (Białek, 2015; Kuru Çolak et al., 2023; Ridderbusch et al., 2018; Ruiz et al., 2023; Weiss et al., 2022). Observation or follow-up can be defined as the evaluation of children with a low calculated risk of progression at certain intervals. However, it should be noted that the curve progresses in patients at risk of progression and who are only followed up with observation (Kuru et al., 2016).

The basic objectives of the comprehensive conservative treatment of idiopathic scoliosis are as follows:

1. to stop curve progression during periods of rapid growth (or possibly even reduce it),
2. to avoid or remedy respiratory problems,
3. to eliminate or cure spinal pain syndromes,
4. to enhance appearance through postural improvement (Negrini et al., 2012).

## Main Body

### Indications for Conservative Treatment

The risk of curve progression varies depending on many factors such as age, maturity, and Cobb angle. Therefore, conservative treatment also depends on these factors. Indications for conservative treatment are based on conservative treatment guidelines that consider the risk of curve progression (Weiss et al., 2006; Weiss et al., 2022).

According to the SOSORT guidelines, indications for conservative treatment of early-onset scoliosis between 6 and 10 years of age without signs of maturity vary according to the extent of the curve.

- In patients with EOS with a *Cobb angle of less than 15°*, it is recommended that the patients be followed up with observation at six to 12 month intervals.
- In patients with EOS with a *Cobb angle between 15-20°*, outpatient physiotherapy with free intervals is recommended. In outpatient physiotherapy, physiotherapy should first be applied in the clinic and then followed up with a home program. Depending on the method applied in the clinic, it can be organized into two or seven sessions per week.
- Physiotherapy and rehabilitation are recommended in patients with EOS with a *Cobb angle of 20-25°*, while the use of a brace in addition to physiotherapy is important in patients with a *Cobb angle above 25°* (Weiss et al., 2006; Dereli et al., 2021; Weiss et al., 2022).

## Physiotherapy and Rehabilitation in Patients with EOS

Physiotherapy and rehabilitation include many parameters such as strengthening, stretching, balance, proprioception, and respiratory exercises that are planned and applied to bring the musculoskeletal system to the optimal level as a result of scoliosis-specific methods and evaluation of the individual (Figure 1).

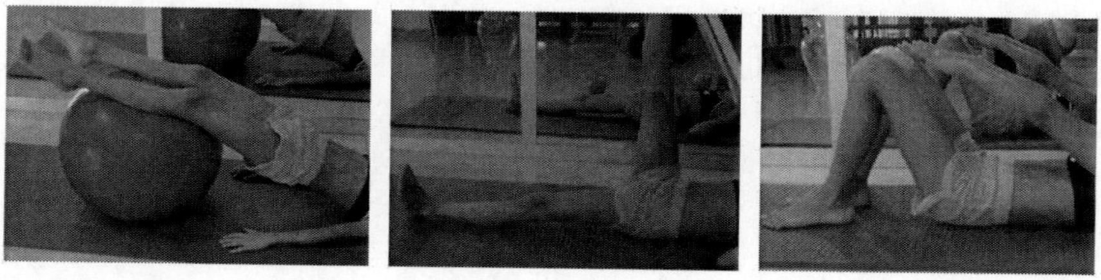

**Figure 1.** General strengthening and stretching exercises for early-onset scoliosis.

In early-onset idiopathic scoliosis, in addition to the goals in the treatment of adolescent idiopathic scoliosis, rehabilitation programs to improve thoracic volume and function, optimize chest and spine mobilization, and delay surgical indication as much as possible are among the treatment goals (Skaggs et al., 2015). This is because the lungs are still developing, and the thorax and spine will continue to grow for longer.

## Scoliosis-Specific Physiotherapy Exercises in Patients with EOS

There are currently different scoliosis-specific physiotherapy concepts developed by physiotherapists around the world. In these concepts, scoliosis-specific exercise approaches are applied for various purposes such as stopping the progression of curvature, reducing the angle of curvature, improving the cosmetic appearance, preventing the side effects of the brace, and pain control in adult individuals.

SOSORT (International Society on Scoliosis Orthopaedic and Rehabilitation Treatment) defines scoliosis-specific exercises as "Scoliosis Specific Physiotherapy Exercises." Scoliosis specific physiotherapy exercises are used in scoliosis treatment in the world: Schroth, Barcelona Scoliosis Physical Therapy School (BSPTS), Schroth Best Practice (SBP), Lyon, Scientific Exercise Approach for Scoliosis (SEAS), Dobomed, Side Shift, and Functional Individual Treatment of Scoliosis (FITS) (Berdishevsky et al., 2016; Kuru Çolak & Akçay, 2020; Negrini et al., 2012).

All these scoliosis-specific physiotherapy exercise approaches should include auto-correction in three dimensions (3D), training in daily living activities (ADL), improving the corrected posture, and patient education (Negrini et al., 2012).

Furthermore, scoliosis specific physiotherapy exercises are applied to prepare the patient for the brace before brace treatment, to increase compliance with brace use during brace treatment, and to maintain trunk stabilization during the brace weaning period and before or after surgical treatment. In addition, scoliosis-specific physiotherapy exercises can be used to reduce pain and increase functionality before and after the operation (Negrini et al., 2018). In addition, it is important to start physiotherapy as early as possible in patients with EOS (Fernandes et al., 2007).

### *The Lyon Approach*

The Lyon approach is one of the oldest scoliosis rehabilitation approaches. Dr. Jean Claude de Mauroy, the head of the orthopedic division at Lyon's "Clinique du Parc," currently serves as its leader. This school is known as one of the scoliosis-specific exercise schools and one of the oldest schools in

France, and unlike other methods, it is integrated into the medical school. The exercises were first applied based on self-elongation. In 1947, physiotherapy was introduced in the Lyon approach with bracing and casts. The brace and cast also apply elongation, postural correction, core stabilization, and respiratory exercises. Cast treatment is mostly preferred in the treatment of congenital or idiopathic early-onset scoliosis. The main features of the Lyon method include improvement of postural balance, learning to correct the spine and adapting it to daily life activities, respiratory control with pelvic stabilization, three-dimensional spinal and iliolumbar mobilization, patient education, improvement of sitting posture, and endurance of deep paraspinal muscles. Symmetrical exercises are performed in the frontal plane. Exercises are repeated daily at home without using complex materials. There are no restrictions for sports activities in the Lyon method. The Ponseti and Lenke classifications are used for treatment protocols (Berdishevsky et al., 2016; Kuru Çolak & Akçay, 2020).

***The Schroth Approach***

The Schroth method is the most widely used method by physiotherapists worldwide among scoliosis-specific exercise methods (Figure 2). Katharina Schroth developed the Schroth method in Germany a hundred years ago (Weiss et al., 2022; Berdishevsky et al., 2016). With the guidance of proprioceptive and exteroceptive stimuli provided by the physiotherapist, the aim is to correct the scoliotic posture. Changes in the sagittal plan are also addressed in the treatment program. A mirror is used to increase exteroceptive stimuli in exercise applications. The mirror aims for the patient to see themselves anteriorly and posteriorly, realize correct correction patterns, and improve body awareness and midline sensation. Under a physiotherapist's supervision, group or individual exercise programs are applied for patients with similar curvature patterns. The main features of the Schroth method include improving the patient's consciousness of the deformity to facilitate self-correction, application of three-dimensional asymmetric spinal corrective exercises with rotational breathing, passive mobilization specific to the scoliosis pattern, active three-dimensional stabilization (mostly isometric contractions are used), improvement of proprioception, an adaptation of postural corrections to daily life activities and easy home programs. Simple materials such as towels, exercise balls, and rice bags can be used in home exercises. Active axial elongation and rotational breathing exercises, which form the basis of the Schroth exercises, are very important during all activities. The Schroth classification system developed by Schroth's daughter is used for scoliosis and treatment. Exercises and treatment protocols are determined according to this classification system (Weiss, 2011; Lehnert-Schroth, 1992).

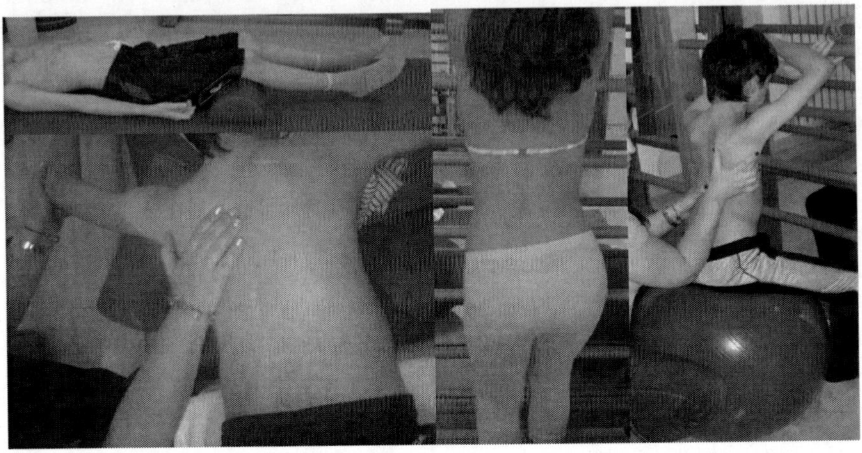

**Figure 2.** Examples of Schroth-based exercises, the most widely used scoliosis-specific exercise method used by physiotherapists in the world.

### *The Schroth Best Practice Approach*

Over time, the Schroth method continued to be developed by Katharina Schroth's daughter, physiotherapist Christa Lehnert-Schroth, and her grandson, Dr. Hans R. Weiss. The Best Practice method is based on the same basic principles as the Schroth method. The Schroth Best Practice method can be defined as an updated, improved, and simplified version of the Schroth method. Multidisciplinary teams implement treatment programs. Physio-logic® exercises for sagittal plane changes, activities of daily living, and active walking exercises were added to the Schroth method by Dr. Weiss. He also developed the Schroth classification and bracing concept defined by his mother and started a comprehensive, up-to-date rehabilitation practice. Today, in addition to exercise therapy, the rigid and asymmetric Gensingen brace, which includes three-dimensional correction principles developed by Dr. Weiss, is used for children and adolescents with indications for brace use (Weiss et al., 2022; Borysov & Borysov, 2012; Weiss et al., 2017).

### *The SEAS (Scientific Exercise Approach to Scoliosis) Approach*

The SEAS method was developed based on the Lyon method, and some updates were added to the method over time. It was introduced in a scoliosis treatment center established in Italy in the early 1960s, and in 2002 the name of the center was changed to "Instituto Scientifico Italiani Colonna Vertebrale (ISICO)," which is still in use today. Today, physiotherapists Michele Romano and Alessandra Negrini are the method's developers, educators, and leaders. They work in a multidisciplinary manner with Dr. Negrini and Dr. Zaina, specialists in their field at the Institute. This method does not primarily aim to apply corrective exercises for curvature. The main thing is to maintain the patient's corrected posture in unstable situations and positions. Through active three-dimensional corrections, it seeks to reestablish spinal balance and postural stability. Active self-correction is applied by educating the patient and increasing awareness of deformity. Posture continuity and spinal stabilization are tried to be maintained with different exercises applied in various positions, such as transitioning from sitting to standing, climbing stairs, and standing on one leg while maintaining balance on a balance board. Exercises train the neuromotor system and reflexively activate the self-correction of posture. These exercises can be performed in an outpatient or as a home program. To classify scoliosis, the location of the curve (thoracic, thoracolumbar, or lumbar) is taken into consideration. In addition to exercises, the less rigid Sibilla and rigid Sforzesco corsets are used in cases where there are more indications (Berdishevsky et al.,2016; Kuru Çolak & Akçay, 2020; Romano et al., 2015; Negrini et al., 2011).

***The BSPTS (Barcelona Scoliosis Physical Therapy School) Approach***

Utilizing Schroth's principles, Spanish physiotherapist Elena Salvá learned the treatment methods from Schroth and Schroth's daughter in the clinic in Bad Sobernheim, and then she established the Barcelona School of Scoliosis Physiotherapy in 1968. The principles of treatment practiced at this school were adapted from the original intensive (inpatient clinic) Schroth rehabilitation. For more than 40 years, Salvá implemented a rehabilitation program for spinal deformities using the Schroth method in her clinic. In 1989, after being granted permission, Gloria Quera-Salvá and Manuel Rigo, the daughter of Elena Salvá, started the training and certification of Spanish physiotherapists in the Schroth method. In 2009, the method was modified and started to be called BSPTS. BSPTS includes Schroth's basic rotational respiratory techniques, three-dimensional postural correction movements, maintenance of corrections with muscle contraction, training of some core muscles, mobilization techniques, and daily living activities. The classification used for scoliosis and treatment is the Schroth method, updated by Dr. Weiss and Dr. Rigo. In addition to exercise therapy, it includes combinations of education, psychosocial support, and a rigid and asymmetric

Rigo system Chêneau model brace used in cases where there is an indication (Berdishevsky et al., 2016; Jelačić et al., 2012; Rigo & Weiss, 2008).

***The Dobosiewicz-Dobo Approach***

The Dobosiewicz method combines crawling exercises (Klapp) and Schroth exercises. It was created in 1979 by Polish physiotherapist and doctor Prof. Dobosiewich by combining the two approaches, and until 1982 it was widely applied in Poland for the conservative management of scoliosis. After 2000, an inpatient rehabilitation program similar to the Schroth method was applied in the Rehabilitation Department of the Medical University of Katowice. It consists of asymmetric respiratory exercises and active rotational correction in the symmetric position of the thoracic spine and the posture of the kyphosis. Unlike other methods, 3D correction of the primary curvature is performed in various closed kinetic chain positions.

Three-dimensional self-correction may be referred to as a biodynamic method based on the mechanical changes observed in idiopathic scoliosis. If necessary, kyphosis is provided for the thoracic region and lordosis for the lumbar region. The pelvis and shoulder girdle are in a fixed position during the exercises. Correction is provided in the sagittal and axial planes. Frontal plane corrections occur spontaneously. Lateral flexion is not applied for the correction of thoracic curvatures. It has its classification system for scoliosis and its treatment protocol. Exercises are used with the Chêneau brace concept in children and adolescents with an indication for bracing (Berdishevsky et al., 2016; Rigo & Weiss, 2008; Dobosiewicz et al., 2002; Dobosiewicz et al., 2006).

***The Side Shift Approach***

Dr. Min Mehta developed the side shift in 1984 at the Royal National Orthopaedic Hospital in London to correct scoliotic curvatures. This method was originally developed for the treatment of congenital scoliosis, but it was later used for other spinal deformities. Tony Betts, a physiotherapist with expertise in spinal problems working in the same hospital, is the person in charge of this strategy today.

This method aims to stabilize a flexible curve with extreme lateral movements. The lateral deviation of the trunk in the coronal plane is corrected by extreme lateral movements.

With these repetitive lateral movements, the formation of structural curvature is prevented. Trunk shifting with muscle activation corrects the lateral curvature, stretches connective tissues, realigns soft tissues, and increases musculoskeletal mobility. At the same time, somatosensory integration is thought to be achieved with repetitive corrective movements, and a more upright and physiologic spinal posture is obtained. Schroth's rotational breathing exercises and the Schroth method's guiding principles are both incorporated into the Side Shift approach. It also includes Maitland's principles and myofascial release techniques. It is especially aimed at providing active correction of the apex of the curve. Along with isometric exercises, core stabilization exercises and strengthening exercises for the scapular muscles are applied. The King and Lenke classifications are used in the classification of scoliosis. When indicated according to the Cobb angle and the age of the child, brace treatment is used in addition to exercise therapy (Berdishevsky et al., 2016; Mamyama et al., 2002; Betts, 2014).

***The FITS (Functional Individual Therapy of Scoliosis) Approach***

The FITS method, like the Dobosiewicz method, was developed in Poland in 2004. During the development process, physiotherapists Marianna Białek and Andrzej M'hango developed the method with the experience of other colleagues in this field. The FITS method continues to develop with the contributions of Prof. Tomasz Kotwicki from the Department of Pediatric Orthopedics, Poznan University of Medical Sciences. This method is defined as a complex and asymmetric treatment for spinal deformities. Techniques have been selected from many different treatment approaches, modified according to the experience of physiotherapists, and adapted to scoliosis rehabilitation.

The technique entails raising awareness of the spinal column and the guidance of scoliosis improvement, as well as training in sensorimotor skills, stability, and posture, relaxation of the myofascial systems in three planes, lumbopelvic stabilization, correction of the primary curvature with stabilization of the secondary curvature in the frontal plane, and self-correction in daily activities.

Myofascial relaxation techniques such as trigger point, passive-active relaxation, post-isometric relaxation, and joint mobilization are applied before the correction exercises to mobilize the spine and ensure flexibility. Asymmetric exercises and respiratory techniques aim to correct the curve and prevent its progression. It involves the use of more elastic bands and exercise balls for correction exercises than other methods. Similar to the Schroth method, patients can receive treatment with a two-week intensive rehabilitation program. The FITS method does not use a special classification system to classify scoliosis. Exercise and other physiotherapeutic interventions can be applied in combination with rigid brace treatment or alone (Berdishevsky et al., 2016; Białek, 2011; Bialek & M'hango, 2008).

To the best of our knowledge, one study has been published in which scoliosis-specific exercises were applied and patients diagnosed with EOS were included. In this study, 41 children with idiopathic EOS were treated with the Functional Individual Therapy for Scoliosis (FITS method) without any other treatment. The youngest child included in the study was four years old and the oldest was nine. The children were followed up for an average of 4.8 years, and progression was found in only one child (1.9%). The mean Cobb angle and the angle of trunk rotation were also reported to be significantly reduced. It has been observed that the FITS method is effective in preventing the progression of curvature in patients with EOS, and body imbalance is improved (Białek, 2015).

Ridderbusch et al. presented retrospective treatment results for 22 patients with EOS. The authors suggest that surgical treatment may be necessary in some patients despite conservative treatment, but conservative approaches, such as physical therapy, casts, and bracing, can postpone the (frequent) need for surgery or even prevent it altogether, especially in cases of idiopathic early childhood scoliosis (Ridderbusch et al., 2018).

Of 34 children with idiopathic EOS, 14 were treated with physiotherapy and 20 with bracing and were followed up for 25 years. The researchers reported that the mean duration of treatment varied between nine and 15 months and in patients with EOS who were followed up for 25 years, there was no significant progression in scoliosis during the growth spurt in any patient with physiotherapy (Diedrich et al., 2002).

Since scoliosis-specific exercises involve three-dimensional correction of the spine and trunk, it is appropriate for very young children to perform the exercises under supervision. Depending on the child's age, ability to stabilize the body, and capacity to learn the exercise, exercises specific to the type of curvature should be selected. The level of evidence that shows the efficacy of physiotherapy in adolescent idiopathic scoliosis is increasing and the Schroth method is reported to be effective in adolescent idiopathic scoliosis at the level of evidence 2. Additionally, physiotherapy studies on EOS are very limited in literature. Randomized controlled and long-term follow-up studies are needed to increase the level of evidence in this field.

## Cardiopulmonary Rehabilitation Approaches in Patients with EOS

As the Cobb angle increases, the rate at which pulmonary function is affected also increases, which is influenced by the age of onset of the deformity. Lung volumes are more affected in patients with EOS than in adolescent idiopathic scoliosis (Muirhead & Conner, 1985). Natural lung compliance, lung volumes, and alveolar growth are affected by the onset of scoliosis, which affects the shape and biomechanics of the rib cage during spinal development. Therefore, as lung compliance decreases, the work of breathing may increase, and the respiratory rate may increase due to the inability to produce sufficient tidal volumes during normal breathing (Fletcher et al., 2012). Respiratory muscle weakness can be seen in children with EOS and is associated with decreased tidal capacity (Redding et al., 2017).

These changes in pulmonary structures also affect alveolar development (Fletcher et al., 2012). This is related to the timing of pulmonary alveolar development and the age of onset of scoliosis. The earlier the onset of scoliosis, the more profound the effect on the normal maturation of the alveoli, and this process is usually completed by the age of eight years (Reid, 1970; Fernandes & Weinstein, 2007). Onset scoliosis before alveolar development can significantly affect pulmonary function (Gillingham et al., 2006). Furthermore, in children with early-onset scoliosis, cardiovascular capacity may be affected in addition to respiratory function depending on the severity of the scoliosis (Scott & Morgan, 1995).

Although there is no clear consensus in the literature on the scope, duration, and intensity of cardiopulmonary rehabilitation in children with EOS, pulmonary training and interventions to increase pulmonary and cardiac capacity constitute an important part of the conservative treatment parameters of scoliosis. Scoliosis-specific physiotherapy exercises aimed at correcting the deformity, targeting the symmetry of the rib cage, and including asymmetric corrective breathing exercises support the positive development of pulmonary functions. Since EOS adversely affects lung function and poses a risk of restrictive pulmonary disease, it is of great importance for the treatment of patients with scoliosis to identify pulmonary problems, evaluate them in terms of pulmonary rehabilitation, and include respiratory exercises in the treatment program. Therefore, it is important to develop EOS-specific parameters for cardiopulmonary rehabilitation, which should play an active role at every stage of scoliosis and may positively affect the prognosis (Akçay, 2016; Negrini et al., 2018).

## Sportive Activities in Patients with EOS

Although there is no information in the literature regarding specific sporting activities for patients with EOS, it is generally stated that sport is not recommended as a treatment option for all patients with idiopathic scoliosis.

Sports activities, in addition to all stages of conservative treatment, may be recommended due to their aerobic capacity and psychological and neuromotor effects (Negrini et al., 2018). However, it should be taken into consideration that the risk of scoliosis is higher in people practicing ballet and rhythmic gymnastics (Tanchev et al., 2000; Longworth et al., 2014).

## Brace Treatment in Patients with EOS

Bracing is currently the treatment approach with the highest level of evidence in the treatment of adolescent idiopathic scoliosis (Weinstein et al., 2013).

However, the number of brace treatment studies for EOS in the literature is still limited. Thometz and Liu performed serial bracing treatment with CAD/CAM technology on nine children between two and six years of age (Thometz & Liu, 2019). They reported that in four of the children who were followed up for at least 24 months, the curve was completely corrected and in five children whose curves were relatively more rigid, there was a decrease from an average of 57° to 21° (Thometz & Liu, 2019). Another study by Thometz et al. also used the brace made with the CAD/CAM system and the authors reported that the juvenile group had 25.7% correction and 42.9% stabilization, while the infantile group had 50% correction and 32.1% stabilization (Thometz et al., 2018). Sauvagnac and Rigo reported an 80% success rate of brace treatment in children with EOS who were followed up for more than 6.5 years (Sauvagnac & Rigo, 2022). Short- and long-term results of brace treatment show that brace treatment of EOS is successful.

## Conclusion

Scoliosis-specific physiotherapy exercises are a physiotherapy approach used to prevent scoliosis progression in children with EOS. Cardiopulmonary rehabilitation should be considered in patients with EOS to improve cardiopulmonary functions at all stages of both operative and non-operative treatments. Although it is observed that studies on physiotherapy in patients with EOS are insufficient in the literature, it is emphasized that physiotherapy should be started at the earliest possible stage in children with EOS.

## References


Akçay, B. (2016). Skolyoz ve Pulmoner Rehabilitasyon [Scoliosis and Pulmonary Rehabilitation]. *Turkiye Klinikleri J Physiother Rehabil-Special Topics*, *2*(2), 78-85.

Berdishevsky, H., Lebel, V. A., Bettany-Saltikov, J., Rigo, M., Lebel, A., Hennes, A., Romano, M., Białek, M., M'hango, A., Betts, T., de Mauroy, J. C., & Durmala, J. (2016). Physiotherapy scoliosis-specific exercises - a comprehensive review of seven major schools. *Scoliosis and spinal disorders*, *11*, 20. https://doi.org/10.1186/s13013-016-0076-9.

Betts, T. (2014). The development of a classification system for the treatment of scoliosis by the side shift. *Scoliosis*, *9*(1), 1-1.

Białek M. (2011). Conservative treatment of idiopathic scoliosis according to FITS concept: presentation of the method and preliminary, short term radiological and clinical results based on SOSORT and SRS criteria. *Scoliosis, 6,* 25. https://doi.org/10.1186/1748-7161-6-25.

Białek M. (2015). Mild angle early onset idiopathic scoliosis children avoid progression under FITS method (Functional Individual Therapy of Scoliosis). *Medicine*, *94*(20), 1-20. e863. https://doi.org/10.1097/MD.0000000000000863.

Bialek, M., & M'hango, A. (2008). "FITS" concept Functional Individual Therapy of Scoliosis. *Studies in health technology and informatics, 135,* 250–261.

Borysov, M., & Borysov, A. (2012). Scoliosis short-term rehabilitation (SSTR) according to 'Best Practice' standards-are the results repeatable?. *Scoliosis*, *7*(1), 1. https://doi.org/10.1186/1748-7161-7-1.

Dereli, E. E., Gong, S., Çolak, T. K., & Turnbull, D. (2021). Guidelines for the conservative treatment of spinal deformities–Questionnaire for a Delphi consensus. *The South African journal of physiotherapy*, *77*(2), 1587. https://doi.org/10.4102/sajp.v77i2.1587.

Diedrich, O., Von Strempel, A., Schloz, M., Schmitt, O., & Kraft, C. N. (2002). Long-term observation and management of resolving infantile idiopathic scoliosis: A 25-year follow-up. *The Journal of Bone and Joint Surgery. British volume*, *84*(7), 1030-1035. https://doi.org/10.1302/0301-620x.84b7.13005.

Dobosiewicz, K., Durmala, J., Czernicki, K., & Jendrzejek, H. (2002). Pathomechanic basics of conservative treatment of progressive idiopathic scoliosis according to Dobosiewicz method based upon radiologic evaluation. *Studies in health technology and informatics*, *91*, 336–341.

Dobosiewicz, K., Durmala, J., Czernicki, K., & Piotrowski, J. (2006). Radiological results of Dobosiewicz method of three-dimensional treatment of progressive idiopathic scoliosis. *Studies in health technology and informatics*, *123*, 267–272.

Fernandes, P., & Weinstein, S. L. (2007). Natural history of early onset scoliosis. *JBJS*, *89*(suppl_1), 21-33. https://doi.org/10.2106/JBJS.F.00754.

Fletcher, N. D., & Bruce, R. W. (2012). Early onset scoliosis: current concepts and controversies. *Current reviews in musculoskeletal medicine*, *5*, 102-110. https://doi.org/10.1007/s12178-012-9116-0.

Gillingham, B. L., Fan, R. A., & Akbarnia, B. A. (2006). Early onset idiopathic scoliosis. *JAAOS-Journal of the American Academy of Orthopaedic Surgeons*, *14*(2), 101-112. https://doi.org/10.5435/00124635-200602000-00005.

Jelačić, M., Villagrasa, M., Pou, E., Quera-Salvá, G., & Rigo, M. (2012). Barcelona Scoliosis Physical Therapy School–BSPTS–based on classical Schroth principles: short term effects on back asymmetry in idiopathic scoliosis. *Scoliosis*, *7*(Suppl 1), O57.

Kuru Çolak, T. & Akçay, B. (2020). Current Exercise Approaches in Scoliosis Treatment. *Archives of health science and research (Online)*, *7*(2), 196-200.

Kuru Çolak, T., Akçay, B., Apti, A., & Çolak, İ. (2023). The Effectiveness of the Schroth Best Practice Program and Chêneau-Type Brace Treatment in Adolescent Idiopathic Scoliosis: Long-Term Follow-Up Evaluation Results. *Children*, *10*(2), 386. https://doi.org/10.3390/children10020386.

Kuru, T., Yeldan, İ., Dereli, E. E., Özdinçler, A. R., Dikici, F., & Çolak, İ. (2016). The efficacy of three-dimensional Schroth exercises in adolescent idiopathic scoliosis: a randomised controlled clinical trial. *Clinical rehabilitation*, *30*(2), 181-190. https://doi.org/10.1177/0269215515575745.

Lehnert-Schroth, C. (1992). Introduction to the three-dimensional scoliosis treatment according to Schroth. *Physiotherapy*, *78*(11), 810-815.

Longworth, B., Fary, R., & Hopper, D. (2014). Prevalence and predictors of adolescent idiopathic scoliosis in adolescent ballet dancers. *Archives of physical medicine and rehabilitation*, *95*(9), 1725-1730. https://doi.org/10.1016/j.apmr.2014.02.027.

Mamyama, T., Kitagawal, T., Takeshita, K., & Nakainura, K. (2002). Side shift exercise for idiopathic scoliosis after skeletal maturity. *Studies in health technology and informatics*, *91*, 361–364.

Muirhead, A., & Conner, A. N. (1985). The assessment of lung function in children with scoliosis. *The Journal of bone and joint surgery. British volume*, *67*(5), 699-702. https://doi.org/10.1302/0301-620X.67B5.4055863.

Negrini, S., Aulisa, A. G., Aulisa, L., Circo, A. B., de Mauroy, J. C., Durmala, J., Grivas, T. B., Knott, P., Kotwicki, T., Maruyama, T., Minozzi, S., O'Brien, J. P., Papadopoulos, D., Rigo, M., Rivard, C. H., Romano, M., Wynne, J. H., Villagrasa, M., Weiss, H. R., & Zaina, F. (2012). 2011 SOSORT guidelines: Orthopaedic and Rehabilitation treatment of idiopathic scoliosis during growth. *Scoliosis*, *7*(1), 3. https://doi.org/10.1186/1748-7161-7-3.

Negrini, S., Donzelli, S., Aulisa, A. G., Czaprowski, D., Schreiber, S., de Mauroy, J. C., Diers, H., Grivas, T. B., Knott, P., Kotwicki, T., Lebel, A., Marti, C., Maruyama, T., O'Brien, J., Price, N., Parent, E., Rigo, M., Romano, M., Stikeleather, L., Wynne, J., & Zaina, F. (2018). 2016 SOSORT guidelines: orthopaedic and rehabilitation treatment of idiopathic scoliosis during growth. *Scoliosis and spinal disorders*, *13*, 3. https://doi.org/10.1186/s13013-017-0145-8.

Negrini, S., Marchini, G., & Tessadri, F. (2011). Brace technology thematic series - The Sforzesco and Sibilla braces, and the SPoRT (Symmetric, Patient oriented, Rigid, Three-dimensional, active) concept. *Scoliosis*, *6*, 8. https://doi.org/10.1186/1748-7161-6-8.

Redding, G., Mayer, O. H., White, K., Bompadre, V., Emerson, J., Krengel, W., & Campbell, R. (2017). Maximal respiratory muscle strength and vital capacity in children with early onset scoliosis. *Spine*, *42*(23), 1799-1804. https://doi.org/10.1097/BRS.0000000000002351.

Reid L. (1970). Lung growth. *Proceedings of the 3rd Symposium of the Institute of Diseases of the Chest.* London, England.

Ridderbusch, K., Spiro, A. S., Kunkel, P., Grolle, B., Stücker, R., & Rupprecht, M. (2018). Strategien in der Behandlung der frühkindlichen Skoliose [Strategies in the treatment of early childhood scoliosis]. *Dtsch Ärztebl Int*, *115*, 371-376. https://doi.org/10.3238/arztebl.2018.0371.

Rigo, M., & Weiss, H. R. (2008). The Chêneau concept of bracing--biomechanical aspects. *Studies in health technology and informatics*, *135*, 303–319.

Romano, M., Negrini, A., Parzini, S., Tavernaro, M., Zaina, F., Donzelli, S., & Negrini, S. (2015). SEAS (Scientific Exercises Approach to Scoliosis): a modern and effective evidence based approach to physiotherapic specific scoliosis exercises. *Scoliosis*, *10*, 3. https://doi.org/10.1186/s13013-014-0027-2.

Ruiz, G., Torres-Lugo, N. J., Marrero-Ortiz, P., Guzmán, H., Olivella, G., & Ramírez, N. (2022). Early-onset scoliosis: a narrative review. *EFORT Open Reviews*, *7*(8), 599. https://doi.org/10.1530/EOR-22-0040.

Sauvagnac, R., & Rigo, M. (2022). Evolution of Early Onset Scoliosis under Treatment with a 3D-Brace Concept. *Journal of Clinical Medicine*, *11*(5), 1186. https://doi.org/10.3390/jcm11051186.

Scott, J. C., & Morgan, T. H. (1955). The natural history and prognosis of infantile idiopathic scoliosis. *The Journal of Bone and Joint Surgery. British volume*, *37*(3), 400-413. https://doi.org/10.1302/0301-620X.37B3.400.

Skaggs, D. L., Guillaume, T., El-Hawary, R., Emans, J., Mendelow, M., & Smith, J. (2015). Early onset scoliosis consensus statement, SRS Growing Spine Committee, 2015. *Spine Deform*, *3*(2), 107.

Tanchev, P. I., Dzherov, A. D., Parushev, A. D., Dikov, D. M., & Todorov, M. B. (2000). Scoliosis in rhythmic gymnasts. *Spine*, *25*(11), 1367-1372. https://doi.org/10.1097/00007632-200006010-00008.

Thometz, J., & Liu, X. C. (2019). Serial CAD/CAM bracing: an alternative to serial casting for early onset scoliosis. *Journal of Pediatric Orthopaedics*, *39*(3), e185-e189. https://doi.org/10.1097/BPO.0000000000001287.

Thometz, J., Liu, X., Rizza, R., English, I., & Tarima, S. (2018). Effect of an elongation bending derotation brace on the infantile or juvenile scoliosis. *Scoliosis and Spinal Disorders*, *13*(1), 1-6. https://doi.org/10.1186/s13013-018-0160-4.

Weinstein, S. L., Dolan, L. A., Wright, J. G., & Dobbs, M. B. (2013). Effects of bracing in adolescents with idiopathic scoliosis. *New England Journal of Medicine*, *369*(16), 1512-1521. https://doi.org/10.1056/NEJMoa1307337.

Weiss H. R. (2011). The method of Katharina Schroth - history, principles and current development. *Scoliosis*, *6*, 17. https://doi.org/10.1186/1748-7161-6-17.

Weiss, H. R., Lehnert-Schroth, C., Moramarco, M., & Moramarco, K. (2022). Schroth therapy advancements in conservative scoliosis treatment. In *Schroth Therapy Advancements in Conservative Scoliosis Treatment (3rd Edition)* (pp. 67-76)., India & United Kingdom: BP International. ISBN 978-93-5547-343-1 (eBook).

Weiss, H. R., Negrini, S., Rigo, M., Kotwicki, T., Hawes, M. C., Grivas, T. B., Maruyama, T., & Landauer, F.; SOSORT guideline committee. (2006). Indications for conservative management of scoliosis (guidelines). *Scoliosis*, *1*, 5. https://doi.org/10.1186/1748-7161-1-5.

Weiss, H. R., Tournavitis, N., Seibel, S., & Kleban, A. (2017). A Prospective Cohort Study of AIS Patients with 40° and More Treated with a Gensingen Brace (GBW): Preliminary Results. *The open orthopaedics journal*, *11*, 1558–1567. https://doi.org/10.2174/1874325001711011558.

# Chapter 17

# Surgical Treatment and Growth-Friendly Implants

**Bilge Kağan Yılmaz*, MD**
Department of Orthopaedics and Traumatology Afyonkarahisar State Hospital, Afyonkarahisar, Turkiye

## Abstract

Early-onset scoliosis (EOS) is defined as childhood spinal curvatures that differ significantly depending on the prognosis and etiology. It is used for the purpose of describing spinal curvatures that occur in the first 10 years of life due to congenital, neuromuscular, syndromic, and idiopathic causes. Its prognosis and natural course vary considerably depending on the etiology. In EOS, the growth rate and ratio of the spine display a rapid increase bimodally with age. Lung capacity and the development of bronchiolar and alveolar structures are formed by 85% by 8 years of age. During this period, the progression and early fusion of the spinal curvature restrict thoracic volume, leading to undesirable effects on pulmonary functions. The objective of treatment in EOS is to stop and correct the progression of the deformity, prevent the development of thoracic insufficiency, avoid early fusion, and increase the quality of life by reducing the adverse effects of treatment and surgical complications while increasing the growth of the spine and thorax.

The treatment methods recommended for EOS include serial castings and braces in the early period and non-fusion surgical applications as the child grows. Serial castings are frequently recommended before spinal instrumentation as a good treatment option for minor curvatures. Bracing can be applied in suitable patients,

---

* Corresponding Author's Email: yilmazbk@gmail.com.

In: Early Onset Scoliosis
Editor: Ahmed Majid Heydar
ISBN: 979-8-89113-600-7

especially after a plaster cast, with the objective of delaying surgical treatment. In treating large curvatures that cannot be controlled with serial casting and bracing, non-fusion surgical applications, named growth-friendly methods, have been developed. Systems with growth, orientation, and compression effects, particularly distraction-based systems, have begun to be widely utilized in the surgical treatment of rapidly progressing EOS. Nowadays, high rates of complication are also reported due to the use of growth-friendly surgical systems. Surgical techniques and implants used to treat scoliosis are still being developed with the advancement of technology.

**Keywords:** early-onset scoliosis, surgical treatment, growth-friendly implants

## Introduction

Early-onset scoliosis (EOS) is defined as childhood spinal curvatures with heterogeneous causes that differ significantly depending on the prognosis and etiology. It is used for the purpose of describing spinal curvatures that occur in the first 10 years of life due to congenital, neuromuscular, syndromic, and idiopathic causes. The natural course of severeprogressive EOS in the growing child is complex and difficult to manage. Moreover, these children may also have pathological syndromic conditions associated with cardiopulmonary and gastrointestinal diseases that increase pulmonary morbidity (Thompson et al., 2016).

In EOS, the growth rate and ratio of the spine display a rapid increase bimodally with age. The first 5 years and 10 years of life and the adolescence period, which lasts until skeletal maturation, are the periods when this increase is the highest (Dimeglio et al., 2006). Lung capacity and the development of bronchiolar and alveolar structures are formed by 85% until the age of 8 (Merkus et al., 1996). In this period, the progression and early fusion of the spinal curvature restrict thoracic volume, leading to undesirable effects on pulmonary functions. The objective of treatment in EOS is to stop and correct the progression of deformity, prevent the development of thoracic insufficiency, avoid early fusion, increase the quality of life by reducing the adverse effects of treatment and surgical complications, while increasing the growth of the spine and thorax (Lenke et al., 2004).

In the treatment of EOS, serial castings, braces, growth-friendly implant systems, and surgical applications have been frequently recommended in the last 2 decades. Serial castings are frequently recommended before spinal instrumentation as a good treatment option for minor curvatures. Bracing can be applied in suitable patients, especially after a plaster cast, with the objective of delaying surgical treatment. Non-fusion surgical applications, named growth-friendly methods, have been developed to treat large curvatures that cannot be controlled with serial casting and bracing. Nowadays, surgical techniques and implants used to treat scoliosis are still being developed with the advancement of technology.

## Main Body

EOS is used to express spinal curvatures occurring in the first 10 years of life due to congenital, neuromuscular, syndromic, and idiopathic causes. In EOS, the growth rate and ratio of the spine display a rapid increase bimodally with age. Since lung capacity and the development of alveolar structures are formed by 85% in the first 8 years, the progression and early fusion of the spinal curvature during this period may lead to undesirable effects on pulmonary functions by restricting the thoracic volume. The objective of treatment in EOS is to stop and correct the progression of deformity, prevent the development of thoracic insufficiency, avoid or limit early fusion, and increase the quality of life by reducing the adverse effects of treatment and surgical complications while increasing the growth of the spine and thorax. The treatment methods recommended for EOS include serial castings and braces in the early period and non-fusion surgical applications as the child grows. Non-fusion surgical applications, named growth-friendly methods, have been developed to treat large curvatures that cannot be controlled with serial casting and bracing.

The effects and side effects of "fusion" therapy, which is used to correct spinal curvatures, are well known nowadays. Fusion performed in the growing spine slows or stops the growth and longitudinal growth of the spinal canal, chest wall, and lungs. Hence, the main purpose of the surgical approach in EBS is to prevent the progression of scoliosis, allow the maximum growth and movement of the vertebral column, and not to hinder thoracopulmonary development (Lenke et al., 2004).

The surgical treatment of EOS is recommended for children with advanced curvatures (Cobb ≥45°) and children who have not reached maturity (Lenke et al., 2004). During the progression of the curvature, the patient's age and maturity determine the type of surgical procedure selected. Skaggs divides growth-friendly spinal implant systems into distraction-based, compression-based, and growth-guided systems according to the correction forces exerted by the implant on the spine (Skaggs et al., 2014) (Table 1).

**Table 1.** Growth-friendly implant systems

| Distraction-Based Systems | Compression-Based Systems | Growth Guided Systems |
|---|---|---|
| Traditional Growing Rod (TGR) | Staples | Luque Trolly |
| Magnetic Growing Rod (MCGR) | Tethers | Shilla |
| VEPTR | | |
| Hybrid Growing Rod | | |

## Distraction-Based Systems of EOS

Distraction-based systems are the most frequently used growth-friendly systems nowadays. The aim of distraction-based systems is to correct spinal deformity by applying mechanical distractive force to the deformed segments through implants. According to the Hueter-Volkmann law, it has been proven that distraction stimulates growth while compression suppresses growth (Mehlman et al., 1997). In the said system, distractive force stimulates the growth rate of the spine with abnormal growth in EOS, providing an advantage in correcting the curvature and contributing to spinal elongation. Furthermore, unlike compression-based systems, it has the advantage of restoring vascular channel volume and disc height in endplates due to compression and disc regeneration by decreasing peripheral pressure (Guehring et al., 2006). The current distraction-based implants are spine-based or rib-based growing rods, vertically expandable titanium rib prostheses (VEPTR), and remotely expandable devices.

Harrington described the non-fusion instrumentation technique for the first time in 1962 when he published the results of the non-fusion internal fixation method applied to 27 post-polio and idiopathic patients. Harrington placed laminar hooks at both ends of the curvature, placed an extendable single rod with subperiosteal dissection on the concave side of the curvature, and attempted to treat it with distraction (Harrington, 1962).

Moe further developed this technique and modified it using subcutaneously. He treated 20 patients with rapidly progressive scoliosis of different etiologies with Harrington threaded rods and hooks. He applied fusion by implementing subperiosteal dissection to the hook edges on a limited basis. He aimed to make the central part of the rod smooth, place it easily, and reduce the formation of scar tissue.

Lengthening treatment with TGR is among the frequently preferred methods in EOS. It requires lengthening at certain intervals to correct the curvature and maintain the position. Studies have demonstrated that skin problems, wound infections, implant-related complications, and anesthesia complications increase considerably with frequently repeated surgeries (Baky et al., 2018). The high number of complications in TGR limits its use, and some surgeons prefer delaying methods, whereas others have started to reduce surgical indications in patients with EOS (Fletcher et al., 2012). Novel methods have been developed accordingly. The MCGR system developed to this end was first reported for the correction of experimentally induced scoliosis in beagle dogs (Takaso et al., 1998). Another study found that MCGRs are safe and effective in achieving physiological spinal growth in a pig model (Akbarnia et al., 2012). The MCGR system has similar results to the TGR in curvature correction and growth success. Its advantage is that it allows lengthening that does not require surgery, which considerably decreases the number of operations planned and therefore reduces the complication rate (Akbarnia et al., 2014).

VEPTR is employed in EOS, particularly in cases of thoracic insufficiency syndrome. Non-fusion is a technique. The aim of treatment and application is to correct thoracic deformity and ensure lung development (Campbell et al., 2004). It is not really an extendable rod system. It corrects the decreased thorax volume in three dimensions.

## Compression-Based Systems of EOS

In compression-based systems, the spinal deformity is corrected by compressing the curvature on the convex side and stopping its growth. Thus, growth continues on the concave side, and scoliosis improves. The preservation of motion and disc vitality and the ability to correct spinal deformity with a single surgical procedure are the potential advantages of the system in question (Newton et al., 2008). Changes in the physis region of the disc and implant problems are its disadvantages (Hunt et al., 2010). Moreover, it is not the most ideal method for children because it can restrict growth.

Spine staples and tethers are examples of compression-based systems. The use of staples to treat scoliosis was first published in 1954 (Smith et al., 1954). Staples coming out of the place of their application is an early implant failure, which has been solved using nitinol staples (Nickel Titanium Naval Ordnance lab). Nitinol staples take the "C" shape and become more stable as their temperature increases with body temperature. Suitable patients recommended for this procedure are those who have at least one year left for growth to complete and who can also be considered for brace treatment. According to Betz et al., thoracic and lumbar curvatures must be less than 45° with minimal rotation. It must also be flexed less than 20°, and the sagittal thoracic curvature must be less than 40° (Betz et al., 2010).

Tethers prevent growth on the convex side of the curvature, similar to stapling. They were described for the first time by Crawford and Lenke in 2010. The system is fixed to the vertebrae with screws or anchors. Theoretically, it causes less damage to the intervertebral discs.

## Growth Guided Systems of EOS

Growth guided systems correct spinal deformities by attaching multiple vertebrae (usually including the apical vertebra) to rods through translation and other mechanical forces during the first implantation. Most anchors are not firmly attached to the rods, and thus slide over the rods over time, allowing for longitudinal growth. A significant advantage is that repetitive surgical lengthening is not required. Additionally, since the same growth takes place at both end points, it does not cause any change in the kyphosis of the patient. Thus, adjacent-segment kyphosis may occur in distraction-based systems. Complications such as wound infection and rod breakage and the risk of spontaneous fusion are shown to be disadvantages of growth guided systems (Mardjetko et al., 1992).

Luque published a series of 47 patients in 1982 using his own technique in which he combined Harrington rods and sublaminar wires (Luque, 1980). The above-mentioned technique was later modified by adding "L"-shaped rods and wires to the system and was named the "Luque trolley technique."

The principle of Shilla instrumentation, which was described by McCarthy in 2008, is to control scoliosis by directing growth in a single posterior procedure without repetitive surgery or bracing. The purpose of this treatment is to direct the treatment by preserving the large center as much as possible. Hence, fewer segments are included in the fusion.

## Conclusion

The treatment of EOS is still one of the most current and discussed topics in pediatric spinal surgery. Follow-up, serial casting, braces, and growth-friendly surgical treatment methods are applied to patients with EOS. Surgical treatments are preferred for patients for whom conservative treatment is inappropriate or who do not respond to these treatments. Nowadays, non-fusion surgical treatment methods using growth-friendly implants allow spinal, lung, and chest wall growth, in addition to providing improvement in the curvature and stopping the progression of the curvature. Nevertheless, in these methods, many operations are required prior to definitive surgery in patients. The primary purpose of applying growth-friendly treatment methods must be to reduce or eliminate the frequency of repetitive surgical interventions without compromising the growth and improvement achieved.

In conclusion, EOS is a difficult-to-treat and time-consuming deformity with fatal consequences because of severe cardio-pulmonary complications if left untreated. Therefore, the objective of treatment in EOS is to stop and correct the progression of deformity, prevent the development of thoracic insufficiency, avoid early fusion, and increase the quality of life by reducing the adverse effects of treatment and surgical complications while increasing the growth of the spine and thorax. Performing a thorough analysis of EOS, managing possible complications, and adhering to the literature will contribute significantly to the development of these children.

## References

Akbarnia, B. A., Mundis, G. M., Salari, P., Yaszay, B., & Pawelek, J. B. (2012). Innovation in growing rod technique: a study of safety and efficacy of a magnetically controlled growing rod in a porcine model. *Spine, 37*(13), 1109–1114. https://doi.org/10.1097/BRS.0b013e318240ff67.

Akbarnia, B. A., Pawelek, J. B., Cheung, K. M. C., Demirkiran, G., Elsebaie, H., Emans, J. B., Johnston, C. E., Mundis, G. M., Noordeen, H., Skaggs, D. L., Sponseller, P. D., Thompson, G. H., Yaszay, B., & Yazici, M. (2014). Traditional Growing Rods Versus Magnetically Controlled Growing Rods for the Surgical Treatment of Early-Onset Scoliosis: A Case-Matched 2-Year Study. *Spine Deformity, 2*(6), 493–497. https://doi.org/10.1016/j.jspd.2014.09.050.

Baky, F. J., Milbrandt, T. A., Flick, R., & Larson, A. N. (2018). Cumulative Anesthesia Exposure in Patients Treated for Early-Onset Scoliosis. *Spine Deformity, 6*(6), 781–786. https://doi.org/10.1016/j.jspd.2018.05.001.

Betz, R. R., Ranade, A., Samdani, A. F., Chafetz, R., D'Andrea, L. P., Gaughan, J. P., Asghar, J., Grewal, H., & Mulcahey, M. J. (2010). Vertebral body stapling: a fusionless treatment option for a growing child with moderate idiopathic scoliosis. *Spine, 35*(2), 169-176. https://doi.org/10.1097/BRS.0b013e3181c6dff5.

Campbell Jr, R. M., Smith, M. D., & Hell-Vocke, A. K. (2004). Expansion thoracoplasty: the surgical technique of opening-wedge thoracostomy: surgical technique. *JBJS, 86*(suppl_1), 51-64. https://doi.org/10.2106/00004623-200403001-00008.

Dimeglio, A. (2006). Growth in pediatric orthopaedics. In Morrissy, R. T., & Weinstein, S. L. (Eds.), *Lovell and Winter's Pediatric Orthopaedics* (6th ed.). Philadelphia: Lippincott Williams & Wilkins.

Fletcher, N. D., McClung, A., Rathjen, K. E., Denning, J. R., Browne, R., & Johnston, C. E. (2012). Serial casting as a delay tactic in the treatment of moderate-to-severe early-onset scoliosis. *Journal of Pediatric Orthopedics, 32*(7), 664–671. https://doi.org/10.1097/BPO.0b013e31824bdb55.

Guehring, T., Unglaub, F., Lorenz, H., Omlor, G., Wilke, H.-J., & Kroeber, M. W. (2006). Intradiscal pressure measurements in normal discs, compressed discs and compressed discs treated with axial posterior disc distraction: an experimental study on the rabbit lumbar spine model. *Eur Spine J, 15*, 597–604. https://doi.org/10.1007/s00586-005-0953-z.

Harrington, P. R. (1962). Treatment of scoliosis: Correction and internal fixation by spine instrumentation. *J Bone Joint Surg Am, 44*(A), 591–610. https://doi.org/10.2106/00004623-196244040-00001.

Hunt, K. J., Braun, J. T., & Christensen, B. A. (2010). The effect of two clinically relevant fusionless scoliosis implant strategies on the health of the intervertebral disc: Analysis in an immature goat model. *Spine, 35*(4), 371–377. https://doi.org/10.1097/BRS.0b013e3181b962a4.

Lenke, L. G., & Dobbs, M. B. (2004). Idiopathic scoliosis. In Frymoyer, J. W., & Wiesel, S. W. (Editors), *The Adult and Pediatric Spine* (3rd Ed., pp. 337-60). Philadelphia: Lippincott Williams & Wilkins.

Luque, E. (1980). Paralytic scoliosis in growing children. *Orthop Trans, 4*, 37.

Mardjetko, S. M., Hammerberg, K. W., & Lubicky, J. P. (1992). The Luque trolley revisited. Review of nine cases requiring revision. *Spine, 17*(582-9). https://doi.org/10.1097/00007632-199205000-00018.

Mehlman, C. T., & Araghi, A. (1997). Hyphenated history: the Hueter-Volkmann law. *Am J Orthop (Belle Mead NJ), 26*, 798-800.

Merkus, P. J., ten Have-Opbroek, A. A., & Quanjer, P. H. (1996). Human lung growth: a review. *Pediatr Pulmonol, 21*, 383–397. https://doi.org/10.1002/(SICI)1099-0496(199606)21:6<383::AID-PPUL6>3.0.CO;2-M.

Newton, P. O., Farnsworth, C. L., Faro, F. D., Mahar, A. T., Odell, T. R., Mohamad, F., Breisch, E., Fricka, K., Upasani, V. V., & Amiel, D. (2008). Spinal growth modulation with an anterolateral flexible tether in an immature bovine model: Disc health and motion preservation. *Spine, 33*(7), 724–733. https://doi.org/10.1097/BRS.0b013e31816950a0.

Skaggs, D. L., Akbarnia, B. A., Flynn, J. M., Myung, K. S., Sponseller, P. D., & Vitale, M. G. (2014). A classification of growth friendly spine implants. *Journal of Pediatric Orthopaedics, 34*(3), 260–274. https://doi.org/10.1097/BPO.0000000000000073.

Smith, A. D., von Lackum, H. L., & White, R. (1954). An operation for stapling vertebral bodies in congenital scoliosis. *J Bone Joint Surg Am., 36*, 342–348. https://doi.org/10.2106/00004623-195436020-00011.

Takaso, M., Moriya, H., Kitahara, H., Minami, S., Takahashi, K., Isobe, K., Yamagata, M., Otsuka, Y., Nakata, Y., & Inoue, M. (1998). New remote-controlled growing-rod spinal instrumentation possibly applicable for scoliosis in young children. *Journal of Orthopaedic Science: Official Journal of the Japanese Orthopaedic Association, 3*(6), 336–340. https://doi.org/10.1007/s007760050062.

Thompson, W., Thakar, C., Rolton, D. J., Wilson-MacDonald, J., & Nnadi, C. (2016). The use of magnetically-controlled growing rods to treat children with early-onset scoliosis: early radiological results in 19 children. *The Bone & Joint Journal, 98*(9), 1240-1247. https://doi.org/10.1302/0301-620x.98b9.37545.

# Chapter 18

# Distraction-Based Systems of Early Onset Scoliosis

## Ahmet Aksoy*, MD

Department of Orthopedics and Traumatology, Alaaddin Keykubat University, Faculty of Medicine, Alanya, Antalya, Turkiye

## Abstract

Treatment of early onset scoliosis (EOS) is a challenge for patients and orthopedic surgeons. The aim of treatment is to expand the respiratory capacity of the lung and to create a good lung cavity.

The main goal of surgical techniques used in the treatment is to correct the deformity without preventing growth. There are treatment algorithms based on distraction and compression. The distraction-based systems include traditional growing rods, magnetically growing rods, vertical expandable prosthesis titanium ribs (VEPTR), and hybrid distraction-based strategy.

If curve progression continues despite nonsurgical management, surgical curve control measures are instituted. The best surgical option is dictated by the overall clinical condition of the individual patient.

**Keywords:** early onset scoliosis, growing rods, Magnetic Controlled Growth Rods (MAGEC), Vertical Expandable Prosthetic Titanium Rib (VEPTR)

---

* Corresponding Author's Email: dr.aksoyahmet@gmail.com.

In: Early Onset Scoliosis
Editor: Ahmed Majid Heydar
ISBN: 979-8-89113-600-7

## Introduction

Early onset scoliosis (EOS), which appears before the age of 10, can occur due to many reasons. Some of these are congenital vertebral anomalies, neuromuscular diseases, scoliosis-related syndromes, or idiopathic causes. In early onset scoliosis patients, undesirable results such as death and permanent deformities may occur due to lung development and insufficient pulmonary volume, as well as cardiac compression and related circulatory defect. Therefore, the treatment of this disease is very important. The treatment of the disease is a very difficult process for the patient and requires experience for the scoliosis surgeon. EOS treatments are very challenging for spine surgeons (El-Hawary & Akbarnia, 2015).

The aim of EOS treatment is to maximize thoracic volume and pulmonary function and minimize spinal deformity. The main goal of treatments is to increase lung volume and improve lung function (Canavese & Dimeglio, 2013; Karol et al., 2008). There are 3 different methods that have been used for years for distraction-based systems in the treatment of EOS and these are; traditional growing rods, magnetically growing rods, vertical expandable prosthesis titanium ribs (VEPTR) (Thompson et al., 2007).

## Growing Rods

This technique was first described by MOE et al. In this surgical method, growing rods were placed on the concave side of the deformity curve and applied. Then lengthening was provided during implantation in order to correct the deformity (Moe et al., 1984). Growing rods or expandable spinal implants are known as the gold standard method used in surgical treatment in children who have not completed their growth (Akbarnia et al., 2005).

The well-known Birmingham approach is to use a double-rod structure in treatment. The procedure is made through four small incisions parallel to the midline, and the rods are then tunneled through the skin bridges. The rods are placed in a submuscular plane. This approach allows the largest part of the curve, including the apex, to remain undisturbed during implantation, and periosteal stripping of the spine is not required.

At regular intervals, every 6 months, the structure is lengthened. The upper rod is then distracted away from the lower construct to lengthen the spine. This process is continued until the maturity is completed. The programming timing should be done in accordance with the child's growth rate. Therefore, the average age for implantation is considered to be about 6. A final fusion procedure is usually recommended when maturity is complete. Growing rods are contraindicated if fixation to the spine will not be sufficient. It is also contraindicated if the patient cannot adapt to the extensions (Thompson et al., 2007).

## Magnetic Controlled Growth Rods

The rods can be extended thanks to the magnetic mechanism. Magnetic Controlled Growth Rods (MAGEC) are a popular technique used in the treatment of EOS and consist of a magnetically controlled system. The use of magnetically controlled systems can be done with a mechanical transmitter without the need for a surgical incision. This method of treatment allows remote controllable lengthening after the first surgical procedure. MAGEC has been used in Europe since 2009 and is a treatment method approved by the FDA. This treatment is indicated for patients with progressive scoliosis that does not respond to medical treatment. However, this method is contraindicated in children under 2 years of age and those with implant allergies. In this method, one or two rods can be used. Rods are available in different diameters and lengths, even with an offset structure. In addition to the advantages of this method, it also has disadvantages such as loss of distraction, rod breakage, economic problems, and metal allergy or increased metal ion concentration in serum due to the metal rods used (Takaso et al., 1998).

## Vertical Expansile Prosthetic Titanium Rib

VEPTR (vertical expanding prosthetic titanium rib) is a method used in the treatment of scoliosis. In addition, this method is a non-fusion technique that aims to correct the deformity while preserving its growth potential. The VEPTR technique is a method that aims to improve clinical and radiological results by correcting the deformity and widening the thorax by distracting the implant located on the concave side of the deformity. VEPTR allows distraction to increase volume for lung development. Distraction is required every 6 months, as in the growing rod treatment. The specific complication of this treatment is that the anchor may cause injury to the brachial plexus. This complication can occur acutely or during lengthening procedures. Nerve monitoring can be performed to monitor this complication. The use of this technique in the treatment of early onset scoliosis, especially in children with severe deformities, makes it easier to place the proximal rib cradle than fixation of the proximal spine, which provides a significant advantage. Rib cradles can also be placed around multiple ribs, thus better stabilizing small and fragile bones that have not completed maturation. Positioning the implant on the concave side of the scoliosis deformity allows better soft tissue coverage, providing ease of surgical coverage, as well as reducing complication rates (Hasler et al., 2010; Konieczny et al., 2017).

## Hybrid

The hybrid distraction-based technique incorporates the VEPTR concept of using ribs as anchor sites, but also uses traditional implants. Traditional hooks are placed proximally along the ribs. As in the traditional rod technique, the distal anchor site is incorporated by fusion. Some of the advantages of using the method are that it does not create fusion in the proximal spine and, as a result, it does not restrict the potential growth of the thorax, and it allows for a larger thorax volume. Additionally, the absence of fusion in the proximal spine allows minimal movement of the implant in the proximal region, reducing the stress on the distraction system. As a result, it is thought that complications such as rod breakage are reduced (Yang et al., 2016).

## Complications of Distraction-Based Implants

Regardless of the method used in the distraction-based treatment of a spine that has not completed its growth phase, all of them involve a high risk and complication rate. Complications such as deformation and erosion of the spinal structure, fractures of the rods used, and implant failure are common. Sagittal plane deformities, such as kyphosis, often appear as a result of implants used due to distraction. Rods placed under the skin can cause wound healing problems and infections due to the young age of the patient and the general weakness of malnourished EOS patients. The most common complications are infections. It has been shown that each lengthening surgery in EOS increases the risk of deep infection by 3.3 times. This is due to repetitive surgical incisions and lengthenings. If there is no response to infection treatment, all implants may need to be removed. Another complication is an implant fracture. This issue is well known in orthopedic surgery. Another complication is sagittal malalignment. It occurs due to excessive elongation of the spine structure and the shortness of the implants compared to the spine. At the end of the growth process, the final fusion procedure is performed. These patients sometimes require surgery. This may be due to pseudoarthroses. In addition to all these complications, there are also innovative developments. Recently, it has been reported that new techniques such as MAGEC are frequently used. These are the use of magnetic field-activated devices that eliminate surgical intervention. In addition, new techniques such as MAGEC, which do not require surgical interventions or lengthening, also minimize exposure to anesthesia. Therefore, anesthesia side effects are minimized. These developments also reduce complications (Akbarnia & Emans, 2010; Yang et al., 2016).

## Conclusion

Scoliosis treatment is a very important issue for orthopedic surgeons. The devices and surgical techniques used in the treatment are developing significantly. In the treatment of EOS, there are different methods, such as traditional growing rods, single or double growing rods, magnetically controlled growing rods, and VEPTR. Different devices and surgical techniques have advantages and disadvantages. The important thing is to use the appropriate surgical option and device for the appropriate patient (Block et al., 2022).

## References

Akbarnia, B. A., & Emans, J. B. (2010). Complications of growth-sparing surgery in early onset scoliosis. *Spine, 35*(25), 2193-2204. https://doi.org/10.1097/BRS.0b013e3181f070b5.

Akbarnia, B. A., Marks, D. S., Boachie-Adjei, O., Thompson, A. G., & Asher, M. A. (2005). Dual growing rod technique for the treatment of progressive early-onset scoliosis: a multicenter study. *Spine, 30*(17S), S46-S57. https://doi.org/10.1097/01.brs.0000175190.08134.73.

Block, A. M., Tamburini, L. M., Zeng, F., Mancini, M. R., Jackson, C. A., Antonacci, C. L., Karsmarski, O. P., Stelzer, J. W., Wellington, I. J., & Lee, M. C. (2022). Surgical Treatment of Pediatric Scoliosis: Historical Origins and Review of Current Techniques. *Bioengineering, 9*(10), 600. https://doi.org/10.3390/bioengineering9100600.

Canavese, F., & Dimeglio, A. (2013). Normal and abnormal spine and thoracic cage development. *World Journal of Orthopedics, 4*(4), 167. https://doi.org/10.5312/wjo.v4.i4.167.

El-Hawary, R., & Akbarnia, B. A. (2015). Early onset scoliosis-time for consensus. *Spine Deformity, 2*(3), 105-106. https://doi.org/10.1016/j.jspd.2015.01.003.

Hasler, C.-C., Mehrkens, A., & Hefti, F. (2010). Efficacy and safety of VEPTR instrumentation for progressive spine deformities in young children without rib fusions. *European Spine Journal, 19*, 400-408. https://doi.org/10.1007/s00586-009-1253-9.

Karol, L. A., Johnston, C., Mladenov, K., Schochet, P., Walters, P., & Browne, R. H. (2008). Pulmonary function following early thoracic fusion in non-neuromuscular scoliosis. *JBJS, 90*(6), 1272-1281. https://doi.org/10.2106/JBJS.G.00184.

Konieczny, M., Ehrlich, A., & Krauspe, R. (2017). Vertical expandable prosthetic titanium ribs (VEPTR) in early-onset scoliosis: impact on thoracic compliance and sagittal balance. *Journal of Children's Orthopaedics, 11*(1), 42-48. https://doi.org/10.1302/1863-2548-11-160222.

Moe, J. H., Kharrat, K., Winter, R. B., & Cummine, J. L. (1984). Harrington instrumentation without fusion plus external orthotic support for the treatment of difficult curvature problems in young children. *Clinical Orthopaedics and Related Research®, 185*, 35-45. https://doi.org/10.1097/00003086-198405000-00006.

Takaso, M., Moriya, H., Kitahara, H., Minami, S., Takahashi, K., Isobe, K., Yamagata, M., Otsuka, Y., Nakata, Y., & Inoue, M. (1998). New remote-controlled growing-rod spinal instrumentation possibly applicable for scoliosis in young children. *Journal of Orthopaedic Science, 3*(6), 336-340. https://doi.org/10.1007/s007760050062.

Thompson, G. H., Akbarnia, B. A., & Campbell Jr, R. M. (2007). Growing rod techniques in early-onset scoliosis. *Journal of Pediatric Orthopaedics, 27*(3), 354-361. https://doi.org/10.1097/BPO.0b013e3180333eea.

Yang, S., Andras, L. M., Redding, G. J., & Skaggs, D. L. (2016). Early-onset scoliosis: a review of history, current treatment, and future directions. *Pediatrics, 137*(1). https://doi.org/10.1542/peds.2015-0709.

## Chapter 19

# Traditional Growing Rods

**Bilal Yekeler[1,*], MD**
**and Umut Doğu Aktürk[2], MD**
[1]Department of Neurosurgery, Bayburt State Hospital, Bayburt, Turkiye
[2]Department of Neurosurgery, Emsey Hospital, Istanbul, Turkiye

## Abstract

The objective of treatment in early onset scoliosis (EOS) is to correct the deformity while allowing thoracic growth for optimal cardiopulmonary functions. Traditional growing rods (TGRs) treatment is a distraction-based and growing friendly method widely used in the treatment of early primary scoliosis with specific indications. It is essential for surgeons to understand and perform this technique since it is used for specific indications, and additionally, in some cases, its use has decreased due to the high complication rate developed due to repetitive operations and the newly emerging distraction-based methods.

**Keywords:** early onset scoliosis, traditional growing rods

## Introduction

Multiple etiological factors, including congenital vertebral anomalies, neuromuscular disease, and syndromic conditions, can lead to children with early onset scoliosis (EOS), a potentially life-threatening condition, or it can be idiopathic. Orthoses or serial castings are usually the first methods of

* Corresponding Author's Email: bilalyekeler@gmail.com.

In: Early Onset Scoliosis
Editor: Ahmed Majid Heydar
ISBN: 979-8-89113-600-7

treatment; however, when treatment failures occur or they are contraindicated, surgical operations need to be considered. Absolute posterior spinal fusion (PSF), using segmental spinal instrumentation techniques, can be effective in realigning the spine, but a short body and disproportionate body structure, if not combined with anterior procedures, can result in possible crankshaft deformity and negatively affect lung development in younger children, which can lead to respiratory failure (Dubousset et al., 1989).

The main basis of the treatment is to correct the deformity and delay any surgical operations as much as possible while allowing thoracic growth for optimal cardiopulmonary functions. Paul Harrington is known for his definition of the first fusion-free instrumentation for the growing spine (Harrington, 1962). Using the hooks as anchor points, he placed a single distraction rod on the concave side of the deformity by subperiosteal dissection. This technique was developed by using a method that reaches the anchorage areas and the submuscular passage of the distraction rod with limited dissection by Moe et al. (Moe et al., 1984). They made an adjustment if more than the degree of scoliosis develops greater than 10°. However, it has been indicated that the complication rates of both of these techniques are approaching 50% (Moe et al., 1984). Morin was the first to use segmental spinal instrumentation with a claw model proximally and/or distally (Morin C., 1991). Claw-modeled instrumentation consists of a supralaminar, or transverse process hook proximally, and a sublaminar hook inserted distally in 1 or 2 vertebral segments. Pedicle screws can also be used distally.

There are three techniques for distraction-based expandable segmental spinal instrumentation currently in use. These implants are a single growing rod with a claw model proximally and/or distally (Blakemore et al., 2001; Thompson et al., 2005), dual growing rods with claw models proximally and distally (Akbarnia et al., 2005), and vertical expandable prosthetic titanium rib (VEPTR) (Campbell, 2005; Campbell & Hell-Vocke, 2003).

In the last 30 years, distraction-based techniques have continued to advance with the development of a growing understanding of the spine. The use of this growing rod technique was developed because of the high rate of complications related to single rod instrumentation performed at an early stage of life. The single traditional growing rod (TGR) technique can be used in cases where the patients are younger, their skin is thin, or the rod may have a greater prominence in the convexity of the curve. However, Akbarnia emphasized that dual rod fixation should be preferred to the single rod as much as possible (Akbarnia et al., 2005). Dual TGR was popularized by Akbarnia et al. in 2005. They controlled the scoliosis curve by maintaining spine growth in patients with EOS of various etiologies (Akbarnia et al., 2005). However, it has been presented that the complication rate with this technique varies between 48% and 58% (Bess et al., 2010).

TGR has been used in EOS patients with different etiologies. Elsebai showed that TGR is also effective in the treatment of EOS patients with congenital deformities (Elsebai et al., 2011). It was observed that there was better deformity correction and fewer catastrophic implant-related complications with dual TGR when the use of single and dual TGR was compared (Xu et al., 2016). Furthermore, a higher rate of wound complications associated with its use has been reported due to the increased implant density and implant prominence in dual TGR (Xu et al., 2016).

TGR techniques were used until the development of magnetically controlled growing rods (MCGR) (Akbarnia et al., 2013; Hosseini et al., 2016). Direct comparisons between TGR and MCGR have shown similar results in terms of controlling the curve and ongoing chest and spine growth (Akbarnia et al., 2014; Erdoğan et al., 2019). The main differences between the two are the need for higher costs for MCGR implants and the need for more surgery operations for TGR. The initial cost situation related to MCGR is significantly more than TGR; however, it may become more cost-effective after 4-6 years by eliminating the need for re-operation for extension procedures such as TGR (Luhmann et al., 2018; Oetgen et al., 2019). Even with the use of MCGR, the chance of re-operation is high due to implant-related complications and extension failure of the implant (Choi et al., 2017; Thakar et al., 2018). Even in the common use of MCGR today, both single and dual TGR techniques continue to be operative options in EOS as a primary or revision surgical approach in various etiologies (neuromuscular, congenital, idiopathic, and syndromic).

Among the challenges related to the use of these systems, ensuring, and maintaining deformity correction, ensuring adequate spine growth, enabling lung development, and reducing the high incidence of complications are included. In this article, the traditional growing rods (TGRs) technique has been focused on, and its current use has been discussed.

## Indications

Surgical planning should be made when the major curve increases above 50°, when there is a hardening curve, and it is considered that the patient continues to grow (Figure 1) (Akbarnia et al., 2005, 2008). Despite an active non-operative treatment, such as bracing or casting, early and thoracic curvatures should be treated earlier to prevent pulmonary complications in patients with progressive deformities (Campbell et al., 2003). Because of the size and deformity of the patient, the use of a dual TGR should typically be preferred to use, except in cases where it is necessary to use a single TGR (Akbarnia et al., 2022). Dual TGR is used in patients with short stature, obesity, difficulty with the follow-up frequency of MCGR, severe kyphosis deformities, or who require periodic MRI (Akbarnia et al., 2022). For patients who have MCGR failure, changing to single or double TGR remains an operative revision option (Akbarnia et al., 2022).

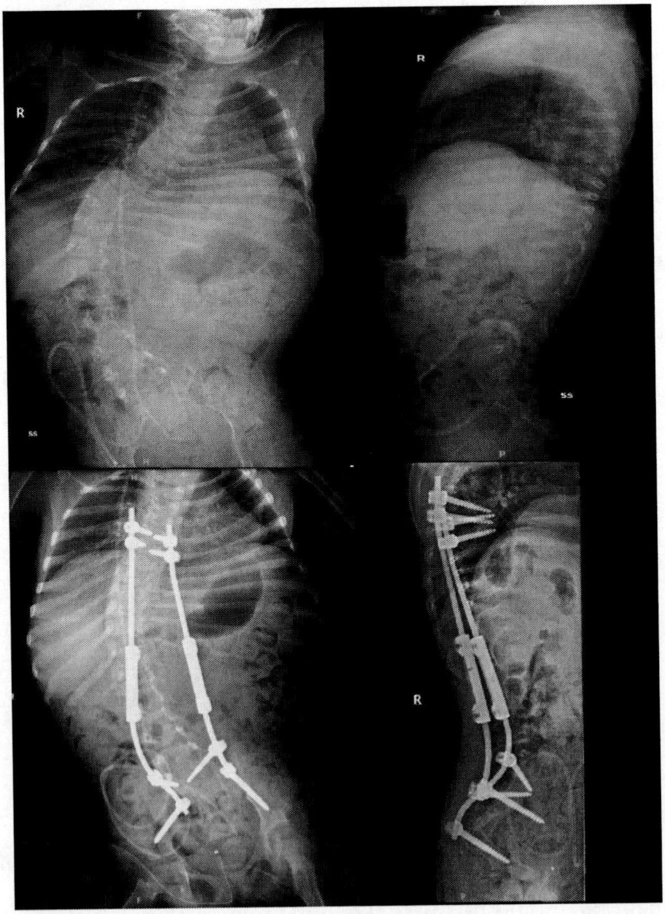

**Figure 1.** Pre-op and post-op images of the TGR operation of an EOS patient with an increase in the curve during follow-up.

## Surgical Technique

The surgical technique includes the preparation of main areas for anchors, rod shape changing, subcutaneous or subfascial rod insert, and the insert of tandem connectors. The skin incision can be one long midline or two separate midline incisions, depending on the length of the child's spine. The head and caudal ruptures made for the insert of the anchors are subperiosteal. The remaining part should be performed subcutaneously or subfascially to prevent adverse fusion.

The choice of anchorage areas depends on the place and type of curve, as well as the age and diagnosis of the child. For example, longer instrumentation is preferred for patients with neuromuscular disorders. The upper part is usually at T2-T4 levels. Hooks and/or screws can be used on both sides (Figure 2). Despite the fact that hooks are generally used depending on the availability of back elements and anatomical variations. In fact, pedicle screws seem to give additional stability to the structure (Mahar et al., 2008). The upper hooks are inserted on top of the transverse process or in a supralaminar region. The lower hooks are positioned upwards in claw style under the facets. If there is concern about the small size of the spinal canal or additional stability is required, hooks can be inserted on both levels. The caudal insertion point is usually two or three levels below the lower vertebra in scoliosis. The insert of local bone or bone graft extenders at the incision levels provides limited fusion and additional stability in the anchor regions.

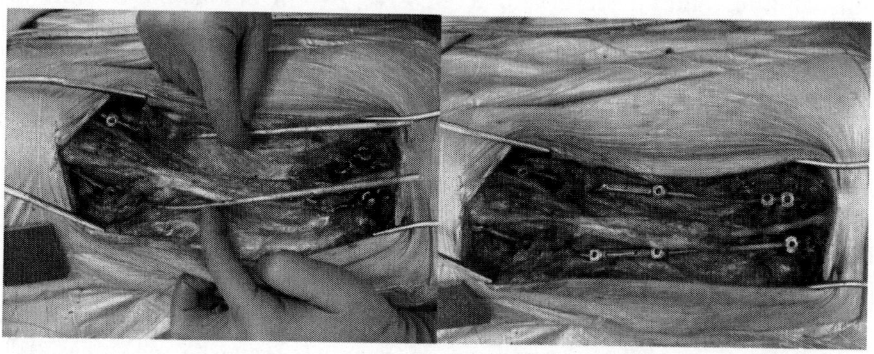

**Figure 2.** Intraoperative image of the patient with TGR and placement of rods.

## Complications

TGRs are growth friendly surgical techniques that require extensions with repeated operations and are associated with a high risk of complications (Akbarnia et al., 2008; Bess et al., 2010; Kabirian et al., 2014). Among these, it can include deep surgical site infections, rod fractures, and proximal fixation failure. Bess et al. indicated that 81 out of 140 children (58%) treated with growing rod instrumentation during at least 5 years of follow-up had at least one complication (Bess et al., 2010). It is revealed that while advanced age and subfascial instrumentation reduced this risk, each surgery increased the risk of complications by 24%. Postponing the growing rod surgery for 1 year has been shown to reduce the risk of complications by 12% (Bess et al., 2010).

### Skin-Related Complications

Multiple surgeries performed primarily through the same incision area for extension purposes can make scar tissues more susceptible to infection and other skin issues. Poor nutritional status can also increase complications, and this condition should be treated before the surgery. During closure, the skin should be under minimal stress. In very weak and small children, implant visibility may be inevitable; implants should not be inserted directly under the incisions. The skin should be carefully monitored for any signs of redness or skin rupture, and, if observed, aggressive treatment should be initiated immediately. It has been shown that inserting rods beneath the muscle reduces wound complications (Bess et al., 2010).

### Mechanical Complications

Rod fracture occurs in at least 15% of cases. Especially in cases of hyperkyphosis, it most often develops near junction points or in an area where the rod is significantly curved. If the diameter of the rod is small or if it is applied as a single rod, the probability of fracture is higher (Yang et al., 2011).

Dislocation of implants occurs at the upper end of the structure in 95% of the cases. It is more likely to develop in hyperkyphosis and can be prevented by enhanced solid fixation using the method of local bone grafts in two or three vertebrae. The screw technique seems to result in the safest proximal anchorage (Mahar et al., 2008), but if the screw fixation fails, neurological complications can result in serious consequences (K. F. Skaggs et al., 2013).

## Sagittal Balance Disorder

The stress applied to the two ends of the rods at the junction point of the rigid and flexible segments may cause adverse deviations in the spine, which increase with each extension session. The most common of these conditions is junctional kyphosis, which develops at the top of the structure. To date, there has been no study that has specifically assessed the impact of surgical intervention on sagittal spinal balance in EOS.

The use of dual TGR, as recommended by Akbarnia, helps reduce the rate of mechanical complications, but increases the number of revision procedures due to subcutaneous complications and increases the risk of spontaneous spinal fusion due to the rigidity of the structure (Akbarnia et al., 2005).

## Infection

Mackenzie reported an infection rate of 6.7% in his patients, and surgical revision was required in 69% of these cases (Mackenzie et al., 2013). It has been shown that the frequency of infection increases as more surgical procedures are performed (Watanabe et al., 2013). Rods should be inserted under the muscle layer to prevent subcutaneous rupture, which is the most common complication in patients with a small and insufficient subcutaneous layer.

## Neurological Complications

During the extension of the rod, no instances of neurological complications have been reported. Intraoperative monitoring has been recommended during the implantation or replacement of instruments or rods (Sankar et al., 2009). Although there is no specific recommendation for systematic monitoring during rod extension procedures, there is a consensus on the importance of performing caution and systematically monitoring high-risk patients with spinal MRI at the beginning of treatment.

## Psychological and Social Complications

Acaroglu reported that the total length of hospital stay between the first surgical procedure and the last fusion was 101 days, and an average of 4.6 sessions of extension sessions were performed on the patient (Acaroglu et al., 2002). This case provides evidence of the possible difficulties and psychological and social consequences of scoliosis care for patients and their families (Matsumoto et al., 2014).

## Absolute Fusion Surgery

This procedure has not yet been standardized and can be challenging due to the presence of fusion areas that develop away from the anchoring points, due to vertebral column hardening, and posterior osteotomy procedures. Several authors removed the growing rods without performing fusion and have observed hardening in the region bridging by the instrumentation and documented that these patients did not require an absolute fusion (Yazici & Olgun, 2013).

## Conclusion

The Dual TGR technique has been proven to be an effective primary distraction-based approach in the treatment of EOS. Additionally, if other growing friendly techniques fail, TGR can be used as a revision technique. Compared to MCGR, the results of curve correction and increased chest height are the same or better than TGR (Akbarnia et al., 2014; Erdoğan et al., 2019).

One of the main advantages of children with EOS who had MCGR is the reduction in physical and psychological stress caused by a limited number of surgical procedures with MCGR compared to TGR. However, several authors have demonstrated that a reduction in surgical burden with MCGR does not necessarily lead to a decrease in patient-reported outcome scores or psychological distress (Aslan et al., 2019; Bauer et al., 2019).

As a result, TGRS is a standard evidence-based surgical technique used in EOS. TGRs allow for reasonable correction of scoliosis and maintenance of adequate spinal growth but require repeated surgeries due to a relatively high risk of complications and repeated surgical prolongations, and the family should fully understand the long-term consequences of treatment before starting treatment. TGR management can cause hardening and autofusion of the spine, and therefore not all patients need a final fusion.

## References

Acaroglu, E., Yazici, M., Alanay, A., & Surat, A. (2002). Three-dimensional evolution of scoliotic curve during instrumentation without fusion in young children. *Journal of Pediatric Orthopedics*, *22*(4), 492–496.

Akbarnia, B. A., Breakwell, L. M., Marks, D. S., McCarthy, R. E., Thompson, A. G., Canale, S. K., Kostial, P. N., Tambe, A., Asher, M. A., & Growing Spine Study Group. (2008). Dual growing rod technique followed for three to eleven years until final fusion: The effect of frequency of lengthening. *Spine*, *33*(9), 984–990. https://doi.org/10.1097/BRS.0b013e31816c8b4e.

Akbarnia, B. A., Cheung, K., Noordeen, H., Elsebaie, H., Yazici, M., Dannawi, Z., & Kabirian, N. (2013). Next Generation of Growth-Sparing Techniques: Preliminary Clinical Results of a Magnetically Controlled Growing Rod in 14 Patients With Early-Onset Scoliosis. *Spine*, *38*(8), 665–670. https://doi.org/10.1097/BRS.0b013e3182773560.

Akbarnia, B. A., Marks, D. S., Boachie-Adjei, O., Thompson, A. G., & Asher, M. A. (2005). Dual Growing Rod Technique for the Treatment of Progressive Early-Onset Scoliosis: A Multicenter Study. *Spine*, *30*(Supplement), S46–S57. https://doi.org/10.1097/01.brs.0000175190.08134.73.

Akbarnia, B. A., Pawelek, J. B., Cheung, K. M. C., Demirkiran, G., Elsebaie, H., Emans, J. B., Johnston, C. E., Mundis, G. M., Noordeen, H., Skaggs, D. L., Sponseller, P. D., Thompson, G. H., Yaszay, B., Yazici, M., & Growing Spine Study Group. (2014). Traditional Growing Rods Versus Magnetically Controlled Growing Rods for the Surgical Treatment of Early-Onset Scoliosis: A Case-Matched 2-Year Study. *Spine Deformity*, *2*(6), 493–497. https://doi.org/10.1016/j.jspd.2014.09.050.

Akbarnia, B. A., Thompson, G. H., Yazici, M., & El-Hawary, R. (Eds.). (2022). *The Growing Spine: Management of Spinal Disorders in Young Children*. Springer International Publishing. https://doi.org/10.1007/978-3-030-84393-9.

Aslan, C., Olgun, Z. D., Ayik, G., Karaokur, R., Ozusta, S., Demirkiran, G. H., Unal, F., & Yazici, M. (2019). Does Decreased Surgical Stress Really Improve the Psychosocial Health of Early-onset Scoliosis Patients?: A Comparison of Traditional Growing Rods and Magnetically-controlled Growing Rods Patients Reveals Disappointing Results. *Spine*, *44*(11), E656–E663. https://doi.org/10.1097/BRS.0000000000002938.

Bauer, J. M., Yorgova, P., Neiss, G., Rogers, K., Sturm, P. F., Sponseller, P. D., Luhmann, S., Pawelek, J. B., & Shah, S. A. (2019). Early Onset Scoliosis: Is there an Improvement in Quality of Life With Conversion From Traditional Growing Rods to Magnetically Controlled Growing Rods? *Journal of Pediatric Orthopaedics*, *39*(4), e284–e288. https://doi.org/10.1097/BPO.0000000000001299.

Bess, S., Akbarnia, B. A., Thompson, G. H., Sponseller, P. D., Shah, S. A., El Sebaie, H., Boachie-Adjei, O., Karlin, L. I., Canale, S., Poe-Kochert, C., & Skaggs, D. L. (2010). Complications of Growing-Rod Treatment for Early-Onset Scoliosis: Analysis of One Hundred and Forty Patients. *The Journal of Bone and Joint Surgery-American Volume*, *92*(15), 2533–2543. https://doi.org/10.2106/JBJS.I.01471.

Blakemore, L. C., Scoles, P. V., Poe-Kochert, C., & Thompson, G. H. (2001). Submuscular Isola rod with or without limited apical fusion in the management of severe spinal deformities in young children: Preliminary report. *Spine*, *26*(18), 2044–2048. https://doi.org/10.1097/00007632-200109150-00021.

Cahill, P. J., Marvil, S., Cuddihy, L., Schutt, C., Idema, J., Clements, D. H., Antonacci, M. D., Asghar, J., Samdani, A. F., & Betz, R. R. (2010). Autofusion in the immature spine treated with growing rods. *Spine*, *35*(22), E1199-1203. https://doi.org/10.1097/BRS.0b013e3181e21b50.

Campbell, R. M. (2005). Operative Strategies for Thoracic Insufficiency Syndrome by Vertical Expandable Prosthetic Titanium Rib Expansion Thoracoplasty. *Operative Techniques in Orthopaedics*, *15*(4), 315–325. https://doi.org/10.1053/j.oto.2005.08.008.

Campbell, R. M., & Hell-Vocke, A. K. (2003). Growth of the thoracic spine in congenital scoliosis after expansion thoracoplasty. *The Journal of Bone and Joint Surgery. American Volume*, *85*(3), 409–420. https://doi.org/10.2106/00004623-200303000-00002.

Campbell, R. M., Smith, M. D., Mayes, T. C., Mangos, J. A., Willey-Courand, D. B., Kose, N., Pinero, R. F., Alder, M. E., Duong, H. L., & Surber, J. L. (2003). The characteristics of thoracic insufficiency syndrome associated with fused ribs and congenital scoliosis. *The Journal of Bone and Joint Surgery. American Volume*, *85*(3), 399–408. https://doi.org/10.2106/00004623-200303000-00001.

Choi, E., Yaszay, B., Mundis, G., Hosseini, P., Pawelek, J., Alanay, A., Berk, H., Cheung, K., Demirkiran, G., Ferguson, J., Greggi, T., Helenius, I., La Rosa, G., Senkoylu, A., & Akbarnia, B. A. (2017). Implant Complications After Magnetically Controlled Growing Rods for Early Onset Scoliosis: A Multicenter Retrospective Review. *Journal of Pediatric Orthopedics*, *37*(8), e588–e592. https://doi.org/10.1097/BPO.0000000000000803.

Dubousset, J., Herring, J. A., & Shufflebarger, H. (1989). The crankshaft phenomenon. *Journal of Pediatric Orthopedics*, *9*(5), 541–550. https://doi.org/10.1097/01241398-198909010-00008.

Elsebai, H. B., Yazici, M., Thompson, G. H., Emans, J. B., Skaggs, D. L., Crawford, A. H., Karlin, L. I., McCarthy, R. E., Poe-Kochert, C., Kostial, P., & Akbarnia, B. A. (2011). Safety and efficacy of growing rod technique for pediatric congenital spinal deformities. *Journal of Pediatric Orthopedics*, *31*(1), 1–5. https://doi.org/10.1097/BPO.0b013e318202c1f0.

Erdoğan, S., Polat, B., Atıcı, Y., Özyalvaç, O. N., & Öztürk, Ç. (2019). Comparison of the Effects of Magnetically Controlled Growing Rod and Tradiotinal Growing Rod Techniques on the Sagittal Plane in the Treatment of Early-Onset Scoliosis. *Journal of Korean Neurosurgical Society*, *62*(5), 577–585. https://doi.org/10.3340/jkns.2019.0094.

Harrington, P. R. (1962). Treatment of scoliosis. Correction and internal fixation by spine instrumentation. *The Journal of Bone and Joint Surgery. American Volume*, *44-A*, 591–610.

Hosseini, P., Pawelek, J., Mundis, G. M., Yaszay, B., Ferguson, J., Helenius, I., Cheung, K. M., Demirkiran, G., Alanay, A., Senkoylu, A., Elsebaie, H., & Akbarnia, B. A. (2016). Magnetically controlled Growing Rods for Early-onset Scoliosis: A Multicenter Study of 23 Cases With Minimum 2 years Follow-up. *Spine*, *41*(18), 1456–1462. https://doi.org/10.1097/BRS.0000000000001561.

Kabirian, N., Akbarnia, B. A., Pawelek, J. B., Alam, M., Mundis, G. M., Acacio, R., Thompson, G. H., Marks, D. S., Gardner, A., Sponseller, P. D., Skaggs, D. L., & Growing Spine Study Group. (2014). Deep Surgical Site Infection Following 2344 Growing-Rod Procedures for Early-Onset Scoliosis: Risk Factors and Clinical Consequences. *The Journal of Bone and Joint Surgery. American Volume*, *96*(15), e128. https://doi.org/10.2106/JBJS.M.00618.

Luhmann, S. J., McAughey, E. M., Ackerman, S. J., Bumpass, D. B., & McCarthy, R. E. (2018). Cost analysis of a growth guidance system compared with traditional and magnetically controlled growing rods for early-onset scoliosis: A US-based integrated health care delivery system perspective. *ClinicoEconomics and Outcomes Research: CEOR*, *10*, 179–187. https://doi.org/10.2147/CEOR.S152892.

Luque, E. R. (1982). Paralytic scoliosis in growing children. *Clinical Orthopaedics and Related Research*, *163*, 202–209.

Mackenzie, W. G. S., Matsumoto, H., Williams, B. A., Corona, J., Lee, C., Cody, S. R., Covington, L., Saiman, L., Flynn, J. M., Skaggs, D. L., Roye, D. P., & Vitale, M. G. (2013). Surgical site infection following spinal instrumentation for scoliosis: A multicenter analysis of rates, risk factors, and pathogens. *The Journal of Bone and Joint Surgery. American Volume*, *95*(9), 800–806, S1-2. https://doi.org/10.2106/JBJS.L.00010.

Mahar, A. T., Bagheri, R., Oka, R., Kostial, P., & Akbarnia, B. A. (2008). Biomechanical comparison of different anchors (foundations) for the pediatric dual growing rod technique. *The Spine Journal: Official Journal of the North American Spine Society*, *8*(6), 933–939. https://doi.org/10.1016/j.spinee.2007.10.031.

Matsumoto, H., Williams, B. A., Corona, J., Comer, J. S., Fisher, P. W., Neria, Y., Roye, B. D., Roye, D. P., & Vitale, M. G. (2014). Psychosocial effects of repetitive surgeries in children with early-onset scoliosis: Are we putting them at risk? *Journal of Pediatric Orthopedics*, *34*(2), 172–178. https://doi.org/10.1097/BPO.0b013e3182a11d73.

Moe, J. H., Kharrat, K., Winter, R. B., & Cummine, J. L. (1984). Harrington instrumentation without fusion plus external orthotic support for the treatment of difficult curvature problems in young children. *Clinical Orthopaedics and Related Research*, *185*, 35–45.

Morin C. (1991). Pediatric Cotrel-Dubousset instrumentation system. In *Bridwell KH, Dewald RL, eds. The Textbook of Spinal Deformity.* (pp. 212–217). JB Lippincott.

Oetgen, M. E., McNulty, E. M., & Matthews, A. L. (2019). Cost-Effectiveness of Magnetically Controlled Growing Rods: Who Really Benefits? *Spine Deformity*, *7*(3), 501–504. https://doi.org/10.1016/j.jspd.2018.09.066.

Patterson, J. F., Webb, J. K., & Burwell, R. G. (1990). The operative treatment of progressive early onset scoliosis. A preliminary report. *Spine*, *15*(8), 809–815.

Sankar, W. N., Skaggs, D. L., Emans, J. B., Marks, D. S., Dormans, J. P., Thompson, G. H., Shah, S. A., Sponseller, P. D., & Akbarnia, B. A. (2009). Neurologic risk in growing rod spine surgery in early onset scoliosis: Is neuromonitoring necessary for all cases? *Spine*, *34*(18), 1952–1955. https://doi.org/10.1097/BRS.0b013e3181afe869.

Skaggs, K. F., Brasher, A. E., Johnston, C. E., Purvis, J. M., Smith, J. T., Myung, K. S., & Skaggs, D. L. (2013). Upper thoracic pedicle screw loss of fixation causing spinal cord injury: A review of the literature and multicenter case series. *Journal of Pediatric Orthopedics*, *33*(1), 75–79. https://doi.org/10.1097/BPO.0b013e318279c31a.

Thakar, C., Kieser, D. C., Mardare, M., Haleem, S., Fairbank, J., & Nnadi, C. (2018). Systematic review of the complications associated with magnetically controlled growing rods for the treatment of early onset scoliosis. *European Spine Journal: Official Publication of the European Spine Society, the European Spinal Deformity Society, and the European Section of the Cervical Spine Research Society*, *27*(9), 2062–2071. https://doi.org/10.1007/s00586-018-5590-4.

Thompson, G. H., Akbarnia, B. A., Kostial, P., Poe-Kochert, C., Armstrong, D. G., Roh, J., Lowe, R., Asher, M. A., & Marks, D. S. (2005). Comparison of single and dual growing rod techniques followed through definitive surgery: A preliminary study. *Spine*, *30*(18), 2039–2044. https://doi.org/10.1097/01.brs.0000179082.92712.89.

Watanabe, K., Uno, K., Suzuki, T., Kawakami, N., Tsuji, T., Yanagida, H., Ito, M., Hirano, T., Yamazaki, K., Minami, S., Kotani, T., Taneichi, H., Imagama, S., Takeshita, K., Yamamoto, T., & Matsumoto, M. (2013). Risk factors for complications associated with growing-rod surgery for early-onset scoliosis. *Spine*, *38*(8), E464-468. https://doi.org/10.1097/BRS.0b013e318288671a.

Xu, G.-J., Fu, X., Tian, P., Ma, J., & Ma, X. (2016). Comparison of single and dual growing rods in the treatment of early onset scoliosis: A meta-analysis. *Journal of Orthopaedic Surgery and Research*, *11*(1), 80. https://doi.org/10.1186/s13018-016-0413-y.

Yang, J. S., Sponseller, P. D., Thompson, G. H., Akbarnia, B. A., Emans, J. B., Yazici, M., Skaggs, D. L., Shah, S. A., Salari, P., Poe-Kochert, C., & Growing Spine Study Group. (2011). Growing rod fractures: Risk factors and opportunities for prevention. *Spine*, *36*(20), 1639–1644. https://doi.org/10.1097/BRS.0b013e31822a982f.

Yazici, M., & Olgun, Z. D. (2013). Growing rod concepts: State of the art. *European Spine Journal*, *22*(Suppl 2), 118–130. https://doi.org/10.1007/s00586-012-2327-7.

# Chapter 20

# Magnetic Growing Rod

**Uğur Yüzügüldü*, MD**
Department of Orthopaedics and Traumatology, Gülhane Education and Research Hospital, Ankara, Turkiye

## Abstract

The high number of complications in traditional growing rods (TGR) limits the use and restricts surgical choices. Magnetically lengthening rod technology with remote-controlled extension has opened a new era in the treatment of patients with early-onset scoliosis (EOS). The technique has similar results to TGR in curve correction and growth success; however, its main advantage over TGR is that it allows lengthening that does not require surgery. The system consists of implantable magnetic rods, a magnet positioner, a manual distractor, and an external remote control. Lengthening is usually done at 3-month intervals. Post-treatment graduation; generally involves removing the growing rod system, correcting residual deformity, and re-instrumentation with arthrodesis, with possible multiple osteotomies.

**Keywords:** scoliosis, early onset, non-invasive lengthening, magnetically controlled growing rods (MCGR)

## Introduction

Multiple lengthening surgeries needed in TGR expose patients to many complications (Bess et al., 2010). These repetitive surgeries cause an increased

---

* Corresponding Author's Email: uguryuzuguldu@gmail.com.

In: Early Onset Scoliosis
Editor: Ahmed Majid Heydar
ISBN: 979-8-89113-600-7

risk of wound infection, skin problems, implant-related complications, and anesthesia complications (Baky et al., 2018; Sankar et al., 2010). In addition, repeated surgeries can profoundly affect children psychologically (Smith & Campbell, 2012), delay children's recovery time, and significantly impact family finances (Teoh et al., 2016b). The high number of complications in conventional growing rods limits their use. While some surgeons prefer delayed methods, others have begun to reduce surgical indications in patients with early-onset scoliosis (Fletcher et al., 2012). As a result of all these developments, the progress of alternative methods that reduce complications and achieve better results has accelerated. The idea of non-invasive multiple lengthening without surgical intervention and complications has become increasingly attractive. Magnetically extendable rod technology with remote-controlled extension has opened a new era in the treatment of these patients.

The use of spinal rods implanted with a remote magnetic distraction system was first reported in 1998 to correct scoliosis in beagles with experimentally induced scoliosis (Takaso et al., 1998). In further studies, magnetically controlled growing rods (MCGR) have been found to be safe and effective for maintaining physiological spine growth in pigs (Akbarnia et al., 2012). The MCGR technique has been available since 2009 in Asia and Europe compared to the USA. In the USA, it was approved and used by the Food and Drug Administration (FDA) in February 2014 (Tsirikos & Roberts, 2020). Cheung et al. first reported the efficacy of MCGRs in 2 patients at a 2-year follow-up without implant-related complications (K. M. C. Cheung et al., 2012). Wick and Konze reported that an MCGR system was implanted in 2 patients simultaneously, and they want to use it in a larger patient population (Wick & Konze, 2012).

The technique has similar results to TGR in growth and curve correction success, with the advantage of allowing non-surgical lengthening, which reduces the number of operations and thus the complication rate (Akbarnia et al., 2014). The MAGEC system (MAGnetic Expansion Control; Nuvasive, SanDiego, USA) is currently the only MCGR system used for the treatment of EOS in the USA and Europe. It consists of an implantable MAGEC wand, MAGEC magnet locator (MML), MAGEC manual distractor (MMD), and external remote controller (ERC) (Figure 1).

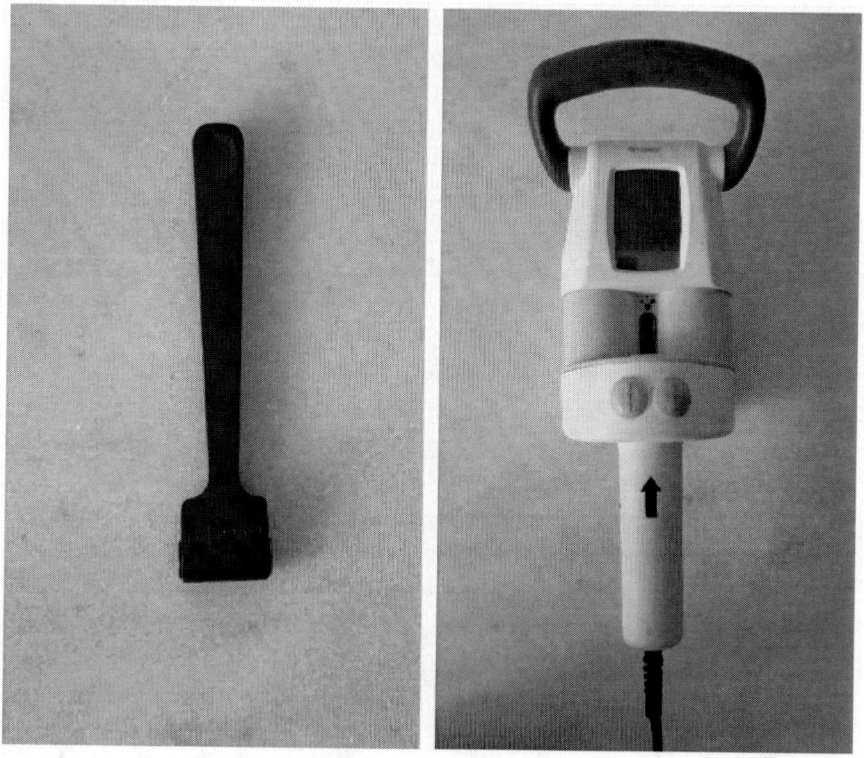

**Figure 1.** MAGEC magnet positioner (MML) view on the left, remote control controller (ERC) view on the right.

## Main Body

### Indications and Contraindications

The indications of MCGR are similar to those of TGR and are indicated for young children at risk for progressive EOS of any etiology; however, the currently accepted contraindications are as follows (Akbarnia & Mundis, 2019):

- Patients with infection or pathological conditions in the bone
- Patients with implant allergy
- Patients not complying with postoperative follow-ups

Magnetic resonance imaging (MRI) compatible pacemakers have been reported to be safe with MCGR by prophylactically returning the pacemaker to vital function prior to magnetic lengthening procedures (Tan et al., 2017). Vivas et al. (Vivas et al. 2017) also showed in their case reports that diaphragmatic pacemakers are compatible with MCGRs.

In the early years, MCGRs were not used in patients requiring MRI during treatment; however, Budd et al. their study reported that MRI had no detrimental effect on MCGR and that head and neck imaging could still be interpreted (Budd et al., 2016). However, due to artifacts, thoracic and lumbar spine MRIs have low clinical utility (Woon et al., 2018). Poon et al. in their study, they stated that MRI, which uses lower magnet power, does not displace the magnetic rods and does not change their length, does not cause significant heating, does not have a negative effect on the extension mechanism, does not damage the surrounding tissue, but causes scattering and artifacts in the imaging of nearby tissues (Poon et al., 2017). Single or double MAGEC rods can be used. It is recommended that the placement of the MCGR actuator is between T10 and L2 during surgery because this region is anatomically flat and is a suitable location (Akbarnia & Mundis, 2019). Screws and hooks can be used depending on the comfort in the proximal region and the difficulty during surgery. The use of screws may have a more substantial biomechanical effect on the operation of the system. Available implant options include 4.5 mm and 5 mm rod diameters, and 70 mm and 90 mm rod lengths. The rods are placed between the upper and lower screws and fixed to the screws (Munigangaiah et al., 2018). Initial lengthening should be performed at the proximal and distal basal levels before final tightening and bone grafting. Follow-up extensions are performed non-invasively via an external remote control. Elongation can be evaluated radiographically or with ultrasound imaging (Yoon et al., 2015), but intermittent radiographs are still recommended to monitor metalware failure (Stokes et al., 2014).

## Rod Extension Procedures

Rod lengthening can be applied more frequently in MCGR than in TGR. MCGR distractions are non-invasive and can be performed while the patient is fully awake. The ideal range for distraction has yet to be discovered. Extensions are usually made at 3-month intervals. During extension, the MML first detects the position of the actuator. (Figure 2) Correct positioning is essential to keep the actuator in motion. Distraction is usually done with the patient in the prone position. Putting a pillow under the navel can help make the distraction appropriate, as it will reduce friction and pressure during extension. A high patient's body mass index can also affect the grip and load created by the actuator for extension. Once the location has been properly found and marked, an ERC performs the actual extension (Figure 3).

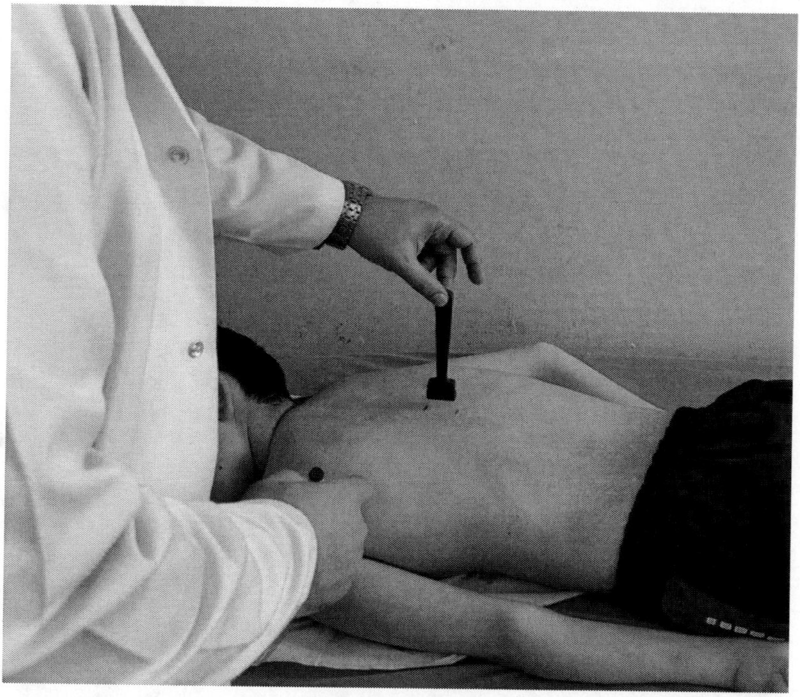

**Figure 2.** Positioning of the activator with MML before the extension.

It has been suggested that more frequent lengthening may reduce the risk of rod breakage by creating less pressure on the rods (Agarwal et al., 2014). Conversely, it was not supported in cases treated with TGR (Hosseini et al., 2017). Cheung et al. (Cheung et al., 2015) stated that lengthening at shorter intervals (from 1 week to 8 weeks) was associated with fewer implant complications, despite the increasing incidence of PJK. Lorenz et al. reviewed a total of 746 lengthening procedures in 40 patients with MCGR. They found a high ratio (0.94) between the length achieved and the expected length. Additionally, the lengthening complication rate was low (4.6%), and complications were correlated with patients with a high BMI. They concluded that the correlation between the resulting implant elongation and the elongation of the spinal column indicates the efficacy of MCGR treatment (Lorenz et al., 2019).

Currently, the preferred imaging modality is the use of ultrasound before and after lengthening. Unless there is a special reason for plain X-rays, they are taken once or twice a year (Figure 4). In a study to validate the application of ultrasound in the evaluation of rod lengthening, Cheung et al. confirmed that ultrasound is a reliable alternative to plain radiographs. Thus, they confirmed that it avoids radiation exposure and potentially harmful effects on the growing child (Cheung et al., 2016).

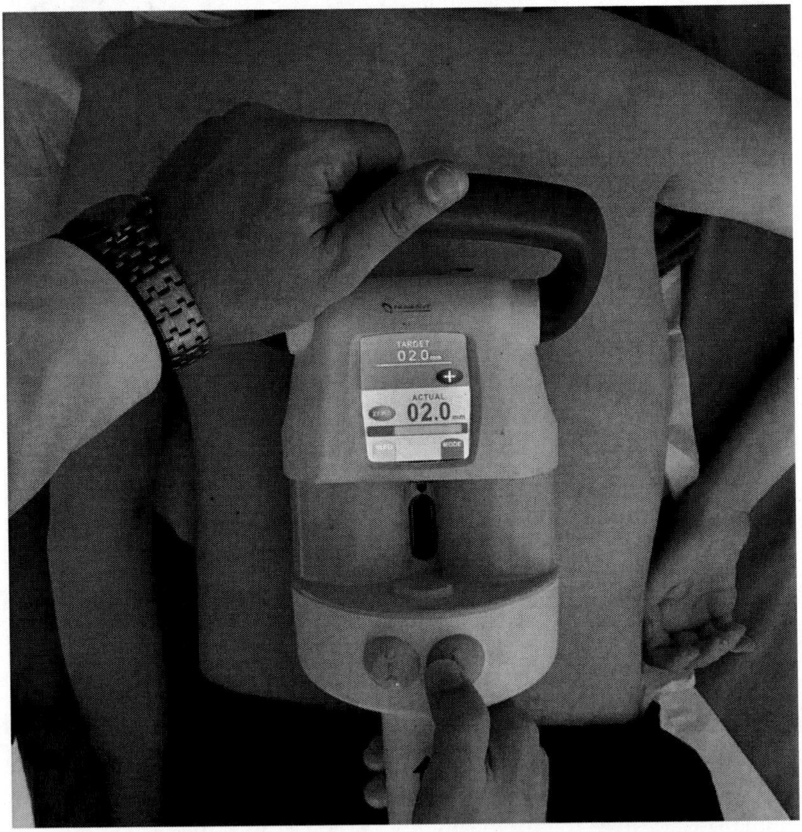


**Figure 3.** Lengthening with ERC after its position is found with the activator.

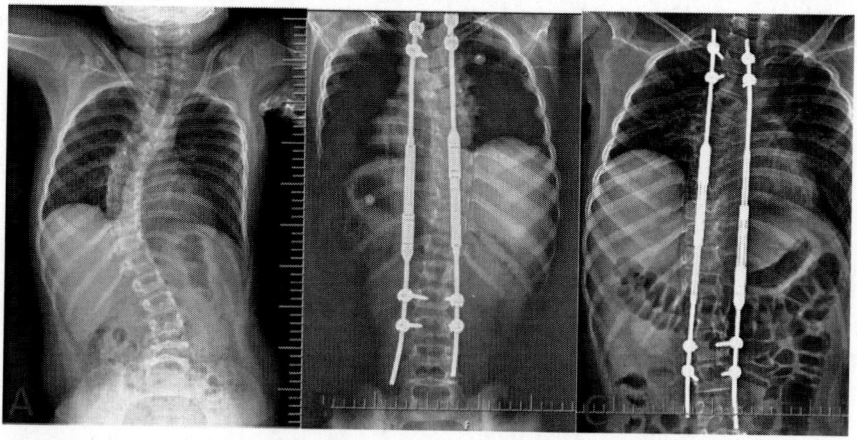

**Figure 4.** A; Pre-op radiograph of an 8-year-old male patient, B; patient's first post-op radiograph, C; X-ray of the patient in the 5th year after extensions.

## Graduation

The endpoint of treatment for children with EOS is controversial. Most authors consider a patient with ongoing treatment who is skeletally mature or has undergone a final spinal fusion to be graduated. Although the authors recommend removal of the implant for final fusion or just observation during graduation, it is traditionally recommended to remove the growing rods, correct residual deformity with osteotomies, and perform arthrodesis with re-instrumentation.

## MCGR Complications

Growing rod surgery is associated with a high rate of complications, from wound infections to implant-related alignment problems (Choi et al., 2017; Watanabe et al., 2013; Yang et al., 2011). Bess et al. have shown that these complications of TGR are directly related to the number of surgical interventions and the age of the patients. According to their study, the risk of complications increases by 24% as the number of surgical interventions increases and decreases by 13% each year as the patient's age at the beginning of treatment increases (Bess et al., 2010).

Implant-related complications include rod breakage, screw withdrawal or loosening, and removal or loosening of the hook (Akbarnia et al., 2005). Proximal junction kyphosis (PJK) and proximal junction failure (PJF) can be examples of complications related to misalignment.

The difficulty in dealing with the complications of EOS therapy is the need for a standard classification system of complications. The classification applies only to planned surgical lengthening methods, such as long-term TGR (Smith et al., 2015).

Compared to the complications mentioned above, a few other complications seem unique to MCGR. For example, rod slippage (Cheung et al., 2018), actuator pin breakage (Kwan et al., 2017), and metallosis (Rushton et al., 2017; Teoh et al., 2016a). In close collaboration between users and industry, it develops MCGR in several versions to overcome these shortcomings. The disruptions seen with each new technique that enters our lives will continue to decrease due to more data and research (Akbarnia & Mundis, 2019).

## Conclusion

MCGR gives similar results to those of TGR in curve correction and spine augmentation. It provides a physiological extension in the growing spine with an effective and safe distraction. The MCGR technique has been shown to reduce the risks associated with repeated general anesthesia and the number of planned surgeries. Patients and their parents are increasingly interested in MCGR instead of traditional techniques requiring frequent surgery. It is logical for countries to prefer cost-effective methods in their health systems. In this context, it is thought that MCGR imposes a less financial burden on the health system in the long run than conventional treatment options (Rolton et al., 2015; Su et al., 2015).

Doany et al. analyzed health-related quality of life data. He reported that overall satisfaction was higher in the MCGR group than in TGR and showed superior financial results. However, as the follow-up period progresses, the superior effects of MCGR decrease (Doany et al. 2018). As a final word, in a recent study, it was stated that the use of TGR, which constitutes approximately 80% of growth-friendly surgeries, has decreased, and the use of MCGR has increased in the last ten years (Klyce et al., 2020).

## References

Agarwal, A., Agarwal, A. K., Jayaswal, A., & Goel, V. (2014). Smaller Interval Distractions May Reduce Chances of Growth Rod Breakage Without Impeding Desired Spinal Growth: A Finite Element Study. *Spine Deformity*, 2(6), 430–436. https://doi.org/10.1016/J.JSPD.2014.08.004.

Akbarnia, B. A., Marks, D. S., Boachie-Adjei, O., Thompson, A. G., & Asher, M. A. (2005). Dual growing rod technique for the treatment of progressive early-onset scoliosis: a multicenter study. *Spine,* 30(17 Suppl). https://doi.org/10.1097/01.BRS.0000175190.08134.73.

Akbarnia, B. A., & Mundis, G. M. (2019). Magnetically controlled growing rods in early onset scoliosis : Indications, timing and treatment. *Der Orthopade*, 48(6), 477–485. https://doi.org/10.1007/S00132-019-03755-0.

Akbarnia, B. A., Mundis, G. M., Salari, P., Yaszay, B., & Pawelek, J. B. (2012). Innovation in growing rod technique: a study of safety and efficacy of a magnetically controlled growing rod in a porcine model. *Spine*, 37(13), 1109–1114. https://doi.org/10.1097/BRS.0B013E318240FF67.

Akbarnia, B. A., Pawelek, J. B., Cheung, K. M. C., Demirkiran, G., Elsebaie, H., Emans, J. B., Johnston, C. E., Mundis, G. M., Noordeen, H., Skaggs, D. L., Sponseller, P. D., Thompson, G. H., Yaszay, B., & Yazici, M. (2014). Traditional Growing Rods Versus Magnetically Controlled Growing Rods for the Surgical Treatment of Early-Onset Scoliosis: A Case-Matched 2-Year Study. *Spine Deformity*, 2(6), 493–497. https://doi.org/10.1016/J.JSPD.2014.09.050.

Baky, F. J., Milbrandt, T. A., Flick, R., & Larson, A. N. (2018). Cumulative Anesthesia Exposure in Patients Treated for Early-Onset Scoliosis. *Spine Deformity*, 6(6), 781–786. https://doi.org/10.1016/J.JSPD.2018.05.001.

Bess, S., Akbarnia, B. A., Thompson, G. H., Sponseller, P. D., Shah, S. A., El Sebaie, H., Boachie-Adjei, O., Karlin, L. I., Canale, S., Poe-Kochert, C., & Skaggs, D. L. (2010). Complications of growing-rod treatment for early-onset scoliosis: analysis of one hundred and forty patients. *The Journal of Bone and Joint Surgery*. American Volume, 92(15), 2533–2543. https://doi.org/10.2106/JBJS.I.01471.

Budd, H. R., Stokes, O. M., Meakin, J., Fulford, J., & Hutton, M. (2016). Safety and compatibility of magnetic-controlled growing rods and magnetic resonance imaging. *European Spine Journal*, 25(2), 578–582. https://doi.org/10.1007/S00586-015-4178-5.

Cheung, J. P. Y., Bow, C., Samartzis, D., Ganal-Antonio, A. K. B., & Cheung, K. M. C. (2016). Clinical utility of ultrasound to prospectively monitor distraction of magnetically controlled growing rods. *The Spine Journal : Official Journal of the North American Spine Society*, 16(2), 204–209. https://doi.org/10.1016/J.SPINEE.2015.10.044.

Cheung, J. P. Y., Yiu, K. K. L., Samartzis, D., Kwan, K., Tan, B. B., & Cheung, K. M. C. (2018). Rod Lengthening With the Magnetically Controlled Growing Rod: Factors Influencing Rod Slippage and Reduced Gains During Distractions. *Spine,* 43(7), E399–E405. https://doi.org/10.1097/BRS.0000000000002358.

Cheung, K. M. C., Cheung, J. P. Y., Samartzis, D., Mak, K. C., Wong, Y. W., Cheung, W. Y., Akbarnia, B. A., & Luk, K. D. K. (2012). Magnetically controlled growing rods for severe spinal curvature in young children: a prospective case series. *Lancet (London, England),* 379(9830), 1967–1974. https://doi.org/10.1016/S0140-6736(12)60112-3.

Cheung (n.d.). *What are the effects of changing the frequency.* Retrieved March 18, 2015.

Choi, E., Yaszay, B., Mundis, G., Hosseini, P., Pawelek, J., Alanay, A., Berk, H., Cheung, K., Demirkiran, G., Ferguson, J., Greggi, T., Helenius, I., La Rosa, G., Senkoylu, A., & Akbarnia, B. A. (2017). Implant Complications After Magnetically Controlled Growing Rods for Early Onset Scoliosis: A Multicenter Retrospective Review. *Journal of Pediatric Orthopedics,* 37(8), e588–e592. https://doi.org/10.1097/BPO.0000000000000803.

Doany, M. E., Deniz Olgun, Z., Kinikli, G. I., Bekmez, S., Kocyigit, A., Demirkiran, G., Ergun Karaagaoglu, A., & Yazici, M. (2018). Health-Related Quality of Life in Early-Onset Scoliosis Patients Treated Surgically: EOSQ Scores in Traditional Growing Rod Versus Magnetically Controlled Growing Rods. *Spine,* 43(2), 148–153. https://doi.org/10.1097/BRS.0000000000002274.

Fletcher, N. D., McClung, A., Rathjen, K. E., Denning, J. R., Browne, R., & Johnston, C. E. (2012). Serial casting as a delay tactic in the treatment of moderate-to-severe early-onset scoliosis. *Journal of Pediatric Orthopedics,* 32(7), 664–671. https://doi.org/10.1097/BPO.0B013E31824BDB55.

Hosseini, P., Pawelek, J. B., Nguyen, S., Thompson, G. H., Shah, S. A., Flynn, J. M., Dormans, J. P., & Akbarnia, B. A. (2017). Rod fracture and lengthening intervals in traditional growing rods: is there a relationship? *European Spine Journal*, 26(6), 1690–1695. https://doi.org/10.1007/S00586-016-4786-8.

Klyce, W., Mitchell, S. L., Pawelek, J., Skaggs, D. L., Sanders, J. O., Shah, S. A., McCarthy, R. E., Luhmann, S. J., Sturm, P. F., Flynn, J. M., Smith, J. T., Akbarnia, B. A., & Sponseller, P. D. (2020). Characterizing Use of Growth-friendly Implants for Early-onset Scoliosis: A 10-Year Update. *Journal of Pediatric Orthopedics*, 40(8), e740–e746. https://doi.org/10.1097/BPO.0000000000001594.

Kwan, K. Y. H., Alanay, A., Yazici, M., Demirkiran, G., Helenius, I., Nnadi, C., Ferguson, J., Akbarnia, B. A., Cheung, J. P. Y., & Cheung, K. M. C. (2017). Unplanned Reoperations in Magnetically Controlled Growing Rod Surgery for Early Onset Scoliosis With a Minimum of Two-Year Follow-Up. *Spine*, 42(24), E1410–E1414. https://doi.org/10.1097/BRS.0000000000002297.

Lorenz, H. M., Braunschweig, L., Badwan, B., Groenefeld, K., Hecker, M. M., Tsaknakis, K., Grote, J., & Hell, A. K. (2019). High Correlation Between Achieved and Expected Distraction Using Magnetically Controlled Growth Rods (MCGR) With Rib to Pelvis Fixation in Pediatric Spine Deformity. *Journal of Pediatric Orthopedics*, 39(5), e334–e338. https://doi.org/10.1097/BPO.0000000000001303.

Munigangaiah, S., Brown, P., Mohamed, M., Bruce, C. E., Trivedi, J. M., & Davidson, N. T. (2018). A novel technique for the subfascial insertion of magnetically controlled growing rods - The Alder Hey technique. *Journal of Craniovertebral Junction & Spine*, 9(4), 250–253. https://doi.org/10.4103/JCVJS.JCVJS_105_18.

Poon, S., Nixon, R., Wendolowski, S., Gecelter, R., Chen, Y. H., DiMauro, J. P., Amaral, T., Graver, A., & Grande, D. A. (2017). A pilot cadaveric study of temperature and adjacent tissue changes after exposure of magnetic-controlled growing rods to MRI. *European Spine Journal*, 26(6), 1618–1623. https://doi.org/10.1007/S00586-016-4918-1.

Rolton, D., Richards, J., & Nnadi, C. (2015). Magnetic controlled growth rods versus conventional growing rod systems in the treatment of early onset scoliosis: a cost comparison. *European Spine Journal*, 24(7), 1457–1461. https://doi.org/10.1007/S00586-014-3699-7.

Rushton, P. R. P., Siddique, I., Crawford, R., Birch, N., Gibson, M. J., & Hutton, M. J. (2017). Magnetically controlled growing rods in the treatment of early-onset scoliosis: a note of caution. *The Bone & Joint Journal,* 99-B(6), 708–713. https://doi.org/10.1302/0301-620X.99B6.BJJ-2016-1102.R2.

Sankar, W. N., Acevedo, D. C., & Skaggs, D. L. (2010). Comparison of complications among growing spinal implants. *Spine*, 35(23), 2091–2096. https://doi.org/10.1097/BRS.0B013E3181C6EDD7.

Smith, J. T., & Campbell, R. M. (2012). Magnetically controlled growing rods for spinal deformity. *Lancet* (London, England), 379(9830), 1930–1931. https://doi.org/10.1016/S0140-6736(12)60528-5.

Smith, J. T., Johnston, C., Skaggs, D., Flynn, J., & Vitale, M. (2015). A New Classification System to Report Complications in Growing Spine Surgery: A Multicenter Consensus Study. *Journal of Pediatric Orthopedics*, 35(8), 798–803. https://doi.org/10.1097/BPO.0000000000000386.

Stokes, O. M., O'Donovan, E. J., Samartzis, D., Bow, C. H., Luk, K. D. K., & Cheung, K. M. C. (2014). Reducing radiation exposure in early-onset scoliosis surgery patients: novel use of ultrasonography to measure lengthening in magnetically-controlled growing rods. *The Spine Journal : Official Journal of the North American Spine Society,* 14(10), 2397–2404. https://doi.org/10.1016/J.SPINEE.2014.01.039.

Su, A. W., Milbrandt, T. A., & Larson, A. N. (2015). Magnetic Expansion Control System Achieves Cost Savings Compared to Traditional Growth Rods: An Economic Analysis Model. *Spine,* 40(23), 1851–1856. https://doi.org/10.1097/BRS.0000000000001077.

Takaso, M., Moriya, H., Kitahara, H., Minami, S., Takahashi, K., Isobe, K., Yamagata, M., Otsuka, Y., Nakata, Y., & Inoue, M. (1998). New remote-controlled growing-rod spinal instrumentation possibly applicable for scoliosis in young children. *Journal of Orthopaedic Science*, 3(6), 336–340. https://doi.org/10.1007/S007760050062.

Tan, K. A., Sewell, M. D., Clarke, A. J., Chan, D., Stokes, O. M., Khan, S. N., & Hutton, M. (2017). Recommendations for Lengthening of Magnetically Controlled Growing Rods in Children With Pacemakers. *Journal of Pediatric Orthopedics*, 37(4), e250–e254. https://doi.org/10.1097/BPO.0000000000000872.

Teoh, K. H., Von Ruhland, C., Evans, S. L., James, S. H., Jones, A., Howes, J., Davies, P. R., & Ahuja, S. (2016a). Metallosis following implantation of magnetically controlled growing rods in the treatment of scoliosis: a case series. *The Bone & Joint Journal*, 98-B(12), 1662–1667. https://doi.org/10.1302/0301-620X.98B12.38061.

Teoh, K. H., Winson, D. M. G., James, S. H., Jones, A., Howes, J., Davies, P. R., & Ahuja, S. (2016b). Do magnetic growing rods have lower complication rates compared with conventional growing rods? *Spine Journal*, 16(4), S40–S44. https://doi.org/10.1016/j.spinee.2015.12.099.

Tsirikos, A. I., & Roberts, S. B. (2020). Magnetic Controlled Growth Rods in the Treatment of Scoliosis: Safety, Efficacy and Patient Selection. *Medical Devices (Auckland, N.Z.)*, 13, 75–85. https://doi.org/10.2147/MDER.S198176.

Vivas, A. C., Hwang, S. W., & Pahys, J. M. (2017). Insertion of magnetically controlled growing rods in a patient with a diaphragmatic pacemaker: case report. *Neurosurgical Focus,* 43(4). https://doi.org/10.3171/2017.7.FOCUS17356.

Watanabe, K., Uno, K., Suzuki, T., Kawakami, N., Tsuji, T., Yanagida, H., Ito, M., Hirano, T., Yamazaki, K., Minami, S., Kotani, T., Taneichi, H., Imagama, S., Takeshita, K., Yamamoto, T., & Matsumoto, M. (2013). Risk factors for complications associated with growing-rod surgery for early-onset scoliosis. *Spine,* 38(8). https://doi.org/10.1097/BRS.0B013E318288671A.

Wick, J. M., & Konze, J. (2012). A magnetic approach to treating progressive early-onset scoliosis. *AORN Journal,* 96(2), 163–173. https://doi.org/10.1016/J.AORN.2012.05.008.

Woon, R. P., Andras, L. M., Noordeen, H., Morris, S., Hutchinson, J., Shah, S. A., Pawelek, J., Johnston, C. E., & Skaggs, D. L. (2018). Surgeon Survey Shows No Adverse Events With MRI in Patients With Magnetically Controlled Growing Rods (MCGRs). *Spine Deformity,* 6(3), 299–302. https://doi.org/10.1016/J.JSPD.2017.10.004.

Yang, J. S., Sponseller, P. D., Thompson, G. H., Akbarnia, B. A., Emans, J. B., Yazici, M., Skaggs, D. L., Shah, S. A., Salari, P., & Poe-Kochert, C. (2011). Growing rod fractures: risk factors and opportunities for prevention. *Spine,* 36(20), 1639–1644. https://doi.org/10.1097/BRS.0B013E31822A982F.

# Chapter 21

# Vertical Expandable Prosthetic Titanium Rib (VEPTR)

**Basri Pür[1,*], MD**
**and Sinan Yılar[2], MD**
[1]The Department of Orthopedics and Traumatology, Erzurum City Hospital, Erzurum, Turkiye
[2]The Department of Orthopedics and Traumatology, Atatürk University, Erzurum, Turkiye

## Abstract

Early onset scoliosis (EOS) is a spinal deformity detected before 10 years old due to any etiology, according to SRS. The treatment algorithm should be managed in the early stages of pulmonary functions, organ dysfunctions, and deformities. Growth-friendly techniques are distinguished in the current literature for EOS. Vertical expandable prosthetic titanium rib (VEPTR) is also actively used for growth-friendly techniques. VEPTR is a non-fusion correction surgical technique that allows physiological growth in rib and spine deformities affecting the thoracic with incomplete skeletal maturation. This technique was improved considering that the correction of the spinal directly positively affects the deformities of the thoracic cage by providing posterior support for the thoracic cage due to the insufficiency of Campbell's traditional spinal correction techniques in the thoracic. The purpose of the VEPTR technique is to correct the spinal deformity while forming a basis for the volumetric and functional development of the lungs. Furthermore, growth is ensured by distraction maneuvers in 6-month periods, in parallel with physiological growth.

* Corresponding Author's Email: basri_pur@hotmail.com.

In: Early Onset Scoliosis
Editor: Ahmed Majid Heydar
ISBN: 979-8-89113-600-7

**Keywords:** VEPTR, EOS, TYS

## Introduction

As an alternative to the classical fusion technique and other methods that enable growth in EOS, the VEPTR technique was developed by Robert Campbell and Melvin Smith for children with thoracic insufficiency syndrome (TIS) with scoliosis. While this technique initially aimed to treat TIS, it began to be actively performed by spine surgeons in scoliosis treatment after receiving FDA approval in 2007(R. M. Campbell, 2013).

The VEPTR technique expands the restricted rib cage on the concave side with a distraction technique while correcting the alignment of vertebrae in the coronal plane (El-Hawary et al., 2017). It enables the correction of deformities by controlling the load transfer of the rib to the spine and/or pelvis (Hasler et al., 2010). The length of the sagittal spine should be taken into account to prevent an increase in the degree of kyphosis in the sagittal plane while providing a correction in the coronal plane (El-Hawary et al., 2016). The VEPTR technique enables extension of up to 15-20 cm in patients with minimally invasive repeated surgeries by performing distraction every 6 months; it allows, in the coronal plane, a correction of 30% in the Cobb angle (54°) and, in the sagittal plane, a correction of 9% in the kyphosis angle (El-Hawary et al., 2016; Hasler et al., 2010; Studer et al., 2019).

It is also known that the VEPTR technique also has correction effects on shoulder imbalance, cervical tilt, and the crankshaft phenomenon in cases of congenital scoliosis (R. M. J. Campbell et al., 2007).

## Main Body

While indications for EOS surgery continue to be researched and debated, VEPTR indications are indicated, particularly in cases of rib fusion and rigid rib cages, by the innovator of the VEPTR technique (R. M. J. Campbell, Smith, & Hell-Vocke, 2004; R. M. J. Campbell, Smith, Mayes, et al., 2004).

Although the issue of contraindications to VEPTR treatment is unclear, VEPTR contraindications can be mentioned in the cases of children younger than 6 months, patients with diaphragm dysfunction, and in the presence of additional conditions where repeated surgical anesthesia is contraindicated.

Additionally, relative contraindications can be mentioned in cases such as patients who had partial fusion before, who had rigid kyphosis, the deficiency of the proximal rib, the presence of inadequate soft tissues, and poor bone stock (osteogenesis imperfecta) (R. M. Campbell, 2013; Hasler et al., 2010).

Among the advantages of this new system, the most significant is its allowance for non-fusion growth of the spine and rib cage, while also allowing a gradual positive change in lung capacities over time during growth. In other growth-friendly systems, traditional growing rods have advantages and disadvantages compared to magnetically controlled growing rods and the Shilla technique. The advantages of this technique include the absence of local fusion, the reduced need for pedicle screws, the greater corrective impact on the thoracic, the allowance for more extension, and the applicability at younger ages. The need for more surgical procedures and more implant insufficiency compared to other techniques, less correction in the coronal plane, and skin problems related to implant irritation suggest the need for further development of this technique (Hasler et al., 2010). The techniques that are growth-friendly in EOS are summarized in the table below (Table 1).

**Table 1.** Non-fusion surgical techniques for early onset scoliosis

| | |
|---|---|
| Preservation and stimulation of growth | • Posterior distraction<br>  • Single-growing rod<br>  • Dual-growing rod<br>  • Magnetically controlled growing rod<br>• Intercostal/costovertebral distraction<br>  • Expansion thoracoplasty<br>  • VEPTR |
| Guidance of growth | • Shilla<br>• Modern Luque Trolley<br>• Sliding growing rod |
| Regulation of growth | • Anterior vertebral stapling<br>• Anterior vertebral tethering |
| Hybrid techniques | • Convex growth arrest + Concave distraction<br>• Limited fusion + Stimulation of growth<br>• Distraction-assisted growth guidance<br>• Non-fusion multi-vertebrae wedge osteotomies |

Even though spinal mobility is relinquished at multiple levels due to fusion, in cases where VEPTR is contraindicated, the Shilla technique can be considered as an alternative (Hasler et al., 2010).

It has been proven that the VEPTR technique has more advantages in the correction of sagittal plane and pelvic obliques compared to dual-growing rods, but dual-growing rods are superior in the correction of coronal angles (Hasler et al., 2010).

When comparing magnetically controlled growing rods with the VEPTR technique, the most significant disadvantage of magnetically controlled rods is the loss of magnetic effectiveness over the rod due to reasons like periosteal coverage, especially when used in younger age groups, along with the high cost of the implants. However, the absence of repeated surgical procedures, performing extension in an upright position without anesthesia, and zero VAS pain score during extension provide advantages for magnetically controlled rods (R. M. Campbell, 2013; Cheung et al., 2012).

Neuromonitoring should be used during the surgical procedure and for each extension process without exception. Not only for the lower extremities but also for the upper extremities, a neuromonitoring technician should place preoperative props for motor and sensory control purposes. Special emphasis should be placed on avoiding brachial plexus injury, particularly during the initial surgical procedure. In order to prevent plexus injuries, the placement of rib hooks on the proximal ribs and excessive correction of curvature should be avoided (Ramirez et al., 2009).

There are three different options during the surgery process. These are rib-rib connections, rib-spine connections, and rib-iliac connections. C-shaped anchors are used for the ribs. For the spine, the spinous process and lamina anchors were previously used, but now they are replaced by pedicle screws; however, in children under 18 months of age with underdeveloped pedicles and experiencing respiratory problems, fixation can still be performed with the spinous process and lamina anchors. An S-shaped McCarthy hook can be used on the crest of the iliac wing. Iliac crest hooks are recommended for lower lumbar curvatures. Titanium rods are connected to each other using distraction-locked attachments. Each hole in the rods has a 5mm gap between them. In minimally invasive techniques, Kelly clamps can be used to guide the placement of the rod. In distraction procedures, a minimum of 5mm to a maximum of 15mm extension can be performed in 6-month intervals. Through the attachment, it reaches the attachment that obtains the connection between the 5 cm incision and two rods. During the extension, a distraction of 2mm should be performed every 3 minutes, and neuromonitoring should be carefully monitored during the distraction process (R. M. Campbell, 2013; R. M. J. Campbell, Smith, & Hell-Vocke, 2004).

C-shaped anchors for the proximal ribs should not be placed on the first and second ribs. While the risk of nerve damage (brachial plexus) increases in the proximal attachments, proximal compensatory curvatures can also occur. Furthermore, anchors placed closer to the midline also have a greater impact on corrective force and long-term durability (Hasler et al., 2010).

There is no spinal support at the rib-rib connections. It is a technique based on rib-based distraction in patients with fused ribs. Hybrid techniques (rib-spine or rib-pelvis) have been developed because this technique used in rib dysmorphisms has the insufficiency of both strength and spinal corrective force in the correction of spinal curvatures. In patients with fused ribs, while separating two ribs with rib elevator assistance, attention should be paid to avoid damaging the ribs and pleura. To avoid disrupting the vascularity of the ribs, soft tissue must be carefully dissected. After performing an osteotomy on the connection between the two ribs, the distraction maneuver can be performed for a maximum of 2 cm and performed slowly. More than this, distractions have been associated with pleural tears. After the surgical procedure, it is essential to ensure that the implants are covered with muscles and soft tissue. The risk of implant irritation should not be overlooked because the profile of the EOS patient is generally cachectic and has less subcutaneous adipose tissue (R. M. Campbell, 2013; Dayer et al., 2014; El-Hawary et al., 2020). Intervention can be performed in isolated thoracic curvatures without fused ribs using newly developed pedicle screws and distraction rods (Figure 1).

If there is no lumbar curvature in the rib-spine hybrid techniques, fixation is achieved with pedicle screws on the lower thoracic vertebrae. In proximal lumbar curvatures, L1 and L2 vertebral pedicle screws can be used, but for more distal curvatures, fixation with S-shaped McCarthy anchors or screws on the iliac crest is recommended. For syndromic and neuromuscular scoliosis, the pelvic-supported bilateral hybrid VEPTR technique is also recommended (Eiffel Tower construct) (Figures 2 and 3) (R. M. Campbell, 2013).

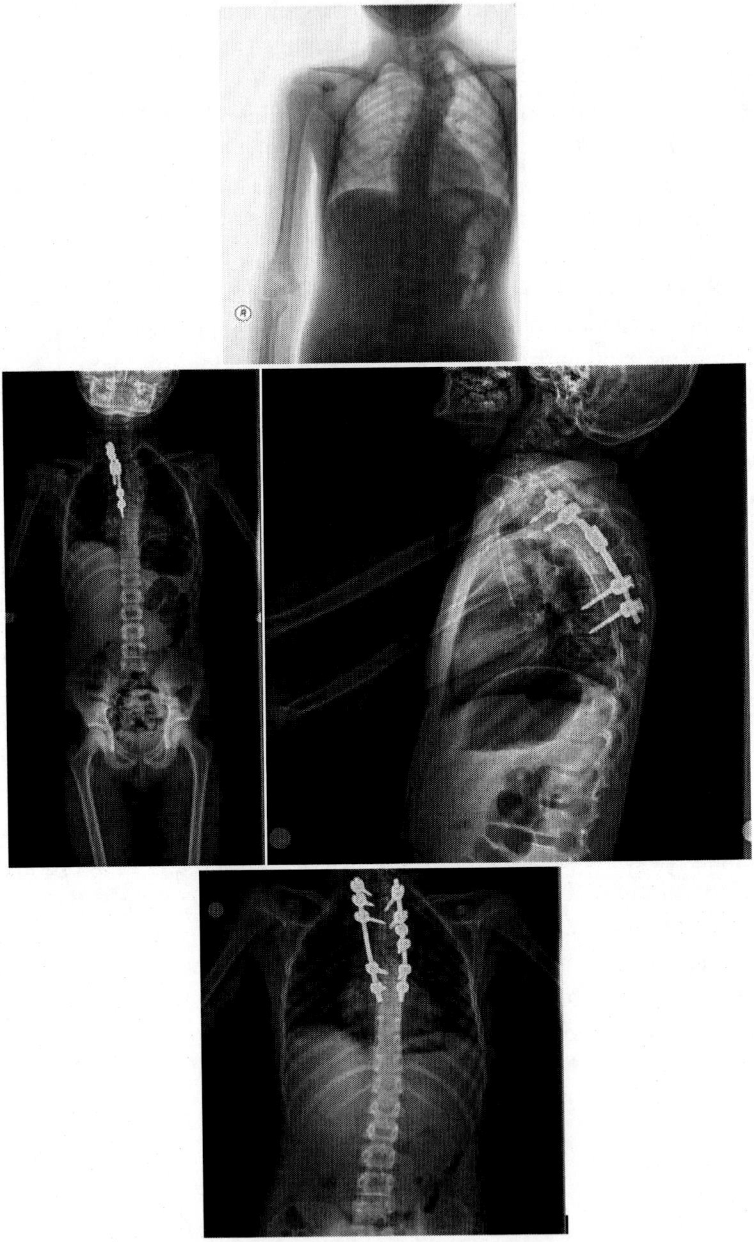

**Figure 1.** The progressive arthrodesis of a patient with thoracic scoliosis (Authors' own archive).

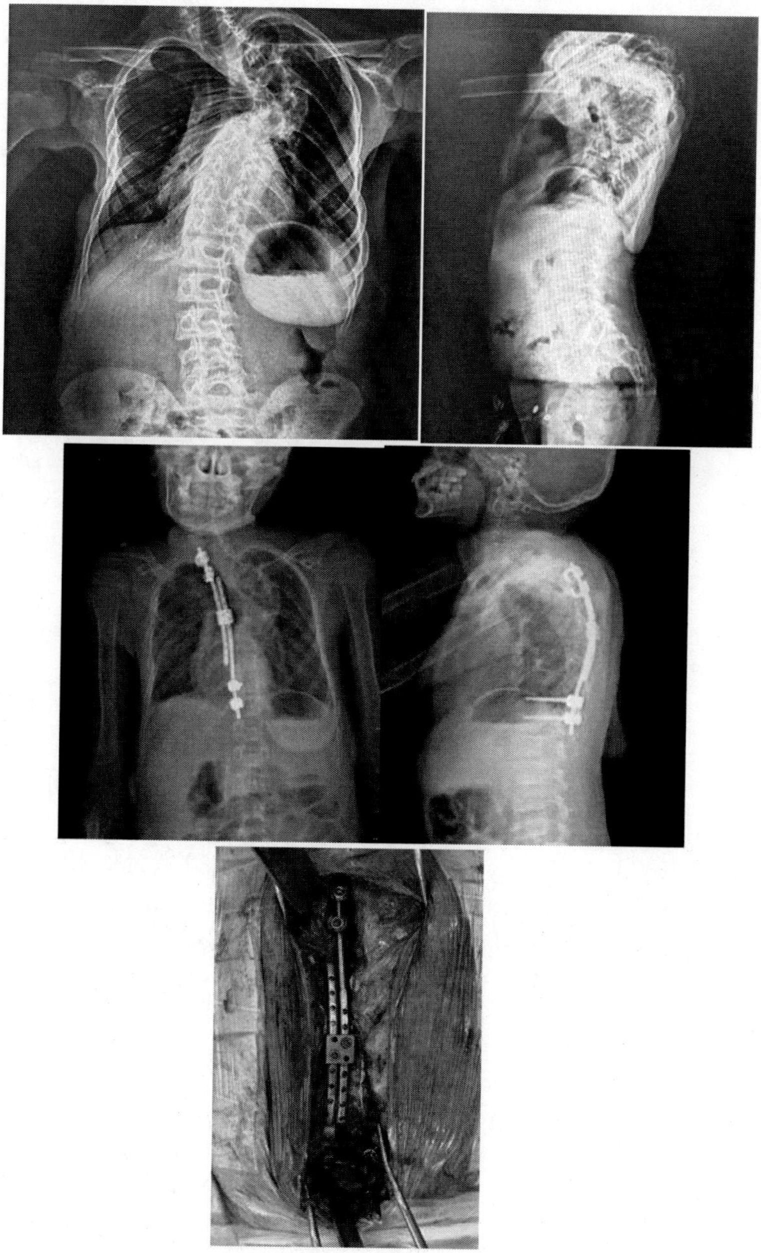

**Figure 2.** VEPTR technique performed with anchors to the third and fourth Costas proximally and pedicle screws to the 11th and 12th vertebrae distally (Authors' own archive).

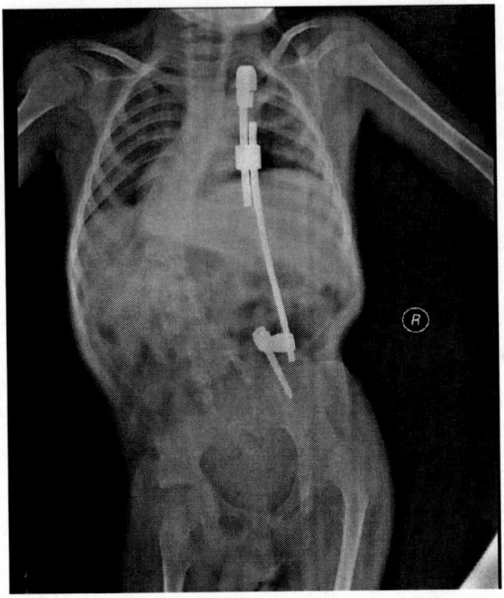


**Figure 3.** The VEPTR technique performed distraction with the iliac screw (Authors' own archive).

## Conclusion

The significant effects of the VEPTR technique on lung capacities and functions are undoubtedly significant. While studies are still ongoing, according to recent research, it is known that in long-term follow-ups, there is an average improvement of around 50% in the FVC calculated by the ratio of average values to predictive values (Thompson et al., 2007). Early surgical intervention is essential in patients with pulmonary problems because it has been reported that the improvement in respiratory functions is inversely proportional to age (Nossov et al., 2019).

It is believed that early intervention in patients at a young age leads in greater results in both respiratory functions and corrective effects on the spine. Additionally, VEPTR prevents the loss of gains proposed by Sankar's "Law of Diminishing Returns" theory through repeated minimal surgical procedures following early intervention (Flynn et al., 2013; Sankar et al., 2011).

Families of patients undergoing VEPTR treatment should be thoroughly informed about the process and repeated surgical procedures. There should be clear and transparent communication between the patient and the surgeon.

Complications can be observed in the extendable spinal systems used for spinal deformities. Although complications can be discussed in patients undergoing the VEPTR technique, most of them are implant-related complications. The patient's relatives should be informed in detail about the entire process, from the initial surgical procedure to the final surgical intervention and fusion surgery. The risk of unplanned surgical procedures and complications should be clarified. It has been reported that hybrid techniques related to the rib-spine connection have lower complication rates. Commonly observed complications are listed below (R. M. Campbell, 2013; El-Hawary et al., 2017; Sankar et al., 2010):

- Implant migration (the most common)
- Skin wounds and infections
- Implant fractures (Figure 4)
- Rib fractures
- Osteopenia
- Neurological injury (brachial plexus)

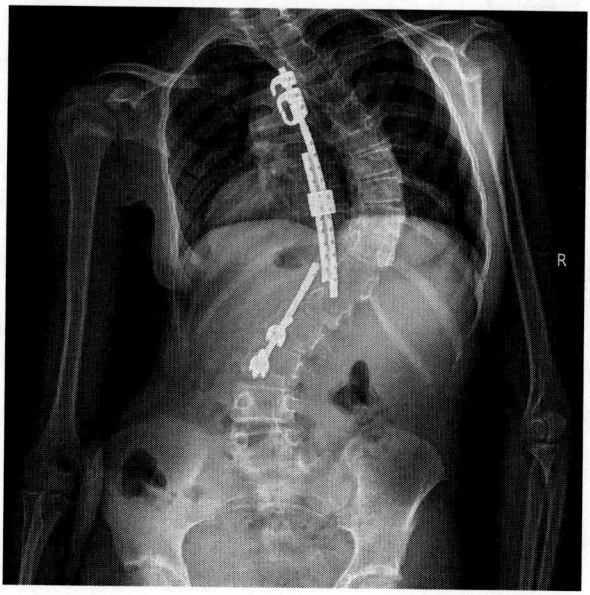


**Figure 4.** A 12-year-old patient with a implant fracture (Authors' own archive).

## References


Campbell, R. M. (2013). VEPTR: Past experience and the future of VEPTR principles. *European Spine Journal*, *22*(Suppl 2), 106-117. https://doi.org/10.1007/s00586-013-2671-2.

Campbell, R. M. J., Adcox, B. M., Smith, M. D., Simmons, J. W. I., Cofer, B. R., Inscore, S. C., & Grohman, C. (2007). The Effect of Mid-Thoracic VEPTR Opening Wedge Thoracostomy on Cervical Tilt Associated With Congenital Thoracic Scoliosis in Patients With Thoracic Insufficiency Syndrome. *Spine*, *32*(20), 2171. https://doi.org/10.1097/BRS.0b013e31814b2d6c.

Campbell, R. M. J., Smith, M. D., & Hell-Vocke, A. K. (2004). Expansion Thoracoplasty: The Surgical Technique of Opening-Wedge Thoracostomy: Surgical Technique. *JBJS*, *86*(suppl_1), 51.

Campbell, R. M. J., Smith, M. D., Mayes, T. C., Mangos, J. A., Willey-Courand, D. B., Kose, N., Pinero, R. F., Alder, M. E., Duong, H. L., & Surber, J. L. (2004). The Effect of Opening Wedge Thoracostomy on Thoracic Insufficiency Syndrome Associated with Fused Ribs and Congenital Scoliosis. *JBJS*, *86*(8), 1659.

Cheung, K. M.-C., Cheung, J. P.-Y., Samartzis, D., Mak, K.-C., Wong, Y.-W., Cheung, W.-Y., Akbarnia, B. A., & Luk, K. D.-K. (2012). Magnetically controlled growing rods for severe spinal curvature in young children: A prospective case series. *The Lancet*, *379*(9830), 1967-1974. https://doi.org/10.1016/S0140-6736(12)60112-3.

Dayer, R., Ceroni, D., & Lascombes, P. (2014). Treatment of congenital thoracic scoliosis with associated rib fusions using VEPTR expansion thoracostomy: A surgical technique. *European Spine Journal*, *23*(4), 424-431. https://doi.org/10.1007/s00586-014-3338-3.

El-Hawary, R., Kadhim, M., Vitale, M., Smith, J., Samdani, A., Flynn, J. M., & Children's Spine Study Group. (2017). VEPTR Implantation to Treat Children With Early-Onset Scoliosis Without Rib Abnormalities: Early Results From a Prospective Multicenter Study. *Journal of Pediatric Orthopedics*, *37*(8), e599-e605. https://doi.org/10.1097/BPO.0000000000000943.

El-Hawary, R., Morash, K., Kadhim, M., Vitale, M., Smith, J., Samdani, A., Flynn, J., & Children's Spine Study Group. (2020). VEPTR Treatment of Early Onset Scoliosis in Children Without Rib Abnormalities: Long-term Results of a Prospective, Multicenter Study. *Journal of Pediatric Orthopedics*, *40*(6), e406-e412. https://doi.org/10.1097/BPO.0000000000001454.

El-Hawary, R., Samdani, A., Wade, J., Smith, M., Heflin, J. A., Klatt, J. W., Vitale, M. G., Smith, J. T., & Group, C. S. S. (2016). Rib-based Distraction Surgery Maintains Total Spine Growth. *Journal of Pediatric Orthopaedics*, *36*(8), 841. https://doi.org/10.1097/BPO.0000000000000567.

Flynn, J. M., Emans, J. B., Smith, J. T., Betz, R. R., Deeney, V. F., Patel, N. M., & Campbell, R. M. (2013). VEPTR to treat nonsyndromic congenital scoliosis: A multicenter, mid-term follow-up study. *Journal of Pediatric Orthopedics*, *33*(7), 679-684. https://doi.org/10.1097/BPO.0b013e31829d55a2.

Hasler, C.-C., Mehrkens, A., & Hefti, F. (2010). Efficacy and safety of VEPTR instrumentation for progressive spine deformities in young children without rib fusions. *European Spine Journal*, *19*(3), 400-408. https://doi.org/10.1007/s00586-009-1253-9.

Nossov, S. B., Curatolo, E., Campbell, R. M., Mayer, O. H., Garg, S., Cahill, A. P. J., & Children's Spine Study Group. (2019). VEPTR: Are We Reducing Respiratory Assistance Requirements? *Journal of Pediatric Orthopedics*, *39*(1), 28-32. https://doi.org/10.1097/BPO.0000000000000986.

Ramirez, N., Flynn, J. M., Serrano, J. A., Carlo, S., & Cornier, A. S. (2009). The Vertical Expandable Prosthetic Titanium Rib in the treatment of spinal deformity due to progressive early onset scoliosis. *Journal of Pediatric Orthopaedics B*, *18*(4), 197. https://doi.org/10.1097/BPB.0b013e32832bf5e0.

Sankar, W. N., Acevedo, D. C., & Skaggs, D. L. (2010). Comparison of Complications Among Growing Spinal Implants. *Spine*, *35*(23), 2091. https://doi.org/10.1097/BRS.0b013e3181c6edd7.

Sankar, W. N., Skaggs, D. L., Yazici, M., Johnston, C. E. I., Shah, S. A., Javidan, P., Kadakia, R. V., Day, T. F., & Akbarnia, B. A. (2011). Lengthening of Dual Growing Rods and the Law of Diminishing Returns. *Spine*, *36*(10), 806. https://doi.org/10.1097/BRS.0b013e318214d78f.

Studer, D., Büchler, P., & Hasler, C. C. (2019). Radiographic Outcome and Complication Rate of 34 Graduates After Treatment With Vertical Expandable Prosthetic Titanium Rib (VEPTR): A Single Center Report. *Journal of Pediatric Orthopedics*, *39*(10), e731-e736. https://doi.org/10.1097/BPO.0000000000001338.

Thompson, G. H., Akbarnia, B. A., & Campbell, R. M. J. (2007). Growing Rod Techniques in Early-Onset Scoliosis. *Journal of Pediatric Orthopaedics*, *27*(3), 354. https://doi.org/10.1097/BPO.0b013e3180333eea.

## Chapter 22

# Hybrid Growing Rods

**Alim Can Baymurat*, MD**
Department of Orthopedics and Traumatology, Gazi University Faculty of Medicine, Ankara, Turkey

## Abstract

Early-onset scoliosis (EOS) is a scoliotic deformity of the spine that develops related to different factors before the age of 10 and is a difficult childhood spinal disease to manage for spinal surgeries. In the surgical treatment of the growing spine, it is important to correct the curvature, as well as protect the growth of the spine at the same time. Spinal fusion surgery should be avoided at an early age to prevent severe iatrogenic thoracic deficiency syndrome depending on the insufficient development of the short body and rib cage. Therefore, growth-friendly surgical methods are preferred in patients with EOS. Among these methods, traditional growing rods (TGRs) are the most widely used method. In rigid and large curvatures, especially in congenital early-onset scoliosis (CEOS), which is a common etiology of EOS, it cannot be adequately corrected by the TGR method. Additionally, complications such as implant failure and correction loss occur. The major residual deformity, limited apex control, the "crankshaft phenomenon," and high risks of mechanical complications have been reported with the TGR used in the treatment of CEOS. Research has been conducted on hybrid methods to overcome these problems. The derotation of the apical region with short segment fusion at the apex of the curvature and correction of the apical vertebral translation (AVT) has promising results in patients with EOS with rigid and large curvatures.

---

* Corresponding Author's Email: alimcanbaymurat@yahoo.com.

In: Early Onset Scoliosis
Editor: Ahmed Majid Heydar
ISBN: 979-8-89113-600-7

**Keywords:** hybrid growing rod, early-onset scoliosis, congenital scoliosis, traditional growing rod

## Introduction

Early-onset scoliosis progresses related to idiopathic, congenital, thoracogenic, neuromuscular, and syndromic etiology. Conservative treatments and surgical interventions are among the treatments practiced for EOS. Although conservative treatments are generally considered, they have certain limitations, and surgical interventions are usually required in patients for whom they have a large number of limitations. The treatment objective of patients with EOS includes minimizing spinal deformity while maximizing thoracic volume and lung function.

Despite great advances in the field of medicine, surgical treatment of EOS is one of the difficult areas in spinal surgery. The reason is that young children with progressive spinal deformities can have life-threatening pulmonary complications. Therefore, it is essential for pediatric spine surgeons to know the development of the lung in children. Lung development grows non-linearly over time, and alveolar-capillary proliferation peaks between the ages of 0 and 2 and ends around the age of 8; the volume of the bronchial tree increases as the child grows (Boyden, 1977). Any deformity and loss of flexibility in the vertebral-costa-sternum complex triggered by the progression of scoliosis distorts the dynamic capacity of the respiratory system and negatively affects the development of the alveoli in terms of number and volume (Canavese and Dimeglio, 2013). This restrictive lung disease can develop into pulmonary arterial hypertension, which is responsible for right heart failure, or pulmonary heart disease, which can be life-threatening at an early stage in adults (Canavese and Dimeglio, 2013; Swank et al., 1982). In the treatment of patients with EOS, spinal fusion surgery should not be avoided to prevent the growth of the rib cage and the development of restrictive lung disease.

Even though the surgical treatment of EOS varies depending on the etiology of the disease, there are traditional and growth-friendly surgical methods. The management of rigid and large CEOS patients may not always be possible with the TGR method, which is majorly used in the surgical treatment of EOS disease. Surgery is practiced with the HGR method to solve these problems.

In this section, the literature review on the HGR method will be conducted, and the HGR method will be mentioned in EOS surgery.

## The Use of Hybrid Growing Rod for EOS Patients

Surgical treatment for patients with EOS varies depending on the etiology of the disease, the extent of the curvature, and flexibility. While the "Crankshaft Phenomenon" is progressing in posterior fusion surgery in the growing spine, it can result in iatrogenic thoracic deficiency in patients practicing anterior-posterior fusion; thus, fusion surgery is avoided in the surgical treatment of patients with EOS, and growth-friendly surgical methods are preferred (Elsebai et al., 2011; Emans et al., 2005; Tang et al., 2019; Ruf, 2022). In curvatures in idiopathic, neuromuscular, and syndromic scoliosis of early-onset, successful outcomes are obtained with traditional growing rods (TGR) (Hardesty et al., 2018; Akbarina, 2005). TGR is a distraction-based and growth-friendly method commonly used in patients with EOS. Even though the TGR results for EOS are promising, severe kyphotic deformities may occur in the sagittal plane with sharp-angle scoliosis related to the congenital formation and segmentation of the spine. It is not always possible to provide correction for spinal deformity at the apex of this type of sharp-angled rigid scoliosis of the spine with the TGR method, which can lead to complications such as implant deficiency and loss of correlation related to poor control of the deformity when TGR is practiced.

Even though dual-growing rods can provide more spine growth and better correction with fewer complications than single rods, it is not possible to control large AVT and apex rotation with the TGR method in patients with severe congenital EOS (CEOS) (Thompson, 2005). When patients with severe CEOS with hard congenital vertebral deformities at the apex and with excessive asymmetric growth potential are used in surgical treatment with growing rods, they have an increased risk of implant failure and residual deformity complications. The HGR technique was introduced to approach these problems. The studies indicate that the HGR technique is a good choice to correct curvatures and reduce complications in patients with rigid and severe CEOS (Wnag et al., 2017; Sun et al., 2019).

Different hybrid or modified growing rod methods have been defined as follows: the method of distraction with a single rod on the concave side by hemiepiphysiodesis on the convex side, the dual-growing rod method by short segment fusion of the apex, and the modified TGR method (insertion of pedicle screws without compressing the rod into the apical areas in addition to the TGR method) (Wang et al., 2014; Sun et al., 2019; Enercan et al., 2017; Demirkiran et al., 2016) (Figure 1a,b,c,d, and Figure 2a,b,c,d).

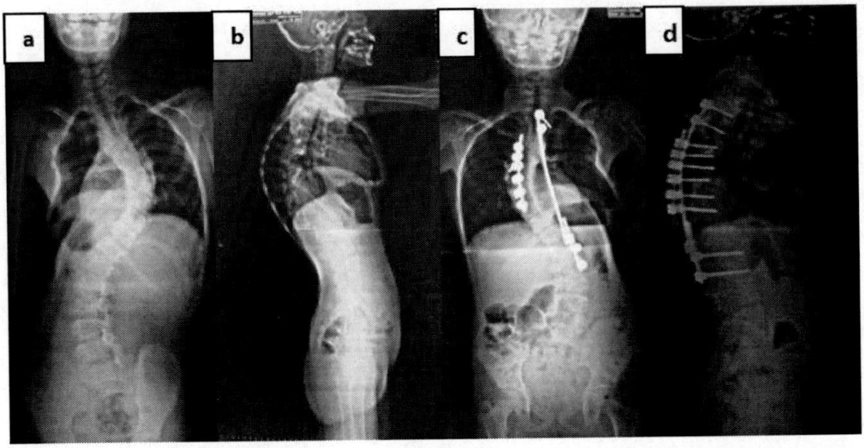


**Figure 1.** Congenital scoliosis. 8-year-old girl. a, b: preoperative posterior-anterior and lateral plain radiography of the spine c. d: postoperative posterior-anterior and lateral plain radiography of the spine.

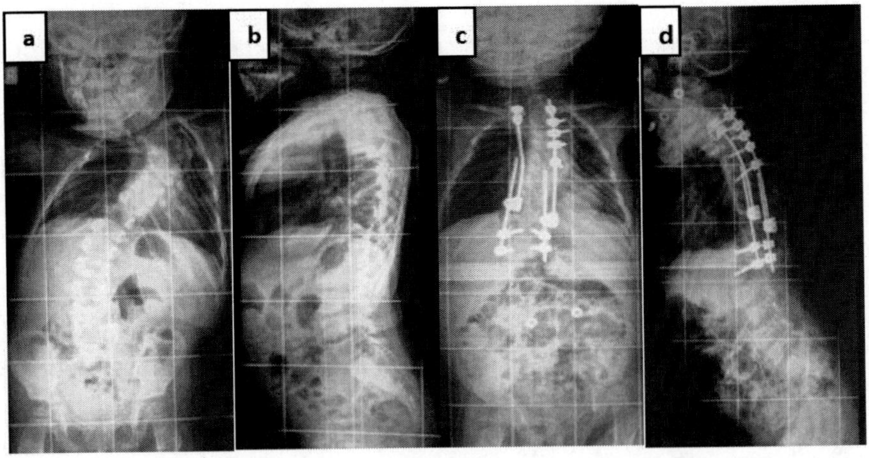


**Figure 2.** Congenital scoliosis. 3.5-year-old girl. a, b: preoperative posterior-anterior and lateral plain radiography of the spine c. d: postoperative posterior-anterior and lateral plain radiography of the spine.

In the study by Wang et al., short-segment fusion with apical vertebrectomy/hemivertebrectomy and dual-growing rods from the cranial and caudal sides of the curvature were practiced. Seven patients with severe CEOS were treated with HGR and the mean curvature improved from 81.4° to 40.1°, and the curvature was 41.0° at the last check-up. They have indicated that the HGR technique may be an option for patients with severe and rigid CEOS (Wang et al., 2014).

As the scoliotic deformity increases in EOS patients with loss of rib cage height, narrowing of the convex hemithorax, and increasing compression of the ribs, it results in hardening of the concave hemithorax, which in the end progresses to lung dysfunction. Rigid and large curvatures severely affect respiratory functions. In these curvatures, the TGR technique may be a choice. However, the asymmetric growth potential caused by sharp deformities at the apex is difficult to prevent and will increase the risk of complications, including implant failures. Various studies have been conducted to approach these problems as "apical fusion" or "apical control" (Enercan et al., 2014; Demirkiran et al., 2016). In the study, which practiced growth procedures with convex hemiepiphysiodesis and a concave distraction technique different from the method of the traditional growing rod, gradual recovery of the primary curvature was defined; however, implant-related complications were known in 8 out of 11 patients (Demirkiran et al., 2016). In this method of convex hemiepiphysiodesis and concave distraction, the control of the apex of curvature also cannot be provided sufficiently.

Because of the possibility of the crankshaft phenomenon, it can only be partially controlled with the TGR technique, even though the biomechanical limitations of simple distraction and serial distraction are used. In advanced deformities, mechanical complications such as rod fracture in the TGR technique, hook dislocation, screw loosening, and stripping, as well as residual deformity and infection have been reported at a rate of more than 50% (Elsebai et al., 2011; Bess et al., 2010).

While apical vertebrectomy/hemivertebrectomy practiced using the HGR technique eliminates the anterior growth potential contributing to the crankshaft phenomenon, the correction can be provided by direct derotation and translation to the apical vertebra of curvatures caused by a defect in the formation or segmentation of the spine. Furthermore, the correction obtained while allowing the spine to grow with the application of TGR with dual rods is protected. Significant recovery in the ratio of lung capacity [space available for lung (SAL)] and AVT in patients with CEOS treated with HGR has been observed in previous studies (Wang et al., 2022).

An important concern with the HGR technique is whether osteotomy and fusion have negative effects on spinal growth. Thompson et al. reported that apical short segmental fusion within growing rods may have a negative effect on spine growth (Thompson et al., 2005). In the study by Wang et al., the annual growth of T1-S1 height was higher in patients with TGR. However, there were no significant differences between patients treated with HGR and TGR at the heights of T1-S1 and T1-12 at their last check-up (Wang et al., 2022).

According to the number of fusion levels practiced in patients with HGR, there can be negative effects on spine growth compared to TGR; however, this relation should be examined in the future with additional patients and long-term follow-ups.

In patients treated with TGR, perioperative neurological complications have rarely been observed. However, when vertebrectomy/ hemivertebrectomy procedures are additionally practiced, it can increase the risk of neurological damage (Wang et al., 2022). Therefore, spinal cord monitoring should be used during initial surgical procedures and growth procedures in patients treated with HGR. In the study by Wang et al., 1 of the 16 patients who had HGR surgery progressed to dura injury, and 1 patient progressed to temporary neurological damage. It is stated that the neurological damage was completely recovered after 1 week of the follow-up of the patients (Wang et al., 2022).

Another concern in patients with EOS treated with the growing rod is whether they can avoid final fusion surgical procedures that may lead to additional complications and revisions (Jain et al., 2016). Autofusion has occurred in most patients treated with TGR, making the spine stiff and relatively stable, and some surgeons have tried to avoid surgical procedures of the final fusion for such patients with acceptable spine alignment (Cahill et al., 2010). They have stopped practicing lengthening procedures and have instead kept growing rods. However, this is not a good option for patients with a large residual curvature and poor spinal alignment by the reason of the limited apex control of the growing rods. In patients treated with HGR, acceptable spine alignment can be achieved and maintained with vertebrectomy/hemivertebrectomy and dual-growing rods. Both short fusions after the osteotomy and autofusion of growing rod-related segments can stabilize the spine. Therefore, final fusion surgical procedures and related complications can be avoided in these patients.

## Conclusion

For EOS patients with severe and rigid curvature, the HGR technique seems to be better than the TGR method in providing correction of spinal deformity. Even though similar results are obtained between HGR and TGR in terms of spine height, the practice of growing rod practiced, in addition to vertebrectomy/hemivertebrectomy, in the apical region in the HGR method will increase the duration of surgery, increase the amount of bleeding, and increase the risk of injury to neurological structures in patients. Therefore, the surgery of the HGR method on EOS patients with severe and rigid curvature should be practiced by experienced spine surgeons.

## Acknowledgments

The figures used in this section are taken from the archive of Professor Dr. Alpaslan Şenköylü, Faculty Member of Orthopedics and Traumatology at the Faculty of Medicine of Gazi University. I would like to express my deepest gratitude to Professor Dr. Alpaslan Şenköylü for his scientific contributions.

## References

Akbarnia, B. A., Marks, D. S., Boachie-Adjei, O., Thompson, A. G., & Asher, M. A. (2005). Dual growing rod technique for the treatment of progressive early-onset scoliosis: a multicenter study. *Spine (Phila Pa 1976), 30*(17), S46–S57. https://doi.org/10.1097/01.brs.0000175190.08134.73.

Bess, S., Akbarnia, B. A., Tu Thompson, G. H., Sponseller, P. D., Shah, S. A., El Sebaie, H., Boachie-Adjei, O., Karlin, L. I., Canale, S., Poe-Kochert, C., Skaggs, D. L. (2010). Complications of growing-rod treatment for early-onset scoliosis: analysis of one hundred and forty patients. *J Bone Joint Surgery Am, 92*(15), 2533–2543. https://doi.org/10.2106/JBJS.I.01471.

Boyden, E. A. (1977). *Development of the lung : Development and growth of the airways.* Marcel Dekker.

Cahill, P. J., Marvil, S., Cuddihy, L., Schutt, C., Idema, J., Clements, D. H., Antonacci, M. D., Asghar, J., Samdani, A. F., Betz, R. R. (2010). Autofusion in the immature spine treated with growing rods. *Spine (Phila Pa 1976), 35*(22), 1199–1203. https://doi.org/10.1097/BRS.0b013e3181e21b50.

Canavese, F., & Dimeglio, A. (2013). Normal and abnormal spine and thoracic cage development. *World J Orthop, 4*(4), 167–174. https://doi.org/10.5312/wjo.v4.i4.167.

Demirkiran, G., Dede, O., Ayvaz, M., Bass, C. E., Alanay, A., Yazici, M. (2016). Convex instrumented hemiepiphysiodesis with concave distraction: a treatment option for long sweeping congenital curves. *J Pediatr Orthop, 36*(3), 226–231. https://doi.org/10.1097/BPO.0000000000000629.

Elsebai, H. B., Yazici, M., Thompson, G. H., Emans, J. B., Skaggs, D. L., Crawford, A. H., Karlin, L. I., McCarthy, R. E., Poe-Kochert, C., Kostial, P., Akbarnia, B. A. (2011). Safety and efficiency of growing rod technique for pediatric congenital spinal deformities. *J Pediatr Orthop, 31*(1), 1–5. https://doi.org/10.1097/BPO.0b013e318202c1dd.

Emans, J. B., Caubet, J. F., Ordonez, C. L., Lee, E. Y, Ciarlo, M. (2005). The treatment of spine and chest wall deformities with fused ribs by expansion thoracostomy and insertion of vertical expandable prosthetic titanium rib: growth of thoracic spine and improvement of lung volumes. *Spine (Phila Pa 1976), 30*(17), S58–S68. https://doi.org/10.1097/01.brs.0000175194.31986.2f.

Enercan, M., Kahraman, S., Erturer, E., Ozturk, C., Hamzaoglu, A. (2014). Apical and intermediate anchors without fusion improve Cobb angle and thoracic kyphosis in early-onset scoliosis. *Clin Orthop Relation Res, 472*(12), 3902–3908. https://doi.org/10.1007/s11999-014-3810-8.

Hardesty, C. K., Huang, R. P., El-Hawary, R., Samdani, A., Hermida, P. B., Bas, T., Balioğlu, M. B., Gurd, D., Pawelek, J., McCarthy, R., Zhu, F., Luhmann, S. (2018). Early-onset scoliosis: updated treatment techniques and results. *Spine Deform, 6*(4), 467–472. https://doi.org/10.1016/j.jspd.2017.12.012.

Jain, A., Sponseller, P. D., Flynn, J. M., Shah, S. A., Tu Thompson, G. H., Means, J. B., Pawelek, J. B., Akbarnia, B. A. (2016). Growing Spine Study Group. Prevention of "Final" Surgical Fusion After Growing-Rod Treatment for Early-Onset Scoliosis. *J Bone Joint Surgery Am, 98*(13), 1073–1078. https://doi.org/10.2106/JBJS.15.01241.

Ruf, M. (2022). *Essentials of Spine Surgery: Congenital Scoliosis.* (Senkoylu, A., & Canavese, F., Eds.). Springer Nature Switzerland AG. https://doi.org/10.1007/978-3-030-80356-8.

Sun, X., Xu, L., Chen, Z., Shi, B., Chen, X., Li, S., Du, C., Zhou, Q., Qiu, Y., Zhu, Z. (2019). Hybrid Growing Rod Technique of Osteotomy with Short Fusion and Spinal Distraction: An Alternative Solution for Long-Spanned Congenital Scoliosis. *Spine (Phila Pa 1976), 44*(10), 707–714. https://doi.org/10.1097/BRS.0000000000002933.

Swank, S. M., Winter, R. B., Moe, J. H. (1982). Scoliosis and cor pulmonale. *Spine (Phila Pa 1976), 7*(4), 343–354.

Tang, N., Zhao, H., Shen, J. X., Zhang, J. G., Li, S. G. (2019). Magnetically controlled growing rod for early-onset scoliosis: systematic review and meta-analysis. *World Neurosurgery, 125*, 593–601. https://doi.org/10.1016/j.wneu.2019.01.153.

Thompson, G. H., Akbarnia, B. A., Kostial, P., Poe-Kochert, C., Armstrong, D. G., Roh, J., Lowe, R., Asher, M. A., Marks, D. S. (2005). Comparison of single and dual growing rod techniques followed through definitive surgery: a preliminary study. *Spine (Phila Pa 1976), 30*(18), 2039–2044. https://doi.org/10.1097/01.brs.0000179082.92712.89.

Wang, S., Zhang, J., Qiu, G., Wang, Y., Weng, X., Guo, J. (2014). One-stage posterior osteotomy with short segmental fusion and dual growing rod technique for severe rigid congenital scoliosis: the preliminary clinical outcomes of a hybrid technique. *Spine (Phila Pa 1976), 39*(4), 294–299.

Wang, S., Zhao, Y., Yang, Y., Lin, G., Shen, J., Zhao, Y., Wu, N., Zhuang, Q., Du, Y., Zhang, J. (2022). Hybrid technique versus traditional dual growing rod technique to treat congenital early-onset scoliosis: a comparative study with more than 3 years of follow-up. *J Neurosurgery of the Spine*, 38_(2), 199–207. https://doi.org/10.3171/2022.8.SPINE22618.

# Chapter 23

# Staple

**Erkan Akgün[1,*], MD**
Department of Etlik City Hospital, Ankara, Türkiye

## Abstract

Treatment of patients with early-onset scoliosis (EOS) still poses considerable challenges for clinicians dealing with spinal diseases. Most patients with EOS are treated with regular follow-up or brace use, accompanied by physiotherapy. Brace treatments such as thoracolumbosacral orthosis (TLSO) represent standard treatment methods in idiopathic scoliosis patients with a Cobb angle of more than 20°. Brace treatment is known to partially correct the deformity, and some studies show that 50% of patients who use braces benefit from treatment. However, problems related to difficulties in the use of brace treatment reduce the effectiveness of the treatment. The fact that patients have to use braces almost all day for years until their skeletal maturation is complete adversely influences the long-term effectiveness of the treatment. This situation has forced clinicians to search for alternative treatment methods. The anterior, unilateral vertebral body stapling (VBS) method, one of these alternative treatment methods, has the potential to correct built-in deformities in the treatment of moderate idiopathic scoliosis (a Cobb angle of 20-40°) and is superior to brace treatment due to the absence of compliance problems with treatment. Moreover, the advantages of VBS compared to other surgical treatments that require fusion are that it allows fusionless growth modulation and is applied as minimally invasive (thoracic vertebrae) and mini-open (lumbar vertebrae). The development of pneumothorax during surgery, implant problems, postoperative wound healing problems, and temporary

* Corresponding Author's Email: akgün@gmail.com.

In: Early Onset Scoliosis
Editor: Ahmed Majid Heydar
ISBN: 979-8-89113-600-7

reduced pulmonary dysfunction can be listed among the disadvantages of VBS treatment.

**Keywords:** scoliosis, growth-friendly, vertebral body staple, brace

## Introduction

EOS is a condition characterized by spinal deformities in the coronal, sagittal, and axial planes that occur before the age of 10. Although the etiology of EOS is not completely understood, it is thought to occur because of different growth rates between the anterior and posterior elements of the spine (Dicson et al., 1984). EOS is etiologically divided into five categories: idiopathic, congenital, neuromuscular, thoracogenic, and syndromic (El-Hawary & Akbarnia, 2015). The objective of treatment in patients with EOS should be to stop the progression of the deformity, preserve the mobility of the spine, and maintain the normal growth and development of the patient. There are two main treatment methods, conservative and surgical, in treating patients with EOS. Follow-up and brace support treatments, such as TLSO, accompanied by physiotherapy, are the most widely used among conservative methods. Various studies have demonstrated that physiotherapy alone is no sufficient in patients with completed skeletal maturation (Zhang & Zhang, 2020; Cyr et al., 2017). Since bracing is a non-invasive method in patients with EOS, it continues to be the main treatment concept (Weinstein et al., 2013). Nevertheless, the success of treatment depends on numerous internal and external factors, which include the state of skeletal maturity, the degree of the Cobb angle, the degree of vertebral rotation, and thoracic scoliosis (Hawary et al., 2019). Therefore, treatment fails in 50% of patients and progression continues in one-third of curvatures (Thometz et al., 2018; Moreau et al., 2014). Difficulties in application represent another important problem in the use of braces. The fact that patients spend years and almost all day using braces causes adaptation problems with time and causes treatment failure in the early period. Creating psychological trauma in children is another negative aspect (Noonan et al., 1996). The negative aspects mentioned above of brace treatments direct researchers and clinicians dealing with spine surgery to alternative treatments. Surgical treatments have been used with increasing frequency in patients with EOS in recent years. Surgical treatments providing long spinal fusion have been observed to cause problems in long-term growth modulation, particularly leading to pulmonary dysfunction in patients with

EOS (Senkoylu et al., 2014; Nathan et al., 2015). These severe complications have brought fusionless, growth-friendly surgical treatments to the agenda. Due to this advantage, fusionless surgical treatments have focused on addressing progressive scoliosis in children with incomplete skeletal maturity, and various techniques have been described. The main purpose of these techniques is to preserve the spine growth of patients, prevent the progression of the disease during growth, and correct the deformity. This is achieved through various mechanisms. The most important of these are compression-based methods, and this mechanism is used in VBS and vertebral body tethering (VBT). Traditional or magnetic growing rods are another method that provides correction with the distraction method. Both methods take their basic scientific foundation from the Hueter-Volkmann law, which states that the compression and distraction forces applied to the epiphyseal growth axis impact growth (Stokes et al., 1996; Roaf, 1960). According to the said law, whereas compression forces suppress epiphyseal growth, distraction forces stimulate growth.

## Main Text

New methods and tools in the diagnosis and treatment of EOS increase every day due to the rapid increase in medical information about EOS. EOS generally describes a spinal deformity and begins under 10 years of age. Etiologically, EOS has five different types: idiopathic, congenital, neuromuscular, thoracogenic, and syndromic (El Hawary & Akbarnia, 2015). There is still no standard treatment algorithm because of the different etiologies in patients with EOS. Different treatment methods are applied alone or in combination depending on the etiology, degree of curvature and progression rate, the presence of kyphosis, and bone maturity (El Hawary & Akbarnia, 2015; Cyr et al., 2017; Williams et al., 2014). Along with recent advancements in patients with EOS, the purpose of treatment should be to maintain lung functions by providing an adequate thoracic volume and reducing the deformity in the spine as much as possible (Karol et al., 2008). Two main treatment methods have been described for EOS patients. The non-operative treatment method, which includes bracing and plaster casting, is the first of them (Gussous et al., 2015; Weinstein et al., 2013). Surgical treatments represent the other treatment option. These are performed using two methods, with and without fusion. Nevertheless, clinical studies have demonstrated that fusion techniques lead to severe pulmonary function disorders in the future

(Gussous et al., 2015; Canavase & Dimeglio, 2013). Hence, techniques known as growth-friendly approaches have become more popular in patients with incomplete skeletal maturity. One of these treatment methods is the VBS method, which has been researched for many years and has been the subject of numerous studies with animal models and clinical studies. The VBS technique applied in EOS patients is based on the Hueter-Volkmann principle and has been applied in animal experiments before scoliosis patients through increased pressure that inhibits epiphyseal enchondral growth or decreased pressure that stimulates growth (Blount, 1971). It is planned that when VBS treatment is applied mechanically to the convex side in scoliosis patients, it stops growth through asymmetric forcing by ensuring an increase in pressure and corrects spinal deformities over time by allowing growth on the opposite concave side (Fletcher & Bruce, 2012). In 1951, Nachlas and Borden applied the VBS technique to 19 models of canine scoliosis and demonstrated that there was an improvement at varying rates in many dogs and progression stopped in some dogs (Nachlas & Borden, 1951). It has been reported that VBS treatment has been applied successfully in bovine and porcine scoliosis models over time (Newton et al., 2008; Braun et al., 2005). In 1954, Smith et al. applied VBS to 3 patients with congenital scoliosis, which resulted in failure because some staples broke or loosened. However, the combination of the design and material content of implants at that time with poor surgical techniques and the fact that all patients enrolled in the study had advanced congenital scoliosis explain why the study failed (Smith et al., 1954). In their next study, Betz et al. applied VBS to 26 patients with thoracic and 15 lumbar curvatures, and the success rate in thoracic curvatures was 77%, whereas this rate was 83% in lumbar curvatures (Betz et al., 2010). VBS treatment has been defined as a treatment method allowing fusionless growth modulation owing to advancements in implant technology and surgical techniques in the last two decades. A dynamic compression shape memory alloy (SMA) staple has become one of the FDA (USA) approved and commonly used VBS implants. The mentioned implants are made of a nickel-titanium alloy called nitinol, have shape memory, are temperature dependent, and are used off-label. The unique feature of these nitinol staples is that the staple ends are flat when cooled, while the ends curl into a C-shape at body temperature. Due to the advantages mentioned above, it leads to an easier application during surgery and creates a tighter compressive effect afterward, and thus implant failure in VBS treatments made with the first stainless steel staples is prevented to a considerable extent (Tis et al., 2012). Some recent animal and biomechanical studies support this opinion. In an animal experiment comparing VBT and

VBS methods, among fusionless scoliosis treatments, fixation failures were compared, and it was demonstrated that staple fixation was 5 times stronger than screw fixation against both cyclic and non-cyclic forces (Yaszay et al., 2017). Spine surgeons have brought VBS treatment to the agenda since the beginning of the 2000s, and it has started to be used more frequently. VBS treatment, a fusionless scoliosis surgery, has become one of the treatment options for clinicians as an alternative, especially in patients with incomplete bone maturation. Nowadays, bracing is still the primary treatment for patients EOS. Nevertheless, fusionless scoliosis surgeries, such as VBS and VBT, are applied in 50% of the patients due to the progression of scoliosis degrees despite the treatment and the difficulty of adaptation to the use of braces or the refusal of families to use braces. Skeletal immaturity is one of the indication criteria, in general, in VBS treatment, although it differs among clinics. Accordingly, patients with skeletal immaturity (a Risser sign of 0 or 1) under the age of 13 among females, under the age of 15 among males, or with idiopathic scoliosis are candidates for fusionless scoliosis surgery. The other indication criteria are as follows; thoracic curvature <35°, lumbar curvature 20-45°, thoracic kyphosis <40°, axial rotation <20°, and flexibility <20° in coronal imaging (Trobisch et al., 2011). Contraindications include patients with congenital scoliosis, scoliosis with thoracic curvature (peak Cobb level) above T4 or below L4, and thoracic kyphosis greater than 40 degrees. In patients with thoracic kyphosis greater than 40 degrees, it can be used in combination with growth-friendly techniques such as vertical expandable prosthetic titanium rib (VEPTR) or magnetic growing rod (MGR) systems (Trobisch et al., 2011; Ahmad, 2020).The most significant advantage distinguishing the VBS technique from other growth-friendly fusionless techniques (VEPRT, MGR, VBT) is that it can be applied minimally invasively (thoracoscopic) in the thoracic region and mini-open retroperitoneally in the lumbar region, and its effectiveness starts immediately after surgery (Trobisch et al., 2011). Betz et al. applied the VBS technique thoracoscopically to a series of 21 patients in 2003 and shared the results. All patients were placed in the lateral decubitus position with the convex side of the deformity. A chest tube was placed in all patients. Then the imaging portals were opened from the 5th and 7th intercostal spaces in the anterolateral of the chest wall under fluoroscopy. Afterward, the researchers described that this procedure could be performed by opening additional portals to place staples along the posterior axillary line, or by performing T4-5 and T9-10-centered mini-thoracotomy instead. They used retroperitoneal mini-incisions at the lumbar level (Betz et al., 2003). As a result, Betz et al. stated that this method was a safe and applicable method that could be compared to brace treatment. Over time, it has been argued that VBS can be an alternative to VBT in treating EOS with changes in techniques and methods. Betz et al. in 2010 and Trobisch et al. in 2011 applied the thoracoscopic VBS technique to their patient series and achieved a success rate above 80% in lumbar curvatures in both series. In the same study, Trobisch et al. reported a success rate of 78% in thoracic curvatures of less than 35°(Trobisch et al., 2011; Betz et al., 2010). Staples used in the VBS technique are made of nitinol (nickel-titanium alloy), a special biocompatible shape memory alloy, and are kept in sterile cold water prior to surgery. Staples with the smallest possible width to cover the disc and epiphyses are determined and placed under fluoroscopy with the help of a guide. Staples with flat ends in the cooled state take the C-shape at body temperature, creating a compressive effect (Laituri et al., 2012). All levels with the main curvature are stapled in this way. It has been reported that anesthesia- and surgery-related complications are among the early complications of the VBS technique (Trobisch et al., 2011; Betz et al., 2010; Laituri et al., 2012). The complications that develop due to the implant and the surgical technique are the most important among them. Various studies have detected implant failures of up to 30%. Some of these patients underwent additional surgical procedures to remove the implant (Trupia et al., 2019; Lavelle et al., 2011). Diaphragmatic injuries and cases of superior mesenteric artery syndrome have been reported, although rarely in patients undergoing thoracoscopic VBS (Trobisch et al., 2011). Surgical wound problems are also among the early postoperative complications. There are few studies on the long-term clinical outcomes of the VBS technique. Smith et al. associated congenital scoliosis and rotational deformities accompanying severe deformities with poor outcomes (Braun et al., 2005). Betz et al. indicated that the deformity was stable in 87% of the patients in their one-year follow-up but did not specify the long-term outcomes (Betz et al., 2003). In a series of 7 patients, Muray et al. (2019) followed up the patients to whom they applied VBS treatment for an average of 83 months, compared the growth rates between the side that was stapled and the side that was not applied, and indicated no significant differences between them (Murray et al., 2020). In another clinical study, Trupia et al. reported the long-term outcomes of the 10-patient series to whom they applied VBS treatment in 2019. According to the study, the researchers concluded that there was no significant difference between VBS treatment and brace treatment. Furthermore, numerous studies have shown that treatments requiring fusion should be applied as scoliosis deformity cannot be stopped long-term after VBS in the treatment of EOS.

This rate can reach up to 30% in some studies, depending on the etiology of scoliosis and the degree of curvature in the selected patients (Bumpass et al., 2015).

## Conclusion

Since EOS patients constitute a heterogeneous group in terms of etiology and deformities, there are still significant difficulties in their treatment and an accepted common treatment algorithm is still absent. Hence, there is a very wide range of treatments. The consensus among clinicians in the treatment of EOS is to use a method that allows thoracic growth without harming pulmonary functions, preserves spinal mobility, can be easily applied by clinicians, and in which patients can easily adapt to treatment (Betz et al., 2010, 36). VBS treatment is used as an alternative treatment method in patients who cannot tolerate treatment with brace methods. With the use of shape-memory staplers, it has started to be applied more easily and reliably, and the problems due to implant failure in the past decreased considerably. Both the development of the thoracic cavity and the preservation of pulmonary functions are provided with its fusionless application. The preservation of spinal mobility is another advantage. Owing to its thoracoscopic (thoracic) and mini-open (lumbar) application, it results in fewer wound problems and incision scars. The VBS technique does not constitute an obstacle to scoliosis surgeries that may be required in the future. If the curvature progresses after VBS surgery, fusion procedures can be applied when necessary. Although short-term outcomes have reported success in thoracic and lumbar curvatures at a rate reaching 80%, there is not much information in the literature on long-term outcomes. However, as a result of clinical studies, fusionless treatments come to the forefront in patients with incomplete skeletal maturity (a Risser sign<2) who cannot adapt to brace treatment. VBS treatment represents a good alternative treatment method in patients with thoracic and lumbar curvatures below 40°, axial rotation below 20°, and thoracic kyphosis below 40°.

## References

Ahmad, A. A. (2020). Early onset scoliosis and current treatment methods. *J Clin Orthop Trauma, 11*(2), 184-190. https://doi.org/10.1016/j.jcot.2019.12.01.

Aldrete, J. A. (1995). The post-anesthesia recovery score revisited. *Journal of Clinical Anesthesia, 7*(1), 89-91. https://doi.org/10.1016/0952-8180(94)00001-k.

Betz, R. R., Kim, J., D'Andrea, L. P., Mulcahey, M. J., Balsara, R. K., & Clements, D. H. (2003). An innovative technique of vertebral body stapling for the treatment of patients with adolescent idiopathic scoliosis: A feasibility, safety, and utility study. *Spine (Phila Pa 1976), 28*(20), 255-65. https://doi.org/10.1097/01.BRS.0000092484.31316.32.

Betz, R. R., Ranade, A., Samdani, A. F., Chafetz, R., D'Andrea, L. P., Gaughan, J. P., Asghar, J., Grewal, H., & Mulcahey, M. J. (2010). Vertebral body stapling: a fusionless treatment option for a growing child with moderate idiopathic scoliosis. *Spine (Phila Pa 1976), 35*(2), 169-76. https://doi.org/10.1097/BRS.0b013e3181c6dff5.

Braun, J. T., Akyuz, E., & Ogilvie, J. W. (2005). The use of animal models in fusionless scoliosis investigations. *Spine (Phila Pa 1976), 30*(17), S35-e45. https://doi.org/10.1097/01.brs.0000175187.61474.9a.

Cyr, M., Hilaire, T. S., Pan, Z., Thompson, G. H., Vitale, M. G., & Garg, S. (2017). Classification of early onset scoliosis has excellent interobserver and intraobserver reliability. *J Pediatr Orthop, 37*, e1-e3. https://doi.org/10.1097/BPO.0000000000000688.

Dicson, R. A., Lawton, J. O., Archer, I. A., & Butt, W. P. (1984). The pathogenesis of idiopathic scoliosis. Biplanar spinal asymmetry. *J Bone Joint Surg Br, 66*(1), 8-15. https://doi.org/10.1302/0301-620X.66B1.6693483.

Eardley, N., Harris, N., Zachary, M., Cundy, P. J., & Gieroba, T. J. (2015). The effectiveness of selective thoracic fusion for treating adolescent idiopathic scoliosis: a systematic review protocol. *JBI Database System Rev Implement Rep, 13*(11), 4-16. https://doi.org/10.11124/jbisrir-2015-2338.

El-Hawary, R., & Akbarnia, B. A. (2015). Early onset scoliosis - time for consensus. *Spine Deform, 3*, 105-106. https://doi.org/10.1016/j.jspd.2015.01.003.

Fletcher, N. D., & Bruce, R. W. (2012). Early onset scoliosis: current concepts and controversies. *Curr Rev Musculoskelet Med, 5*(2), 102-10. https://doi.org/10.1007/s12178-012-9116-0.

Hawary, R. E., Zaaroor-Regev, D., Floman, Y., Lonner, B. S., Alkhalife, Y. I., & Betz, R. R. (2019). Brace treatment in adolescent idiopathic scoliosis: risk factors for failure-a literature review. *Spine J, 19*(12), 1917-1925. https://doi.org/10.1016/j.spinee.2019.07.008.

Jackson, L. M. (2019). *The psychology of prejudice: From attitudes to social action* (2nd ed.). American Psychological Association. https://doi.org/10.1037/0000168-000.

Kim, Y. M., Kang, C., Joo, Y. B., & Lee, S. H. (2019). The role of ultrasound-guided single-shot femoral and sciatic nerve blocks on pain management after total knee arthroplasty. *Knee, 26*(4), 881-888. https://doi.org/10.1016/j.knee.2019.05.002.

Laituri, C. A., Schwend, R. M., & Holcomb, G. W. (2012). Thoracoscopic vertebral body stapling for treatment of scoliosis in young children. *J Laparoendosc Adv Surg Tech A, 22*(8), 830-3. https://doi.org/10.1089/lap.2011.0289.

Lavelle, W. F., Samdani, A. F., Cahill, P. J., & Betz, R. R. (2011). Clinical outcomes of nitinol staples for preventing curve progression in idiopathic scoliosis. *J Pediatr Orthop, 31*(1), S107-13. https://doi.org/10.1097/BPO.0b013e3181ff9a4d.

Moreau, S., Lonjon, G., Mazda, K., & Ilharreborde, B. (2014). Detorsion night-time bracing for the treatment of early onset idiopathic scoliosis. *Orthop Traumatol Surg Res, 100*, 935-939. https://doi.org/10.1016/j.otsr.2014.05.024.

Motoyama, E. K., Deeney, V. F., Fine, G. F., Yang, C. I., Mutich, R. L., Walczak, S. A., & Moreland, M. S. (2006). Effects on lung function of multiple expansion thoracoplasty in children with thoracic insufficiency syndrome: a longitudinal study. *Spine, 31*, 284–290. https://doi.org/10.1097/01.brs.0000197203.76653.d0.

Murray, E., Tung, R., Sherman, A. I., & Schwend, R. M. (2020). Continued vertebral body growth in patients with juvenile idiopathic scoliosis following vertebral body stapling. *Spine Deform, 8*(2), 221-226. https://doi.org/10.1007/s43390-019-00019-x.

Nachlas, I. W., & Borden, J. N. (1951). The cure of experimental scoliosis by directed growth control. *J Bone Joint Surg Am, 33*, 24–34.

Newton, P. O., Farnsworth, C. L., Faro, F. D., Shapiro, G. S., Mohamad, F., Parent, S., & Fricka, K. (2008). Spinal growth modulation with an anterolateral flexible tether in an immature bovine model. *Spine (Phila Pa 1976), 33*, 724–733. https://doi.org/10.1097/01.brs.0000188267.66847.bf.

Noonan, K. J., Weinstein, S. L., Jacobson, W. C., & Dolan, L. A. (1996). Use of the Milwaukee brace for progressive idiopathic scoliosis. *J Bone Joint Surg Am, 78*(4), 557-67. https://doi.org/10.2106/00004623-199604000-00009.

Rattan, A. (2019). How lay theories (or mindsets) shape the confrontation of prejudice. In R. K. Mallett & M. J. Monteith (Eds.), *Confronting prejudice and discrimination: The science of changing minds and behaviors* (pp. 121-140). Academic Press. https://doi.org/10.1016/B978-0-12-814715-3.00008-4.

Senkoylu, A., Luk, K. D., Wong, Y. W., & Cheung, K. M. (2014). Prognosis of spontaneous thoracic curve correction after the selective anterior fusion of thoracolumbar/lumbar (Lenke 5C) curves in idiopathic scoliosis. *Spine J, 14*(7), 1117-24. https://doi.org/10.1016/j.spinee.2013.07.467.

Smith, A. D., Von Lackum, W. H., & Wylie, R. (1954). An operation for stapling vertebral bodies in congenital scoliosis. *J Bone Joint Surg Am, 36*, 342–348. https://doi.org/10.2106/00004623-195436020-00011.

Thometz, J., Liu, X., Rizza, R., English, I., & Tarima, S. (2018). Effect of an elongation bending derotation brace on the infantile or juvenile scoliosis. *Scoliosis Spinal Disord, 13*, 13. https://doi.org/10.1186/s13013-018-0160-4.

Tis, J. E., Karlin, L. I., Akbarnia, B. A., Blakemore, L. C., Thompson, G. H., McCarthy, R. E., Tello, C. A., Mendelow, M. J., & Southern, E. P. (2012). Early onset scoliosis: modern treatment and results. *J Pediatr Orthop, 32*, 647–657. https://doi.org/10.1097/BPO.0b013e3182694f18.

Trobisch, P. D., Samdani, A., Cahill, P., & Betz, R. R. (2011). Vertebral body stapling as an alternative in the treatment of idiopathic scoliosis. *Oper Orthop Traumatol, 23*, 227–231. https://doi.org/10.1007/s00064-011-0032-z.

Trupia, E., Hsu, A. C., Mueller, D. J., Matsumoto, H., Bodenstein, L., & Vitale, M. (2019). Treatment of Idiopathic Scoliosis with Vertebral Body Stapling. *Spine Deform, 7*(5), 720-728. https://doi.org/10.1016/j.jspd.2019.01.006.

Weinstein, S. L., Dolan, L. A., Wright, J. G., & Dobbs, M. B. (2013). Effects of bracing in adolescents with idiopathic scoliosis. *N Engl J Med, 369*, 1512–1521. https://doi.org/10.1056/NEJMoa1307337.

Yaszay, B., Doan, J. D., Parvaresh, K. C., Farnsworth, C. L. (2017). Risk of Implant Loosening After Cyclic Loading of Fusionless Growth Modulation Techniques: Nitinol Staples Versus Flexible Tether. *Spine (Phila Pa 1976), 42*(7), 443-449. https://doi.org/10.1097/BRS.0000000000001809.

Zhang, Y. B., & Zhang, J. G. (2020). Treatment of early-onset scoliosis: techniques, indications, and complications. *Chinese Medical Journal (Engl), 133*(3), 351-57. https://doi.org/10.1097/CM9.0000000000000614.

# Chapter 24

# Anterior Vertebral Body Tethering

**Abdülhalim Akar***, **MD**
Department of Orthopedics and Traumatology, Private Emsey Hospital, Istanbul, Turkiye

## Abstract

The purpose of the treatment of scoliosis is to correct the 3-dimensional deformity without disturbing the development of the spine and chest. Especially at early ages, fusion surgery restricts lung development and height increase and irreversibly reduces the mobility of patients. For this reason, growth-friendly methods have been developed. Anterior vertebral body tethering (AVBT) may be a good option in these patients. AVBT surgery has become widespread in recent years, as patients return to sport quickly and maintain mobility. Discussions about surgical indications continue. In general, it is recommended to be used in skeletally immature patients with a Risser score of 0-2, a Sanders score of 2-4 and a Cobb angle between 35° and 65°. Many complications have been reported in the literature. Thread breakage is the most common mechanical complication. Thread breaks, especially in the first 12 months, cause loss of correction. Pulmonary complications are the most common non-mechanical complications. Although pulmonary complications are common, it has been reported that these complications are not permanent. However, since it is a relatively new technique, long-term studies are needed.

**Keywords:** vertebral body tethering, indications, complications, surgical technique

* Corresponding Author's Email: ahalimakar@gmail.com.

In: Early Onset Scoliosis
Editor: Ahmed Majid Heydar
ISBN: 979-8-89113-600-7

## Introduction

Early-onset scoliosis (EOS) is defined as curvatures of the spine that are seen in patients under 10 years of age and have a tendency to increase rapidly. When looking at etiology, causes such as idiopathic, syndromic, congenital, or neuromuscular have been shown (Williams et al., 2014). Scoliosis is a 3-dimensional deformity in which lateral deviation, reduced kyphosis, and rotation are seen together. As a general approach, it is predicted that the curvature will increase in curves exceeding 40 degrees, and surgical treatment is recommended (Weinstein et al., 1981). It has been reported that lung capacity decreases in patients with thoracic curves of more than 50° (Newton et al., 2005). In the treatment of EOS, brace, physical therapy, and angulation methods are used as conservative treatment. Surgical treatments may be required, especially in patients with advanced curvature or in cases where conservative treatment is insufficient. The gold standard in the treatment of scoliosis is posterior spinal fusion surgery (Ghandhari et al., 2018). Fusion surgery performed at an early age limits spinal growth, lung development, and trunk growth. Additionally, the limitation of spinal movements that will occur after fusion causes concern in patients and their families (Marks et al., 2012). Compared to the normal population, patients undergoing spinal fusion have decreased functional results (Helenius et al., 2019). Therefore, surgeries that both correct scoliosis and preserve movement have been developed in recent years. AVBT is a new technology that was approved by the FDA in August 2019 as a treatment for scoliosis in skeletally immature patients.

Anterior vertebral body tethering has been used for the last 20 years as fusion-free surgery that allows the patient to grow. It has been reported that patients return to their daily activities and sports in the early period after surgery (Baroncini et al., 2021). AVBT surgery is basically based on the Heuter Volkmann principle (Mehlman et al., 1997). The tension is applied to the convex side of the curve with a rope and screw system, thereby restricting the growth of the convex side. The concave side continues to grow normally, thus reducing the curvature (Bonsignore-Opp et al., 2019; Stokes et al., 1996).

## Indications

AVBT surgical indications are still controversial in the literature, and there is no definite consensus. AVBT should be administered to patients aged 8 to 16 years, regardless of gender. There is no definitive method to show the growth potential or final height of patients. Predictions can be made from the pelvis, hand, shoulder, and elbow radiographs from patients. The Risser scoring system based on pelvis apophysis ossification and the Sanders scoring system based on the development of hand bones are the most commonly used methods. These two methods are the most commonly used and reliable methods for estimating the growth potential of the patient. Patients with a Risser score of 0-2 and a Sanders score of 2-4 are considered to have ideal bone development for AVBT surgery (Risser, 1958; Sanders et al., 2008a). In particular, the Sanders scoring has been shown to be very effective in determining the growth potential of the patient and the progression of the curvature (Sanders et al., 2008b; Sitoula et al., 2015). The timing of surgery is of critical importance. In early surgeries, overcorrection may occur, and rope breakage may occur in late surgeries (Senkoylu et al., 2020).

Patients whose cobb angle is between 45-65° in measurements taken on standing scoliosis radiographs, whose bending radiographs are flexible with an absolute improvement of more than 30%, and whose rib hump is less than 20° are suitable for AVBT surgery (Newton, 2020a; Takahashi et al., 2021).

## Surgical Procedure

We administer total intravenous anesthesia to patients in our own clinic. All patients are connected to a neuromonitor and followed up throughout the surgery. The use of a neuromonitor is very effective in preventing possible neurological damage. A double-lumen intubation tube that allows ventilation of one lung is used and the patients are placed in the lateral decubitus position with the apex of the curve on the upper side. In patients who need double-side VBT, we start at the thoracic level first (Figure 1). The patient's height, underarm, knees, and elbows are supported by soft silicone pillows. We make sure that there is no pressure. Before starting the surgery, the spinal levels of the patient are confirmed by fluoroscopy and marked on the skin. The ribs in the surgical area are palpated by hand and drawn on the skin with the help of a marker. AVBT surgery is a surgery that requires a thoracotomy or a thoracoscopy (Figure 2). We mostly prefer the thoracoscopy method in our own clinic. Usually, 3 or 4 portals are used; anterolateral portals are used for imaging, and posterolateral portals are used as working portals. After the lung is deflated, the vertebral bodies appear. All segmental vessels are seen and first compressed with the help of a clamp. If there is no change in the neuromonitor, the segmental vessels are coagulated. The rib heads are used as a benchmark for the ideal screw entry point. Staples are placed just anterior to the rib heads, and then screws are placed. The length of the screws is determined by a feeler and checked with fluoroscopy. A suitable size and screw size are preferred for each patient. Both the monitor and fluoroscopy control are provided at every stage of implantation. Care is taken to ensure that the screws are especially parallel to the endplates. In cases where the diaphragm is passed, it is opened by leaving a distance of approximately 1 cm from the vertebral body so that the diaphragm can be repaired after the procedure. After the Cobb-to-Cobb screws are placed, starting from the most distal, the thread is stretched and advanced towards the proximal. After being made parallel to the endplates, it is checked with fluoroscopy. After the correction is achieved, the lung on the operating side is ventilated again.

In patients with both thoracic and lumbar curvature, double-side AVBT surgery is preferred. If double-side AVBT is to be performed, the patient is turned to the other side and placed in the lateral decubitus position again. Using the mini-open retroperitoneal approach, the external oblique, internal oblique, and transverse fascia are passed. After the psoas muscle is passed, the vertebral corpuscles are reached. After the Cobb-to-Cobb screws are placed, the stretching process is performed again, and the correction is checked with a fluoroscopy. After the chest tube is placed, the closure is started. The chest tube is inserted through a different incision than the skin incision. First, the pleura is repaired and then the layers are closed anatomically. Care is taken to avoid including the intercostal nerves in the suture. After the skin is repaired, the surgery is terminated.

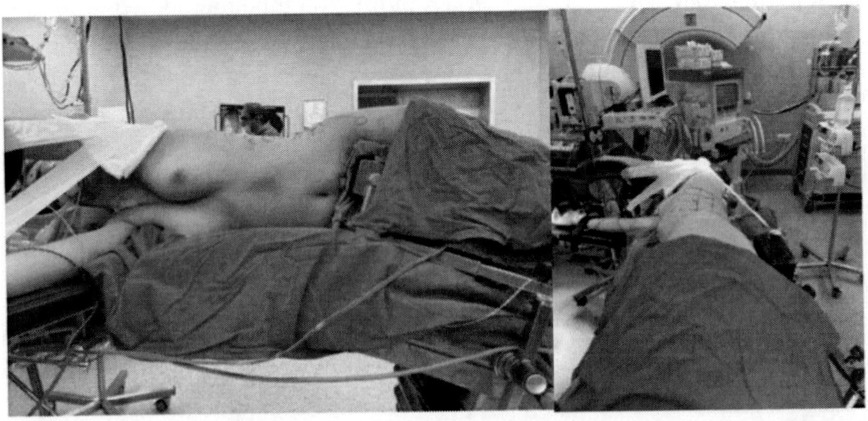

**Figure 1.** Positioning of the Patient and Operation Table (Author's own archive).

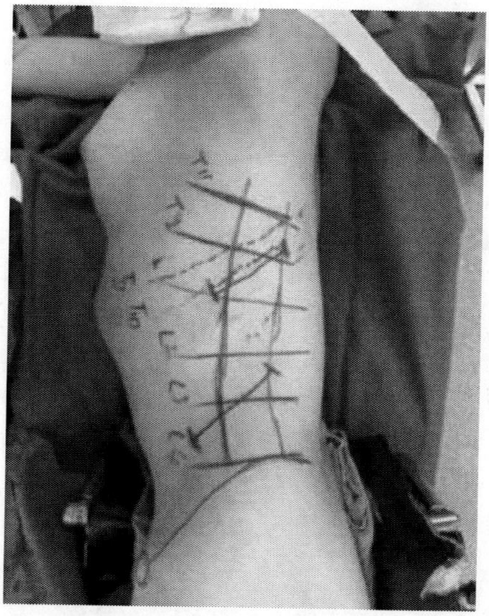

**Figure 2.** Vertebral Levels and Ribs Marked on the Skin (Author's own archive).

## Post-Operative Rehabilitation

In our own clinic, we provide detailed information for patients about the pre-operative and post-operative process and prepare patients mentally for the post-operative period. We started triflow exercises before the surgery and continued until the 6th week after the surgery. Patients are mobilized on the 1st day after surgery by a physiotherapist who is specialized in the spine. Patients with a chest tube are evaluated with a daily chest X-ray. The patient should be closely followed in the first days in terms of pulmonary complications. The chest tube is kept until there is less than 100 cc coming from the tube. After the tube is removed, we discharge the patients. We do not allow the patient to do sport activies or receive physical therapy for the first 3 months. After the 3rd month, the patient can start exercises such as swimming and non-contact sports. We take scoliosis radiographs every month for the first 6 months. After the 6th month, the 1st year radiograph is taken, and then the annual follow-ups continue.

## Case Examples

Examples of two cases with appropriate indications for AVBT;

Case 1: A 12-year-old female patient. The preoperative evaluation revealed isolated thoracic curvature. The Cobb angle is 43°, and the curvature is flexible. Preoperative and 2-year follow-up radiographs are as follows (Figure 3).

Case 2: An 11-year-old female patient had flexible curvature in the double major pattern. Preoperatively, the thoracic Cobb angle was 44° and the lumbar Cobb angle was 57°. The pre-operative and most recent 3rd year follow-up radiographs are as follows (Figure 4).

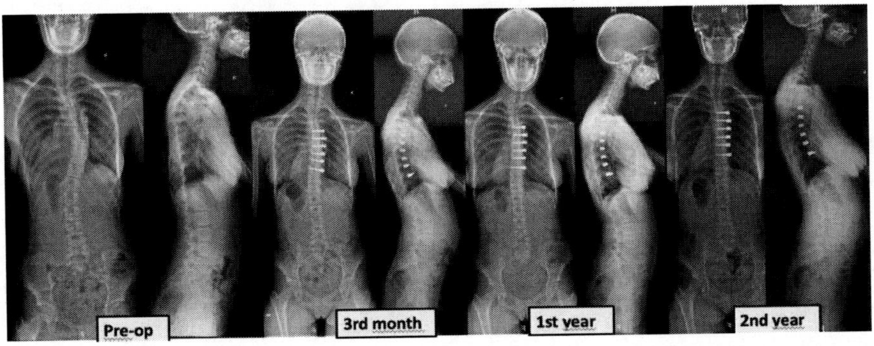


**Figure 3.** Case 1; 2-year follow-up radiographs of a 12-year-old female patient who underwent thoracic VBT (Author's own archive).

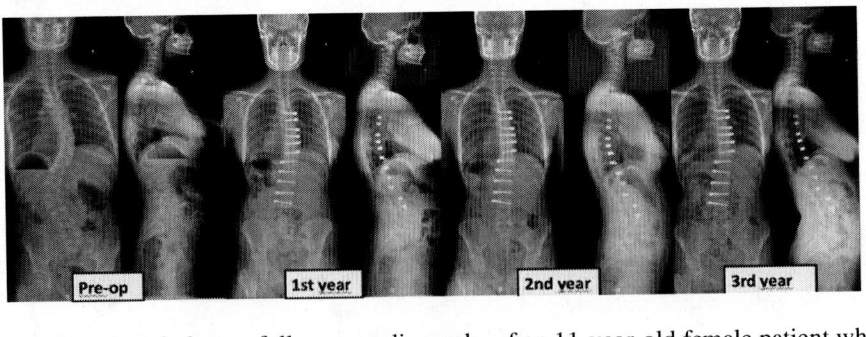


**Figure 4.** Case 2; 3-year follow-up radiographs of an 11-year-old female patient who underwent double-sided VBT (Author's own archive).

## Outcomes

Since AVBT surgery is a relatively new technique, data in the literature is still limited. Samdani et al. reported 2-year results of 11 patients in their study. The mean pre-operative curves were 44°, 20.3° post-operatively, and 13.5° at the end of the second year. A 70% improvement in curvature has been reported (Samdani et al., 2014). In 2018, Newton et al. examined the results of 2 to 4 years of patients in a study of 17 patients. Patients with a post-operative Cobb angle of less than 35° were defined as successful. Accordingly, a success rate of 59% was reported (Newton et al., 2018). In their study, Pehlivanoğlu et al. reported 2-year results of 21 patients treated with thoracoscopic VBT. The Cobb angles, which were 48° before the operation, were measured as 10° in the 2nd year post-operatively (Pehlivanoglu et al., 2020). In another study with 13 patients, 2-year results of patients with thoracic and thoracolumbar-lumbar curvatures were reported. The patients underwent double-sided AVBT. An 80% improvement (48° to 9.7°) in the thoracic curves and an 82% (45.3-8.2%) improvement in the thoracolumbar-lumbar curves were reported (Pehlivanoglu et al., 2021).

Especially in the literature, there are many studies that evaluate the follow-up results of AVBT surgery. Considering these studies, high success rates have been reported in mid-term results. However, more studies are needed on this subject to evaluate the long-term results.

## Complications

AVBT surgery is a relatively new surgical technique that has become widespread in recent years. Mechanical complications have been reported quite frequently in studies. Furthermore, these complications may be related to patient selection (Alanay et al., 2020; Baker et al., 2021; Samdani et al., 2014). Considering mechanical complications, tether breakage is the most common complication. Thread breakage can usually cause loss of correction after surgery. In a study, thread breakage that develops within the first 12 months is observed to cause a loss of correction. The results of the ruptures seen after 12 months and the patients who did not experience any thread rupture were compared, and the results were found to be similar (Baroncini et al., 2022a). A coronal angulation of more than 5° between screws in two consecutive vertebrae can be considered a thread break (Pehlivanoglu et al.,

2020). When the results of the 2-year follow-up are examined, rates of between 5% and 7% have been reported (Pehlivanoglu et al., 2020; Shin et al., 2021). At the end of the 5-year follow-up, 52% of tether rupture has been reported (Newton et al., 2020b). Considering the literature, the rates may have been seen as low, as long-term studies are few. Studies have shown that the use of twin screws and twin threads reduces the ruptures that occur within the first year (P. D. Trobisch & Baroncini, 2021). Overcorrection and adding-on are other common mechanical complications to prevent thread breakage. Rare complications such as ureteral damage and iatrogenic dural tear have been reported (Rathbun et al., 2019; Shen & Parent, 2021).

Considering non-mechanical complications, the most common complication is pulmonary complications. Rates of 10-15% have been reported in the literature. It is thought that patients who underwent surgery beyond the diaphragm and had low FVC values in the pre-operative period are prone to pulmonary complications (P. Trobisch et al., 2022). Among pulmonary complications, pleural effusion is the most common complication. Pleural effusion usually occurs within the first month and most of them regress with conservative treatment. The chest tube should be applied in patients who develop persistent pleural effusion. Hemithorax and phyllotaxy are rare complications and are generally thought to be the result of the surgical procedure. In the early post-operative period, atelectasis to the mucus plug may develop, and these patients may require bronchoscopy. Although AVBT surgery is prone to pulmonary complications, it has been reported that patients fully recovered and their pulmonary problems resolved in long-term follow-ups. Considering the relationship between respiratory function and VBT, Baroncini et al. included 51 patients with VBT in their study and found results close to preoperative PFT values at 1 year post-operatively (Baroncini et al., 2022b). In the studies of Alanay et al. and Samdani et al., a significant improvement was observed in respiratory function tests compared to the pre-operative period (Alanay et al., 2021; Samdani et al., 2021).

## Conclusion

AVBT is an encouraging and promising technique for treating scoliosis in patients who are skeletally immature. Although there is no consensus on indications, patients with a Risser score of 0-2 and a Sanders score of 2-4 were considered suitable for this surgery. Compared to fusion surgery, AVBT is a very effective method in terms of patient mobility. After surgery, patients can quickly return to their daily activities. Although high complications have been reported in studies on AVBT, these complications heal without sequelae in patients. However, studies are needed to examine the longer-term outcomes of complications.

## References

Alanay, A., Yucekul, A., Abul, K., Ergene, G., Senay, S., Ay, B., Cebeci, B. O., Yalinay Dikmen, P., Zulemyan, T., Yavuz, Y., & Yilgor, C. (2020). Thoracoscopic Vertebral Body Tethering for Adolescent Idiopathic Scoliosis. *Spine*, *45*(22), E1483–E1492. https://doi.org/10.1097/BRS.0000000000003643.

Alanay, A., Yucekul, A., Abul, K., Karaman, I., Durbas, A., Zulemyan, T., Ergene, G., Senay, S., Balci, S. T., Dikmen, P. Y., Yavuz, Y., & Yilgor, C. (2021). 173. Two to five years follow up results after thoracoscopic VBT: a single surgeon's experience. *The Spine Journal*, *21*(9), S86–S87. https://doi.org/10.1016/j.spinee.2021.05.201.

Baker, C. E., Milbrandt, T. A., & Larson, A. N. (2021). Anterior Vertebral Body Tethering for Adolescent Idiopathic Scoliosis. *Orthopedic Clinics of North America*, *52*(2), 137–147. https://doi.org/10.1016/j.ocl.2021.01.003.

Baroncini, A., Migliorini, F., Eschweiler, J., Hildebrand, F., & Trobisch, P. (2022). The timing of tether breakage influences clinical results after VBT. *European Spine Journal*, *31*(9), 2362–2367. https://doi.org/10.1007/s00586-022-07321-9.

Baroncini, A., Trobisch, P., Blau, C., Golias, C., Kobbe, P., Eschweiler, J., Tingart, M., & Migliorini, F. (2022). Analysis of the pulmonary function in patients undergoing vertebral body tethering for adolescent idiopathic scoliosis. *European Spine Journal*, *31*(4), 1022–1027. https://doi.org/10.1007/s00586-021-07029-2.

Baroncini, A., Trobisch, P. D., Berrer, A., Kobbe, P., Tingart, M., Eschweiler, J., da Paz, S., & Migliorini, F. (2021). Return to sport and daily life activities after vertebral body tethering for AIS: analysis of the sport activity questionnaire. *European Spine Journal*, *30*(7), 1998–2006. https://doi.org/10.1007/s00586-021-06768-6.

Bonsignore-Opp, L., Murphy, J., Skaggs, D., Cahill, P., Blakemore, L., Parent, S., Samdani, A., St.Hilaire, T., & Vitale, M. (2019). Growth Modulation for Childhood Scoliosis: Where Have We Come From and Where Are We Going? *Journal of the Pediatric Orthopaedic Society of North America*, *1*(1). https://doi.org/10.55275/JPOSNA-2019-9.

Ghandhari, H., Ameri, E., Nikouei, F., Haji Agha Bozorgi, M., Majdi, S., & Salehpour, M. (2018). Long-term outcome of posterior spinal fusion for the correction of adolescent idiopathic scoliosis. *Scoliosis and Spinal Disorders*, *13*(1), 14. https://doi.org/10.1186/s13013-018-0157-z.

Helenius, L., Diarbakerli, E., Grauers, A., Lastikka, M., Oksanen, H., Pajulo, O., Löyttyniemi, E., Manner, T., Gerdhem, P., & Helenius, I. (2019). Back Pain and Quality of Life After Surgical Treatment for Adolescent Idiopathic Scoliosis at 5-Year Follow-up. *Journal of Bone and Joint Surgery*, *101*(16), 1460–1466. https://doi.org/10.2106/JBJS.18.01370.

Marks, M., Newton, P. O., Petcharaporn, M., Bastrom, T. P., Shah, S., Betz, R., Lonner, B., & Miyanji, F. (2012). Postoperative Segmental Motion of the Unfused Spine Distal to the Fusion in 100 Patients With Adolescent Idiopathic Scoliosis. *Spine*, *37*(10), 826–832. https://doi.org/10.1097/BRS.0b013e31823b4eab.

Mehlman, C. T., Araghi, A., & Roy, D. R. (1997). Hyphenated history: the Hueter-Volkmann law. *American Journal of Orthopedics (Belle Mead, N.J.)*, *26*(11), 798–800.

Newton, P. O. (2020a). Spinal growth tethering: indications and limits. *Annals of Translational Medicine*, *8*(2), 27–27. https://doi.org/10.21037/atm.2019.12.159.

Newton, P. O., Bartley, C. E., Bastrom, T. P., Kluck, D. G., Saito, W., & Yaszay, B. (2020b). Anterior Spinal Growth Modulation in Skeletally Immature Patients with Idiopathic Scoliosis. *Journal of Bone and Joint Surgery*, *102*(9), 769–777. https://doi.org/10.2106/JBJS.19.01176.

Newton, P. O., Faro, F. D., Gollogly, S., Betz, R. R., Lenke, L. G., & Lowe, T. G. (2005). Results of Preoperative Pulmonary Function Testing of Adolescents with Idiopathic Scoliosis. *The Journal of Bone & Joint Surgery*, *87*(9), 1937–1946. https://doi.org/10.2106/JBJS.D.02209.

Newton, P. O., Kluck, D. G., Saito, W., Yaszay, B., Bartley, C. E., & Bastrom, T. P. (2018). Anterior Spinal Growth Tethering for Skeletally Immature Patients with Scoliosis. *Journal of Bone and Joint Surgery*, *100*(19), 1691–1697. https://doi.org/ 10.2106/JBJS.18.00287.

Pehlivanoglu, T., Oltulu, I., Erdag, Y., Korkmaz, E., Sarioglu, E., Ofluoglu, E., & Aydogan, M. (2021). Double-sided vertebral body tethering of double adolescent idiopathic scoliosis curves: radiographic outcomes of the first 13 patients with 2 years of follow-up. *European Spine Journal*, *30*(7), 1896–1904. https://doi.org/10.1007/s00586-021-06745-z.

Pehlivanoglu, T., Oltulu, I., Ofluoglu, E., Sarioglu, E., Altun, G., Korkmaz, M., Yildirim, K., & Aydogan, M. (2020). Thoracoscopic Vertebral Body Tethering for Adolescent Idiopathic Scoliosis: A Minimum of 2 Years' Results of 21 Patients. *Journal of Pediatric Orthopaedics*, *40*(10), 575–580. https://doi.org/10.1097/BPO.0000000000001590.

Rathbun, J. R., Hoernschemeyer, D. S., Wakefield, M. R., Malm-Buatsi, E. A., Murray, K. S., & Ramachandran, V. (2019). Ureteral injury following vertebral body tethering for adolescent idiopathic scoliosis. *Journal of Pediatric Surgery Case Reports*, *46*, 101219. https://doi.org/10.1016/j.epsc.2019.101219.

Risser, J. C. (1958). The Iliac apophysis; an invaluable sign in the management of scoliosis. *Clinical Orthopaedics*, *11*, 111–119.

Samdani, A. F., Ames, R. J., Kimball, J. S., Pahys, J. M., Grewal, H., Pelletier, G. J., & Betz, R. R. (2014). Anterior Vertebral Body Tethering for Idiopathic Scoliosis. *Spine*, *39*(20), 1688–1693. https://doi.org/10.1097/BRS.0000000000000472.

Samdani, A. F., Pahys, J. M., Ames, R. J., Grewal, H., Pelletier, G. J., Hwang, S. W., & Betz, R. R. (2021). Prospective Follow-up Report on Anterior Vertebral Body Tethering for Idiopathic Scoliosis. *Journal of Bone and Joint Surgery*, *103*(17), 1611–1619. https://doi.org/10.2106/JBJS.20.01503.

Sanders, J. O., Khoury, J. G., Kishan, S., Browne, R. H., Mooney, J. F., Arnold, K. D., McConnell, S. J., Bauman, J. A., & Finegold, D. N. (2008a). Predicting Scoliosis Progression from Skeletal Maturity: A Simplified Classification During Adolescence. *The Journal of Bone and Joint Surgery-American Volume*, *90*(3), 540–553. https://doi.org/10.2106/JBJS.G.00004.

Sanders, J. O., Khoury, J. G., Kishan, S., Browne, R. H., Mooney, J. F., Arnold, K. D., McConnell, S. J., Bauman, J. A., & Finegold, D. N. (2008b). Predicting Scoliosis Progression from Skeletal Maturity: A Simplified Classification During Adolescence. *The Journal of Bone and Joint Surgery-American Volume*, *90*(3), 540–553. https://doi.org/10.2106/JBJS.G.00004.

Senkoylu, A., Riise, R. B., Acaroglu, E., & Helenius, I. (2020). Diverse approaches to scoliosis in young children. *EFORT Open Reviews*, *5*(10), 753–762. https://doi.org/10.1302/2058-5241.5.190087.

Shen, J., & Parent, S. (2021). Iatrogenic dural tear after growth modulation in AIS: an unusual complication and its management. *Spine Deformity*, *9*(6), 1699–1703. https://doi.org/10.1007/s43390-021-00368-6.

Shin, M., Arguelles, G. R., Cahill, P. J., Flynn, J. M., Baldwin, K. D., & Anari, J. B. (2021). Complications, Reoperations, and Mid-Term Outcomes Following Anterior Vertebral Body Tethering Versus Posterior Spinal Fusion. *JBJS Open Access*, *6*(2). https://doi.org/10.2106/JBJS.OA.21.00002.

Sitoula, P., Verma, K., Holmes, L., Gabos, P. G., Sanders, J. O., Yorgova, P., Neiss, G., Rogers, K., & Shah, S. A. (2015). Prediction of Curve Progression in Idiopathic Scoliosis. *Spine*, *40*(13), 1006–1013. https://doi.org/10.1097/BRS.0000000000000952.

Stokes, I. A. F., Spence, H., Aronsson, D. D., & Kilmer, N. (1996). Mechanical Modulation of Vertebral Body Growth. *Spine*, *21*(10), 1162–1167. https://doi.org/10.1097/00007632-199605150-00007.

Takahashi, Y., Saito, W., Yaszay, B., Bartley, C. E., Bastrom, T. P., & Newton, P. O. (2021). Rate of Scoliosis Correction After Anterior Spinal Growth Tethering for Idiopathic Scoliosis. *Journal of Bone and Joint Surgery*, *103*(18), 1718–1723. https://doi.org/10.2106/JBJS.20.02071.

Trobisch, P. D., & Baroncini, A. (2021). Preliminary outcomes after vertebral body tethering (VBT) for lumbar curves and subanalysis of a 1- versus 2-tether construct. *European Spine Journal*, *30*(12), 3570–3576. https://doi.org/10.1007/s00586-021-07009-6.

Trobisch, P., Migliorini, F., Vanspauwen, T., & Baroncini, A. (2022). Pulmonary Complications after Vertebral Body Tethering: Incidence, Treatment, Outcomes and Risk Factor Analysis. *Journal of Clinical Medicine*, *11*(13), 3778. https://doi.org/10.3390/jcm11133778.

Weinstein, S. L., Zavala, D. C., & Ponseti, I. v. (1981). Idiopathic scoliosis: long-term follow-up and prognosis in untreated patients. *The Journal of Bone and Joint Surgery. American Volume*, *63*(5), 702–712.

Williams, B. A., Matsumoto, H., McCalla, D. J., Akbarnia, B. A., Blakemore, L. C., Betz, R. R., Flynn, J. M., Johnston, C. E., McCarthy, R. E., Roye, D. P., Skaggs, D. L., Smith, J. T., Snyder, B. D., Sponseller, P. D., Sturm, P. F., Thompson, G. H., Yazici,

M., & Vitale, M. G. (2014). Development and Initial Validation of the Classification of Early-Onset Scoliosis (C-EOS). *Journal of Bone and Joint Surgery*, *96*(16), 1359–1367. https://doi.org/10.2106/JBJS.M.00253.

# Chapter 25

# Growth Guided Systems – Luqué Trolley

**Göker Utku Değer***, **MD**
Department of Orhopaedics and Traumatology, Beykoz State Hospital, Istanbul, Turkiye

## Abstract

The aim of surgical treatment in early-onset progressive spinal curvatures is to correct the spinal curvature, ensure lung development, and preserve the growth potential of the spine. Guided growth systems are one of the useful techniques used for EOS surgery. These systems correct the spinal deformity by using implants that anchor, fixed (screws) and non-fixed (screws and sublaminar wires), and multiple vertebrae to rods to direct the growing spine along with the spinal implant. The advantages of these procedures are that they avoid common concerns in other systems such as infections, repeated surgical lengthening, hardware failure, or exposure to anesthesia. The Luqué Trolley technique is the first described guided growth procedure. The procedure is relatively quick and can be performed in just a few hours. However, the use of the Luqué Trolley system has gradually decreased due to low growth rates in the spine, high spontaneous fusion rate, and implant-related complications. This method was modified by Oullet in 2011 and guided growth systems were popularized again under the name of the modified Luqué Trolley (MLT).

**Keywords:** luqué trolley, guided growth, scoliosis, early-onset scoliosis

---

* Corresponding Author's Email: gokerdeger@hotmail.com.

In: Early Onset Scoliosis
Editor: Ahmed Majid Heydar
ISBN: 979-8-89113-600-7

## Introduction

The aim of surgical treatment in early-onset progressive spinal curvatures is to correct the spinal curvature, ensure lung development, and preserve the growth potential of the spine. The patient's age and maturity during the progression of the curve will determine the type of surgical procedure chosen. Non-fusion surgical methods applied in this group of patients are examined in three groups.

In this grouping, growth-friendly spinal implant systems have been divided into three by Skaggs, based on the correction forces exerted by the implant on the spine, as distraction-based (extensible rods and VEPTR), compression-based (vertebral staples-tethers), and guided growth systems (Skaggs et al., 2014).

The use of guided growth systems in scoliosis surgery is an effective and minimally invasive option to treat scoliosis. It has been shown to be effective both in reducing the curvature of the spine and in preventing the further progression of scoliosis. Implants can be adjusted as needed over time, allowing for the growth and development of the spine without compromising the integrity of the spine. Guided growth systems have been used for several decades and have proven to be a safe and effective way to treat scoliosis. Guided growth systems correct the spinal deformity by attaching multiple vertebrae (usually including the apical vertebra) to the rods through translation and other mechanical forces during initial implantation. Most anchors are not firmly attached to the rods and thus slide over the rods over time, allowing for longitudinal growth. The most important advantage of guided growth systems is that there is no need for repetitive surgery for elongation. Since the growth occurred evenly at both ends, it is expected that no change in the sagittal alignment would arise, unlike distraction-based systems in which proximal junctional kyphosis is a concern. Other advantages are lower infection rates and implant-related complications. The guided growth systems are the Luque trolley and Shilla (Figure 1).

The most important disadvantage of guided growth systems is that repetitive surgical lengthening may be required. It does not cause any change in the kyphosis of the patient, as growth occurs at the same rate at both endpoints. As a matter of fact, the adjacent segment kyphosis may occur in distraction-based systems. Although the main goal of using these systems is to leave the patient without an implant at the end of the treatment, it cannot be predicted in advance which patient will require fusion after treatment or from which patient the implants will be removed.

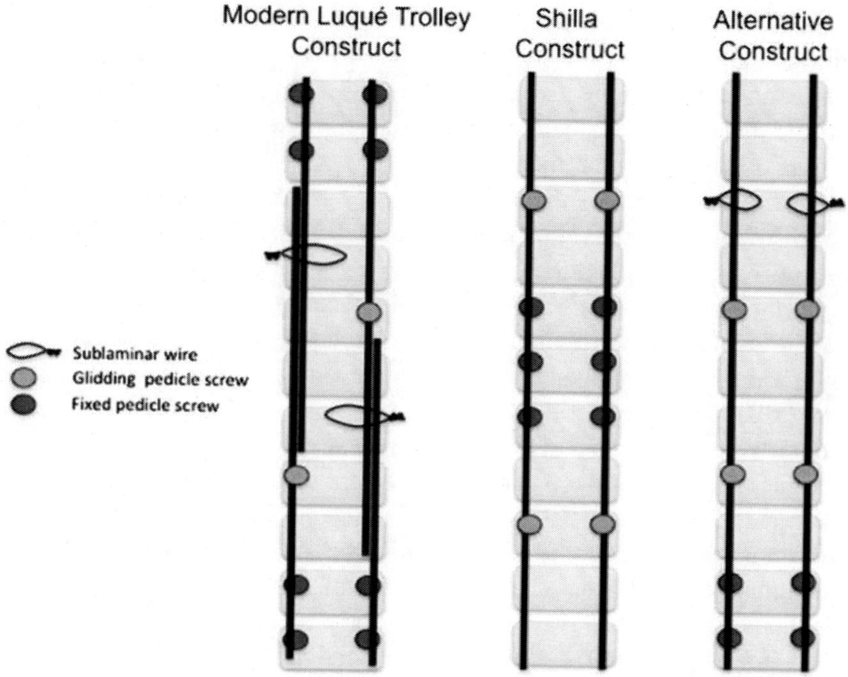


**Figure 1.** The schematization of growth-guided constructs (Oullet, 2011).

## Luqué Trolley

The first and pioneer of guided growth system was the Luqué Trolley method. During the development of this method, Luque and Cardosa described segmental spinal fusion without fusion in 1977 (Luque, 1977) and published a series in which they operated on 47 patients using combined Harrington rods and sublaminar wires (Luque, 1982). It was reported that an average lengthening of 2.6 cm and a 78% improvement in curvature were obtained in the instrumented spine with the technique used in this series. Later, this technique was modified as the "Luque Trolley" technique by adding 'L' shaped rods and wires. In this technique, sublaminar wires were placed with minimal subperiosteal dissection to reduce the risk of fusion. Then, the placed sublaminar wires were passed through the rods, and mechanical pulling was applied. Thus, it was seen that while allowing both the correction of the curvature during the operation and the lengthening of the spine, it also guided the spine. It can be said that the system attracted a lot of attention at that time due to its minimally invasive and rapid applicability and allowing growth compared to other methods applied in scoliosis surgery. In this technique, there is no need for repetitive surgical intervention as the implants can slide over the rods during elongation. Due to the strong technique, there is no need for post-operative immobilization.

However, the use of the Luqué Trolley system has gradually decreased due to low growth rates in the spine, a high spontaneous fusion rate, and implant-related complications. Rod breakage or patient non-compliance with lengthening procedures are the most common complications of this technique. In addition, it is very difficult to apply sublaminar wires without subperiosteal exploration, and spontaneous fusion can sometimes occur in young patients despite all efforts. In a series in which revisions of the Luqué Trolley surgical method were reported, it was reported that at least 1 revision surgery was performed for each of the 9 patients who were operated on at an average age of 9 years (Mardjetko et al., 1992). Spontaneous fusion was reported in all patients in this study. They stated that the revisions included technical difficulties due to fibrosis and weakening of the sublaminar bone. Spinal growth at instrumented levels was 35% of the predicted normal spinal growth. As a result of their studies, the authors reported that fusion-free surgery in the treatment of scoliosis both failed to control the deformity and was not a successful method because the predicted growth could not be achieved in the implanted segments. There are also studies with similar poor results resulting in spontaneous fusion. In another study reporting the results of the Luqué Trolley method, Pratt et al. reported that 32% of the expected growth in the spine could be achieved as a result of the 5-year follow-up of 18 patients (Pratt et al., 1999). It was reported that the Cobb angle deteriorated in the follow-up of all patients to whom only the Luqué Trolley technique was applied. In another study conducted in the same center, they reported that half of 25 patients with 12-year follow-up underwent revision surgery, and restrictive lung disease developed in 76% of them (Scheuler et al., 2008).

This method was modified by Oullet in 2011, and guided growth systems were popularized again under the name of the modified Luqué Trolley (MLT) (Ouellet, 2011). The modification made by Oullet aimed to prevent the weakness of the previous method in the initial rotational correction and implant failures in the follow-up by using titanium rods to increase the stabilization of the system, applying screws to the proximal and distal end vertebrae, and applying screws to the apex of the deformity. In the system, sublaminar wires are used, and guided growth is achieved by means of screws applied to the apex with these wires, which do not tighten the rods. The technique uses modern anchors (pedicular screws) and a surgical approach that preserves soft tissue. The sliding anchors are placed transmuscularly to limit the risk of spontaneous fusion. In this study they published, they reported that as a result of the modern method they applied in 5 early-onset scoliosis patients with an average age of 4.5 years, the deformity was reduced from 60° to 21° on average, with lower implant-related complication rates compared to the previously reported classical method in an average of 3.6 years of follow-up, and remained at 21° in 21 follow-ups. Two of the five cases outgrew the structure, requiring a lengthening of the rods. A patient had a gradual recurrence of the deformity that required revision surgery after 4 years. However, MLT is a new technique and has not been officially approved in most areas. Concerns regarding spinal fusion may remain, but the study reported fewer implant failures when compared to the original trolley results.

The modern Luqué Trolley procedure is typically performed under general anesthesia. Oullet describes their surgical procedure; in the prone position, the modern Luqué construct involved a midline incision spanning the segment of the spine to be instrumented. Fixed spinal anchors (screws or hooks locked to the rods) and gliding spinal anchors (screws or sublaminar wire free to travel along the rods) were inserted through multiple "keyhole" dissections. Since fixed segments will be fused at the proximal and distal ends, it is performed with a classical subperiosteal dissection. Sliding anchor points at the apex of the deformity should be applied with screws or sublaminar cables to the most suitable points to provide apical tension. It is very important not to perform subperiosteal dissection in this region in order to prevent fusion. Pedicle screws were applied with the free hand technique from appropriate entry points with the help of fluoroscopy imaging. These gliding screws captured a 5-mm rod with a locking cap and nut designed for 6-mm rods, thus permitting motion. At the segments where sublaminar titanium cables were to be passed, the dissection was carried from the midline to the medial border of the facet. Care should not be taken to remove the periosteum, and even a muscle layer should be left on it. It is necessary to carefully cut the spinous processes and apply the sublaminar wires without damaging the periosteum. Two pairs of 5-mm titanium rods were tunneled in a subfascial/intramuscular fashion (below the fascia, above the periosteum) from the opened proximal and distal ends. Each of the rods is rigidly fixed to the spine at its proximal or distal endpoints. In the apex section, screws and sublaminar wires, which act as sliding anchors, ensure that the rods are parallel and connected. Thus, the growth is achieved by sliding the rod from the rigid fixation end to the other end. A classic apical translation reduction maneuver was performed to correct the deformity. The number of implants that will act as a sliding anchor in the apex region should be low enough to keep the risk of spontaneous fusion to a minimum, but it should also be sufficient to provide the strength to correct the deformity and protect the spinal alignment afterwards. An average of 10 vertebrae (range, 8–13) was between the fixed anchors (Figure 2).

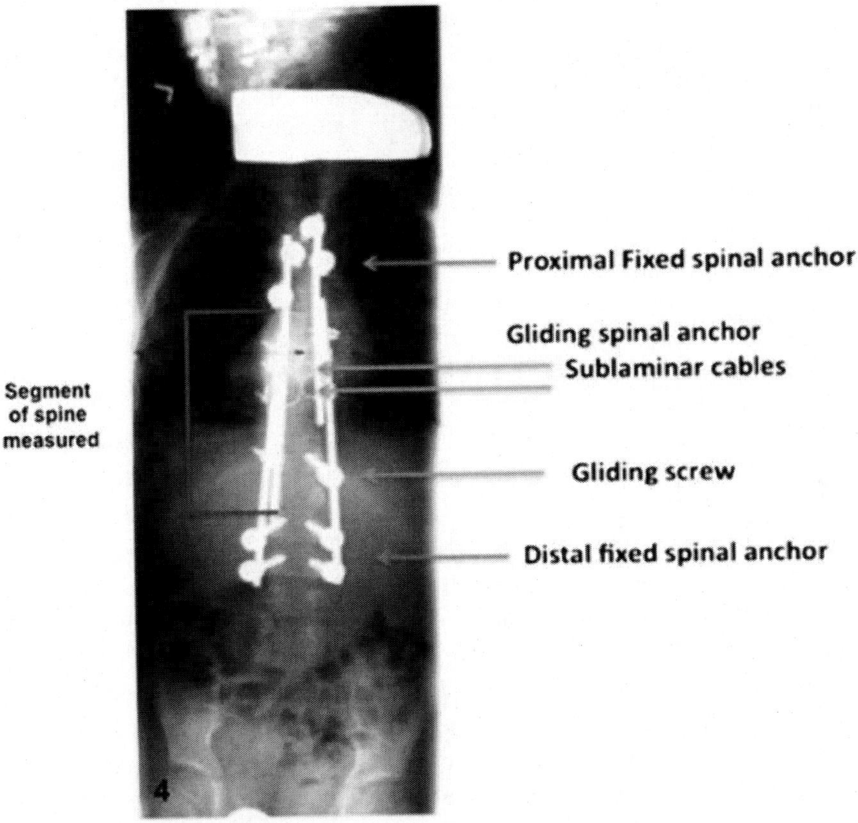


**Figure 2.** Modern Luqué Trolley design (Ouellet, 2011).

After the modern Luqué Trolley procedure, the patient will typically be required to wear a back brace for several months. This helps to ensure that the rods remain in place and reduces the risk of them becoming loose or shifting. The patients were able to ambulate on day 2. During this time, the patient should also attend physical therapy sessions to help strengthen their back muscles. This will help to reduce the risk of the spine becoming curved again in the future. The patient should also avoid activities that may put a strain on their back, such as heavy lifting or strenuous exercise, until 6 months after surgery.

As with any surgical procedure, there are risks associated with the Luqué Trolley technique. These include infection, bleeding, nerve injury, and allergic reactions to anesthesia. There is also a risk of the spine not being successfully corrected, or the rods becoming loose or shifting over time.

In their recently reported study, Mehdian et al. described the mid-term results of the modified method they used (Mehdian et al., 2020). They reported that the modified Luqué Trolley method applied was very successful, especially in cases of hypotonic non-ambulatory EOS based on myopathy. However, they reported that it should be used carefully, especially in cases of scoliosis at the thoracolumbar junction, due to the high implant failure rates in patients with EOS on the background of idiopathic EOS and cerebral palsy. In another retrospective study, Odent et al. reported that they applied modified Luqué Trolley and modified VEPTR methods in 13 patients with early-onset scoliosis, and as a result, guided extension systems were generally successful in correcting and maintaining the Cobb angle (Odent et al., 2015). They emphasized the importance of balanced sagittal balance and avoidance of junctional kyphosis, although 50% of the expected growth rate could only be achieved. It also highlights the importance of avoiding at least 83 procedures (7 per patient) compared to standard techniques that require lengthening every 6 months.

The cost of the Luqué Trolley procedure will vary depending on the patient's insurance coverage and the specific details of the surgery. The average cost of the Luqué Trolley procedure is around $20,000 in the USA, although this can vary depending on the specific details of the patient's case.

## Conclusion

The Luqué Trolley technique is considered one of the most successful treatments for scoliosis. It is a minimally invasive procedure that avoids the need for large incisions or cutting of the rib cage. Although the mechanism is the first example of guided growth surgery to avoid repetitive lengthening surgeries, it has not been as popular as expected. The reason for this is that the growth is less than expected and the need for a revision is greater than expected due to implant-related complications. After forty years the modern Luqué Trolley surgery has developed and given a new popularity to this procedure. However, it still has not succeeded in becoming one of the most preferred methods in the treatment of EOS. It seems that there is a need to report long-term results from large patient series in this area. Making improvements with new implant developments will also enable a more effective use of the procedure in the future.

## References


Luque, E. R. (1982). Paralytic scoliosis in growing children. *Clinical Orthopaedics and Related Research*, *163*, 202–209. https://doi.org/10.1097/00003086-198203000-00030.

Luque E. R. (1977). Treatment of scoliosis without arthrodesis or external support, preliminary report. *Orthop Trans.*, *1*, 37–38.

Mardjetko, S. M., Hammerberg, K. W., Lubicky, J. P., & Fister, J. S. (1992). The Luque trolley revisited. Review of nine cases requiring revision. *Spine*, *17*(5), 582–589. https://doi.org/10.1097/00007632-199205000-00018.

Mehdian, H., Haddad, S., Pasku, D., & Nasto, L. A. (2020). Mid-term results of a modified self-growing rod technique for the treatment of early-onset scoliosis. *The Bone & Joint Journal*, *102-B*(11), 1560–1566. https://doi.org/10.1302/0301-620X.102B11.BJJ-2020-0412.R3.

Odent, T., Ilharreborde, B., Miladi, L., Khouri, N., Violas, P., Ouellet, J., Cunin, V., Kieffer, J., Kharrat, K., & Accadbled, F. (2015). Fusionless surgery in early-onset scoliosis. *Orthopaedics & Traumatology, Surgery & Research : OTSR*, *101*(6 Suppl), S281–S288. https://doi.org/10.1016/J.OTSR.2015.07.004.

Ouellet, J. (2011). Surgical technique: modern Luqué trolley, a self-growing rod technique. *Clinical Orthopaedics and Related Research*, *469*(5), 1356–1367. https://doi.org/10.1007/S11999-011-1783-4.

Pratt, R. K., Webb, J. K., Burwell, R. G., & Cummings, S. L. (1999). Luque trolley and convex epiphysiodesis in the management of infantile and juvenile idiopathic scoliosis. *Spine*, *24*(15), 1538–1547. https://doi.org/10.1097/00007632-199908010-00007.

Scheuler, A., Steele, N., Medhian, S., Grevitt, M., Freeman, B., Webb, J., & Kiely, P. (2008). Long-Term Spınal And Respıratory Functıon In Early Onset Scolıosıs Managed Wıth Selectıve Epıphysıodesıs And Posterıor 'Luque Trolley' Growıng Instrumentatıon. *Orthopaedic Proceedings*, *90-B*(SUPP_III), 481–481. https://doi.org/10.1302/0301-620X.90BSUPP_III.0900481C.

Skaggs, D. L., Akbarnia, B. A., Flynn, J. M., Myung, K. S., Sponseller, P. D., & Vitale, M. G. (2014). A classification of growth friendly spine implants. *Journal of Pediatric Orthopedics*, *34*(3), 260–274. https://doi.org/10.1097/BPO.0000000000000073.

# Chapter 26

# Shilla

**Abdülhalim Akar[*], MD**
Department of Orthopaedics and Traumatology, Emsey Hospital, Istanbul, Turkiye

## Abstract

Early onset scoliosis (EOS) is a complex condition with many aspects. The aim of treating this multifaceted deformity of the growing spine is to try to prevent the progression of the deformity and correct it with the least necessary intervention. Intervention in this complex situation should allow the spine to grow while correcting the deformity. The Shilla growth guiding system (SGG) is a system that guides the rest of the spine by focusing on correction at the apex of the curve, allowing the spine to grow. Selective bilateral fusion is performed to the apex of the curve, and minimally invasive instrumentation is performed below and above the apex, allowing spine augmentation. Looking at the literature, the results of the SGG system are promising. The Shilla system allows for natural growth of the pediatric spine while correcting the scoliotic deformity with a minimally invasive method.

**Keywords:** early onset scoliosis (EOS), shilla, guiding growth, growth friendly instrumentation

[*] Corresponding Author's Email: ahalimakar@gmail.com.

In: Early Onset Scoliosis
Editor: Ahmed Majid Heydar
ISBN: 979-8-89113-600-7

## Introduction

Early onset scoliosis (EOS) is a challenging pediatric deformity that presents before the age of 10 (El-Hawary & Akbarnia, 2015; Williams et al., 2014), which can negatively affect respiratory and cardiac development, lead to severe progressive deformity, and generally lead to poor outcomes if left untreated (Pehrsson et al., 1992). The wide variety of etiologies involved, variable manifestations of deformities, and associated syndromes pose many problems in early treatment (Thompson et al., 2007). The main purpose of correcting a deformity in the growing spine is to allow the spine to continue growing unhindered. Achieving healthy heart and respiratory development by achieving adequate thoracic development is intricately related to spinal growth. Impaired thoracic volume is closely associated with morbidity and mortality in these patients (Williams et al., 2014). For this reason, the goal of surgery in these patients is to allow adequate correction of the deformity while allowing continued spinal growth.

Traditional growing rod (TGR) instrumentation produces a distracting force between the ends of the scoliotic curve in patients with EOS and typically requires repetitive manual surgical distraction every 6 months. The purpose of TGR is to continue this distraction process throughout the juvenile and early adolescence until a time when adequate growth of the vertebral column has been completed. At this point, the implants are replaced with permanent implants, and a final spinal fusion is performed. The direct and indirect economic costs of these surgeries, the autofusion state that occurs iatrogenically and complicates the absolute fusion surgery procedure, and the morbidity of repeated surgeries and hospitalizations during childhood, constitute the shortcomings of TGR. Magnetically controlled growing rods (MCGR) provide non-surgical distraction and have lower complication rates compared to TGR (Akbarnia et al., 2014; Hosseini et al., 2016). Although there are no repeated surgical procedures, regular hospital visits are required in MCGR. In addition, MCGR requires a sufficient straight spine area and a specific patient size to accommodate the actuator. The vertical expandable prosthetic titanium rib (VEPTR) acts directly on the chest wall in EOS by expanding the thoracic space capacity. In this procedure, direct thoracic closure is tried to increase by osteotomies and intercostal muscle lysis methods. However, in this system, an operation is required to expand the system every 6 to 12 months (Thompson et al., 2007). For these reasons, the Shilla technique was developed in 2004 (McCarthy et al., 2014; McCarthy & McCullough, 2015).

The pedicle screw trolley instrumentation (Shilla) places fixed screws in the apical segment to improve the deformity, and there is a sliding rod system on these screw heads. Thus, it guides the growing spine passively without the need for regular distraction (McCarthy et al., 2010). Shilla instrumentation does not require regular surgical planning, and patients do not need frequent follow-up. Many comparisons of shilla and growing rods have been reported in the literature (Andras et al., 2015; Luhmann et al., 2017; Luhmann & McCarthy, 2017).

In Shilla growth guidance (SGG) system, we focus on correcting the apex of the deformity while allowing other parts of the spinal column to continue to grow in their natural order. Focusing only on correcting the apex, the rest of the spine is protected from damage to the apophysis for further growth.

## Materials and Methods

The Shilla "growing" polyaxial screw has a locking plug in the screw head, and this plug does not fix the rod to the screw. Thus, the rod can be easily moved up and down. The polyaxial head of the screw allows the rod to move several degrees during normal spinal movement, thereby reducing tension between the vertebra and the screw. These growing screws are placed superior and inferior to the apical region of the deformity. To achieve maximum correction in all planes, pedicle screws are placed bilaterally on the spine at the apex of the curvature (Akbarnia et al., 2022).

## Preoperative Planning

The criteria for selecting patients for this procedure include the extent of the curvature (>50°), the amount of remaining growth of the spine, and whether the patient's state of health would allow a 4-5 hour procedure. The family should be carefully informed about the benefits and risks of this procedure. In order for the procedure to be successful, the surgical team should cooperate with the anesthesiology team (Akbarnia et al., 2022). These patients often have other comorbidities as well as cardiopulmonary problems, which may affect preoperative planning and the benefits of the surgery.

Whole spine X-rays, including bending films, help evaluate the correctability of spinal deformities. The determination of the apical segment is one of the most important evaluations. The apical three or four vertebral segments that recover the least with the flexibility test indicate the segments that require maximum correction and stimulation. The aim is to bring these segments into anatomical alignment in all planes. Magnetic resonance imaging of the entire spine in children under 10 years of age is required preoperatively to exclude intrathecal abnormalities. Due to the length and stress of the surgery, an assessment of pulmonary status is also necessary (Akbarnia et al., 2022). An evaluation of pulmonary status should be performed, and the child should be closely evaluated by a pediatric pulmonologist. In addition, it is important to identify remaining growth. To determine bone age and assess potential growth, wrist and hand films are taken.

## Surgical Technique

The apex of scoliosis directs the forces affecting the entire spine, so the primary corrective forces initially applied to align any spinal level with a coronal, sagittal, and axially neutral alignment are focused on the apex of the deformity (McCarthy et al., 2014). To create a permanent fix with the Shilla technique, enough bilateral pedicle screws are placed at the apex to overcome the crankshaft phenomenon, attached to the rods, and fixed (Burton et al., 2000; Dubousset et al., 1989; Sanders et al., 1997). In all cases, ponte osteotomies are performed between three or four posterior apical levels, and in case of rigid curvature (cannot be bent more than 50° on the bending graph), anterior discectomy is added to provide maximum posterior mobility (Diab et al., 2011; Lewis et al., 2014; Sucato, 2010). Rarely are larger posterior-based osteotomies may be needed to restore mobility of the apex. In addition, arthrodesis is required to ensure permanent apical correction and fix screws to rods by preventing the rods from slipping at the apex (McCarthy et al., 2014). The number of segments selected for inclusion at the apex depends on the flexibility of the curve.

The growing screw anchors are placed between the fluoroscopic guide and the muscle layer to avoid disrupting the periosteum or inhibiting growth. The screw head is polyaxial, and the cap surrounds the rod without being attached to the rod. In ambulatory patients, the child's functional level should be adjusted by avoiding lower lumbar levels (below L3 and rarely below L4). In most patients, the lumbar screws are located bilaterally and in the same vertebra, and the thoracic screws are often alternately located level by level.

## Complications

Problems with implants of the Shilla system include loosening/extraction of the pedicle screw, protrusion of the implant, and rod breakage. These problems may require implant revisions depending on the clinical picture. However, the rate of reoperation after TGR surgery is three to four times higher than after Shilla surgery (Luhmann et al., 2017; Luhmann & McCarthy, 2017). SGG complication rates have been reported as 38-73% (Haapala et al., 2020; Luhmann & McCarthy, 2017; McCarthy & McCullough, 2015).

Loosening most often occurs in the most superior and inferior pedicle screws and couses symptoms. Implant prominence can be seen in the proximal system, and this is the most common reason for revision surgery. If partial pullout is noted radiologically, but the patient has no symptoms or the system is not particularly prominent, it can be waited until symptoms occur in the patient, as the screws do their job, controlling the coronal deformity and allowing growth (Akbarnia et al., 2022). If a revision is made, the screw diameter should be increased by 0.5–1.0 mm. If a stepped structure was used initially, the unused contralateral pedicle at the vertebral level can be used to insert the revision screw.

Rod breakage usually occurs 2 years after surgery (Cryar et al., 2017). When a rod breakage occurs, the surgical procedure can be performed as a partial replacement of the broken rod or as a complete replacement of the unilateral or bilateral rod. When a single rod is broken, it is the surgeon's choice to completely replace both rods. In a single rod breakage, it is suggested that the tired but unbroken rod is also replaced. This prevents possible contralateral rod breakage in the future.

## Results

SGG has been used successfully in scoliosis of 40° or greater (up to 115°, typically 60–80°) in patients in whom spine growth is expected for at least 3 years postoperatively (McCarthy & McCullough, 2015). The most common and easiest to control types of scoliosis are single curve patterns. This curve pattern is governed by a prototypical structure consisting of bilateral apical fusion (three to four vertebral levels) and growth-guiding cephalic and caudal Shilla pedicle screws. The SGG concept has been proven to be multi-purpose in the treatment of deformities in idiopathic, congenital, neuromuscular, and syndromic EOS patients (Luhmann & McCarthy, 2017; McCarthy et al., 2014).

Five-year follow-up results from 33 SGG patients showed that the preoperative mean scoliosis curve of 69° (range, 40–115°) decreased to a mean of 38° (range, 16–74°) (McCarthy & McCullough, 2015). Although many patients could not adapt to the pulmonary function test, it has been shown that the average usable area for the lung, measured on radiography using the Campbell technique, increased by 28% in the right lung and by 31% in the left lung (McCarthy & McCullough, 2015).

## Conclusion

The Shilla growth guiding system is an innovative method in the treatment of EOS deformities and offers a natural growth option in patients without the need for regular intervention. Its early results are comparable to other systems, as Shilla patients need less surgery. The SGG focuses primarily on the apex of the scoliotic curve and guides the growth of the compensatory curves. Compared to other methods, this procedure is much less invasive and allows the child to grow naturally without intervention. The frequency of early complications decreases with the experience of the surgeon and the improvement of techniques.

## References

Akbarnia, B. A., Pawelek, J. B., Cheung, K. M. C., Demirkiran, G., Elsebaie, H., Emans, J. B., Johnston, C. E., Mundis, G. M., Noordeen, H., Skaggs, D. L., Sponseller, P. D., Thompson, G. H., Yaszay, B., Yazici, M., & Growing Spine Study Group. (2014). Traditional Growing Rods Versus Magnetically Controlled Growing Rods for the Surgical Treatment of Early-Onset Scoliosis: A Case-Matched 2-Year Study. *Spine Deformity*, *2*(6), 493–497. https://doi.org/10.1016/j.jspd.2014.09.050.

Akbarnia, B. A., Thompson, G. H., Yazici, M., & El-Hawary, R. (Eds.). (2022). *The Growing Spine: Management of Spinal Disorders in Young Children*. Springer International Publishing. https://doi.org/10.1007/978-3-030-84393-9.

Andras, L. M., Joiner, E. R. A., McCarthy, R. E., McCullough, L., Luhmann, S. J., Sponseller, P. D., Emans, J. B., Barrett, K. K., Skaggs, D. L., & Growing Spine Study Group. (2015). Growing Rods Versus Shilla Growth Guidance: Better Cobb Angle Correction and T1-S1 Length Increase But More Surgeries. *Spine Deformity*, *3*(3), 246–252. https://doi.org/10.1016/j.jspd.2014.11.005.

Burton, D. C., Asher, M. A., & Lai, S. M. (2000). Scoliosis Correction Maintenance in Skeletally Immature Patients With Idiopathic Scoliosis: Is Anterior Fusion Really Necessary? *Spine*, *25*(1), 61. https://doi.org/10.1097/00007632-200001010-00012.

Cryar, K. A., Bumpass, D. B., McCullough, L., & McCarthy, R. E. (2017). Rod Breakage in Shilla Growth Guidance Constructs: When, Where, and Why? *The Spine Journal*, *17*(10), S107. https://doi.org/10.1016/j.spinee.2017.07.091.

Diab, M. G., Franzone, J. M., & Vitale, M. G. (2011). The role of posterior spinal osteotomies in pediatric spinal deformity surgery: Indications and operative technique. *Journal of Pediatric Orthopedics*, *31*(1 Suppl), S88-98. https://doi.org/10.1097/BPO.0b013e3181f73bd4.

Dubousset, J., Herring, J. A., & Shufflebarger, H. (1989). The crankshaft phenomenon. *Journal of Pediatric Orthopedics*, *9*(5), 541–550. https://doi.org/10.1097/01241398-198909010-00008.

El-Hawary, R., & Akbarnia, B. A. (2015). Early Onset Scoliosis—Time for Consensus. *Spine Deformity*, *3*(2), 105–106. https://doi.org/10.1016/j.jspd.2015.01.003.

Haapala, H., Saarinen, A. J., Salonen, A., & Helenius, I. (2020). Shilla Growth Guidance Compared With Magnetically Controlled Growing Rods in the Treatment of Neuromuscular and Syndromic Early-onset Scoliosis. *Spine*, *45*(23), E1604–E1614. https://doi.org/10.1097/BRS.0000000000003654.

Hosseini, P., Pawelek, J., Mundis, G. M., Yaszay, B., Ferguson, J., Helenius, I., Cheung, K. M., Demirkiran, G., Alanay, A., Senkoylu, A., Elsebaie, H., & Akbarnia, B. A. (2016). Magnetically controlled Growing Rods for Early-onset Scoliosis: A Multicenter Study of 23 Cases With Minimum 2 years Follow-up. *Spine*, *41*(18), 1456–1462. https://doi.org/10.1097/BRS.0000000000001561.

Lewis, S. J., Zamorano, J. J., & Goldstein, C. L. (2014). Treatment of severe pediatric spinal deformities. *Journal of Pediatric Orthopedics*, *34 Suppl 1*, S1-5. https://doi.org/10.1097/BPO.0000000000000293.

Luhmann, S. J., & McCarthy, R. E. (2017). A Comparison of SHILLA GROWTH GUIDANCE SYSTEM and Growing Rods in the Treatment of Spinal Deformity in Children Less Than 10 Years of Age. *Journal of Pediatric Orthopaedics*, *37*(8), e567–e574. https://doi.org/10.1097/BPO.0000000000000751.

Luhmann, S. J., Smith, J. C., McClung, A., McCullough, F. L., McCarthy, R. E., Thompson, G. H., & Growing Spine Study Group. (2017). Radiographic Outcomes of Shilla Growth Guidance System and Traditional Growing Rods Through Definitive Treatment. *Spine Deformity*, *5*(4), 277–282. https://doi.org/10.1016/j.jspd.2017.01.011.

McCarthy, R. E., Luhmann, S., Lenke, L., & McCullough, F. L. (2014). The Shilla growth guidance technique for early-onset spinal deformities at 2-year follow-up: A preliminary report. *Journal of Pediatric Orthopedics*, *34*(1), 1–7. https://doi.org/10.1097/BPO.0b013e31829f92dc.

McCarthy, R. E., & McCullough, F. L. (2015). Shilla Growth Guidance for Early-Onset Scoliosis: Results After a Minimum of Five Years of Follow-up. *The Journal of Bone and Joint Surgery. American Volume*, *97*(19), 1578–1584. https://doi.org/10.2106/JBJS.N.01083.

McCarthy, R. E., Sucato, D., Turner, J. L., Zhang, H., Henson, M. A. W., & McCarthy, K. (2010). Shilla Growing Rods in a Caprine Animal Model: A Pilot Study. *Clinical Orthopaedics & Related Research*, *468*(3), 705–710. https://doi.org/10.1007/s11999-009-1028-y.

Pehrsson, K., Larsson, S., Oden, A., & Nachemson, A. (1992). Long-term follow-up of patients with untreated scoliosis. A study of mortality, causes of death, and symptoms. *Spine*, *17*(9), 1091–1096. https://doi.org/10.1097/00007632-199209000-00014.

Sanders, J. O., Little, D. G., & Richards, B. S. (1997). Prediction of the crankshaft phenomenon by peak height velocity. *Spine*, *22*(12), 1352–1356; discussion 1356-1357. https://doi.org/10.1097/00007632-199706150-00013.

Sucato, D. J. (2010). Management of severe spinal deformity: Scoliosis and kyphosis. *Spine*, *35*(25), 2186–2192. https://doi.org/10.1097/BRS.0b013e3181feab19.

Thompson, G. H., Lenke, L. G., Akbarnia, B. A., McCarthy, R. E., & Campbell, R. M. (2007). Early onset scoliosis: Future directions. *The Journal of Bone and Joint Surgery. American Volume*, *89 Suppl 1*, 163–166. https://doi.org/10.2106/JBJS.F.01513.

Williams, B. A., Matsumoto, H., McCalla, D. J., Akbarnia, B. A., Blakemore, L. C., Betz, R. R., Flynn, J. M., Johnston, C. E., McCarthy, R. E., Roye, D. P., Skaggs, D. L., Smith, J. T., Snyder, B. D., Sponseller, P. D., Sturm, P. F., Thompson, G. H., Yazici, M., & Vitale, M. G. (2014). Development and initial validation of the Classification of Early-Onset Scoliosis (C-EOS). *The Journal of Bone and Joint Surgery. American Volume*, *96*(16), 1359–1367. https://doi.org/10.2106/JBJS.M.00253.

# Chapter 27

# Hemivertebra Resection in Congenital EOS

**Fatih Emre Topsakal[1,*], MD**
**and Mehmet Demir[2], MD**
[1,2]Department of Orthopedics and Traumatology, Erzurum City Hospital, Erzurum, Turkiye

## Abstract

Hemivertebra is a congenital spinal abnormality that occurs between the 8th and 12th weeks of embryological development. Most hemivertebrae have normal growth plates; thus, they develop deformities that display asymmetric growth. The internal organs are also affected because of the progressive spinal deformity. Therefore, treatment should be planned in the early stages to prevent progression of the deformity. Hemivertebra resection will eliminate the deformity and stop its progression. The best result of the hemivertebra resection is achieved between 1.5 and four years old. Indications for hemivertebra resection are patients with deformities in the thoracolumbar, lumbar, or lumbosacral areas.

**Keywords:** early onset scoliosis, hemivertebra, resection, segmentation anomaly, surgical treatment

## Introduction

Congenital spinal deformities are anomalies that develop depending on the congenital formation and segmentation defects of the spine. The incidence of

* Corresponding Author's Email: Drfatihtopsakal@hotmail.com.

In: Early Onset Scoliosis
Editor: Ahmed Majid Heydar
ISBN: 979-8-89113-600-7

spinal anomaly is stated to be 1/1000 (Akalan, 2014). Delays in diagnosis and treatment can lead to complex spinal deformities in later years.

Hemivertebra abnormality is the most common cause of vertebral anomaly leading to deformity (Weinstein, 1994). As single and multiple hemivertebra anomalies can occur, they can become complex with accompanying bar formations. Depending on individual growth potential, most hemivertebrae develop a progressing wedge-shaped deformity during spinal growth. The rate of deformity and the final severity of the curvature depend on the type of anomaly and the area where it occurs. The level of deformity is another factor that affects the prognosis.

The patient's growth potential, the type, and localization of the anomaly are important prognostic factors in the treatment. In the cases of a poor prognosis, the curvature can become rigid, and secondary structural curvatures can develop to maintain body balance. In such patients, early surgery becomes crucial to prevent the development of compensatory curvatures and to prevent it from becoming structural. In addition to the shorter segmented fusion performed with early surgery, the unaffected spine can develop more healthily.

Treatment options include posterior fusion, combined anterior and posterior fusion, guided growth surgeries, posterior or anterior hemarthrosis, and short segment fusion surgeries with hemivertebra resection (Callahan et al., 1997). The hemivertebra resection becomes prominent because it is performed with a short segment fusion and provides an almost complete correction.

## Etiology

Congenital scoliosis does not commonly occur in a family history. Although isolated hemivertebrae do not show a risk of genetic inheritance, genetic inheritance is observed in 5-10% of cases in complex abnormalities (Callahan et al., 1997). The spine develops during the first six weeks. During this period, fetal hypoxia, exposure to carbon monoxide, smoking, diabetes, and the use of epilepsy medications can lead to formation defects.

## Classification

Congenital spinal abnormalities can be in the formation, segmentation, or mixed types. Winter's classification is based on the developmental pattern of the disease (Winter et al., 1968) (Figure 1).

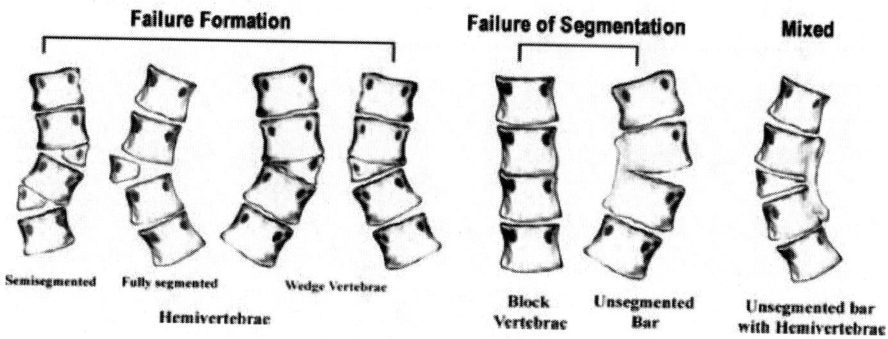


**Figure 1.** Winter's classification (Winter et al., 1968).

The hemivertebra can be considered as an example of a formation defect. In the bar formation related to segmentation defects, one side of the vertebra has normal segmentation, and the other side has a segmentation defect.

The Kawakami classification (Kawakami et al., 2009)

- Type I Single simple (compatible) type
  - Hemivertebra
  - Wedge vertebra
  - Butterfly vertebra
  - Defective type
- Type II Multiple simple (compatible) type
  - Combination of hemivertebra, wedge vertebra, or butterfly vertebra
  - Separated, fused, or other
- Type III Complex (non-compatible) type
  - Non-contiguous complex type
  - Non-mixed complex anomaly type
- Type IV - Formation type
  - Pure segmentation defect

## History and Physical Examination

In patients with the hemivertebra spine, congenital abnormalities can be observed in other organs and systems. A detailed musculoskeletal examination should be performed to detect developmental dysplasia of the hip, vertical talus, pes cavus, and limb anomalies. Congenital heart anomalies are observed in approximately 20% of patients with scoliosis. Sensory, motor, and reflex tests should be considered in neurological examinations.

## Radiological Examination

The anteroposterior and lateral radiographs of the spine are examined with direct radiographs. The balance of the trunk and spine, the type of scoliosis, differences in lower extremity lengths (pelvic tilt), and skeletal maturation (Risser sign) are evaluated. The contours of the lumbar and sagittal spine are examined in the full-lateral radiograph (Figure 2).

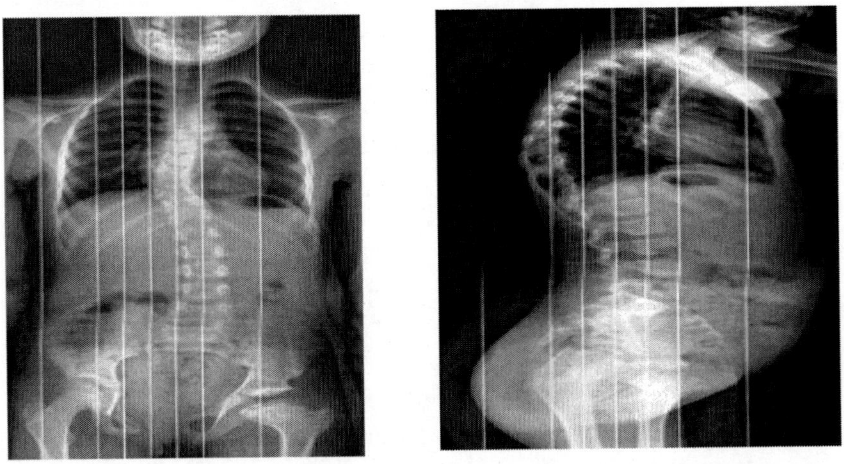

**Figure 2.** Anterior-posterior and lateral radiographs of the full-spine (McMaster & Ohtsuka, 1982).

The Cobb method is used to measure the angle of scoliosis. On the AP radiograph, the angle is measured between the lower surface of the caudal end vertebrae axes and the upper plate of the cephalic end vertebrae axes. The segmental Cobb angle is also used to measure the segmental curvature caused by the hemivertebra (Figure 3).

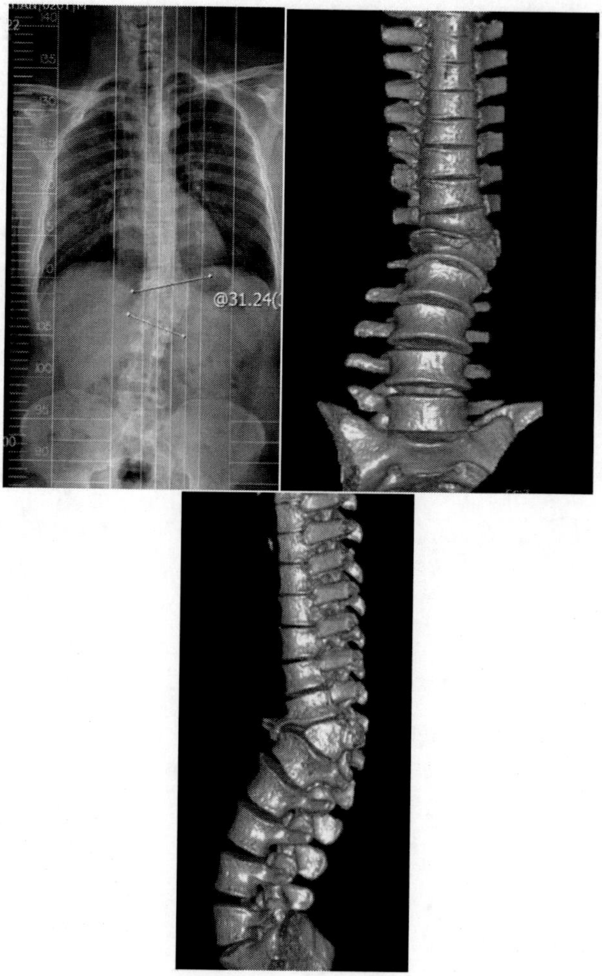

**Figure 3.** Measurement of the segmental Cobb angle and its three-dimensional radiograph (McMaster & Ohtsuka, 1982).

Intraspinal and extraspinal anomalies can accompany congenital scoliosis. Because of the possibility of restricting spinal cord movement, a complete spinal MRI should be performed for detection. Without correcting an intraspinal anomaly, the correction of the deformity could lead to the risk of neurological deficits. Diastematomyelia is a commonly observed pathology that causes tension in the spinal cord; furthermore, syringomyelia, diplomyelia, and Arnold-Chiari malformation can also be seen (Figure 4).

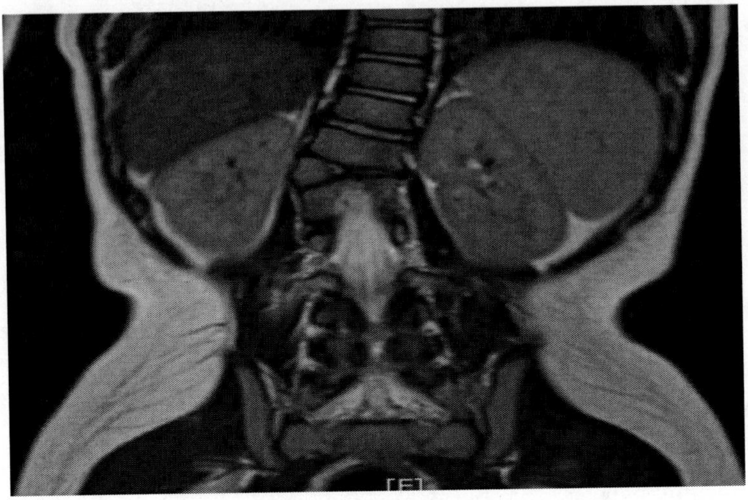

**Figure 4.** Coronal radiography of a complete segmented hemivertebra located in the thoracolumbar area (Nasca et al., 1975).

## Differential diagnosis

Hemivertebra is a congenital failure of formation. In the differential diagnosis, vertebral segmentation failures, tumors, and infections should be considered.

## Treatment

The main goal of treatment is to achieve a balanced growing spine and prevent the progression of the deformity. Non-segmental vertebrae and block vertebrae can be conservatively monitored without showing progression. Cases with low progression potential can be conservatively monitored with radiographs every 6 to 12 months.

Bilateral hemivertebra on the same side, lumbosacral region anomalies, single unilateral unsegmented bar, and unilateral unsegmented bar with hemivertebra are poor prognostic types and should be performed early surgery.

## Surgical Treatment

In patients with non-multiple hemivertebrae and short segment deformities, short segment instrumentation-fusion surgery is commonly added to hemivertebra resection. Principally, the affected posterior elements of the vertebral segment, such as the lamina, transverse processes, and facet joints, are carefully dissected on the convex side of the rib head in the thoracic area (Figure 5).

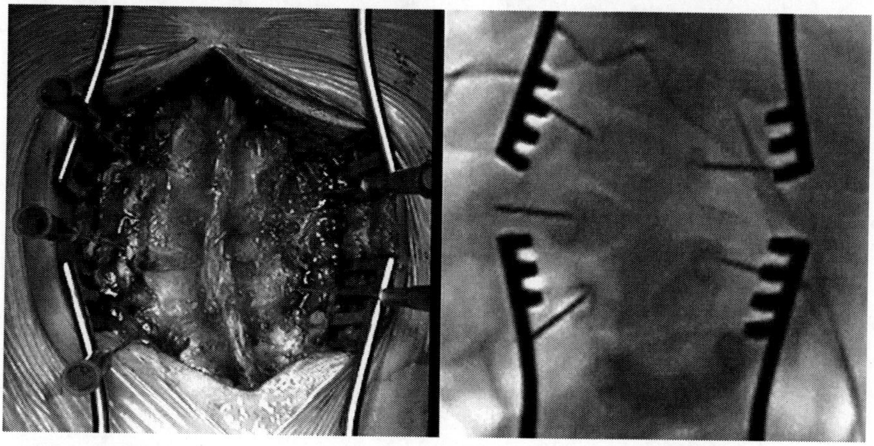

**Figure 5.** Marking the entry points for pedicle screws (Ruf et al., 2009).

The nerve roots above and below the hemivertebra pedicle and the spinal cord should be visible. In the thoracic vertebrae, the rib head on the convex side should be resected. After resection of the rib head and transverse process, the anterior and lateral sides of the hemivertebra can be reached with blunt dissection. In the thoracic area, extrapleural exploration is performed, and in the lumbar area, retroperitoneal exploration is operated. The posterior of the hemivertebra corpus is reached after removing the pedicle. The upper and lower discs of the hemivertebra are cut, and the hemivertebra is removed.

Residual disc remnants are completely removed from the upper and lower vertebral endplates until bleeding is observed. In patients with significant kyphosis, cages can be used to support the anterior column (Ruf et al., 2009).

After the instrumentation is performed after the resection, compression is conducted to the convex side until the gap is closed. The cancellous bone obtained from the resected hemivertebra can be used to support fusion. Especially in cases with kyphosis, if a high amount of compressive force is required to correct the deformity, adding one or two vertebrae to the fusion area can help prevent potential pedicle fractures (Figure 6).

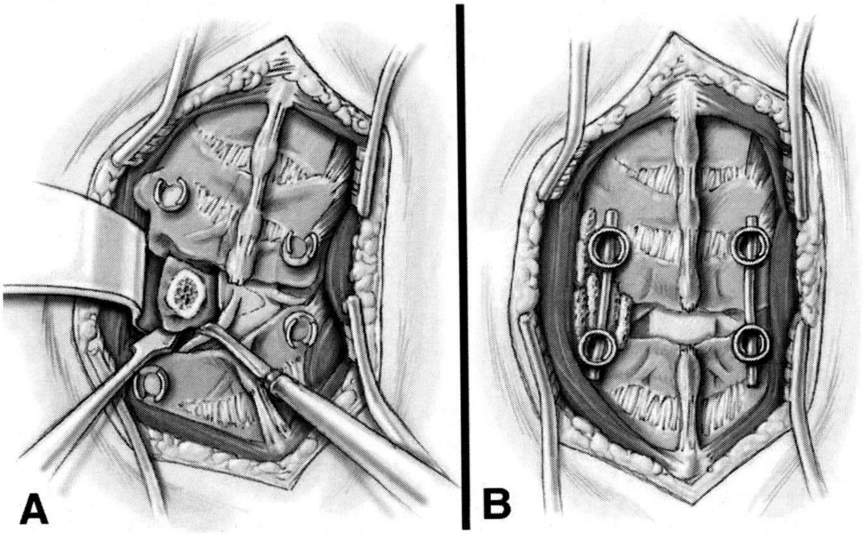


**Figure 6.** Adhesion discs into the hemivertebra are resected, and after being mobilized, the body of the hemivertebra is removed. A. A blunt spatula preserves the anterior vessels. B. The gap is closed with compression on the convex side, and the deformity is corrected. Cancellous bone can be added to facilitate fusion (Ruf et al., 2009).

In the presence of rib head synostosis and the formation of contralateral bar, the bar formation and the proximal parts of the costas causing the synostosis should be removed. The facet joints of the vertebrae involved in synostosis on the concave side should be removed, and the roots on this side should also be carefully preserved. After the removal of the transverse processes and costa heads, the lateral part of the pathological vertebra is exposed with blunt dissection (Figure 7).

The spinal cord should be completely visualized. The bar formation should be osteotomized for the correction. If necessary, the fusion area can be expanded based on the amount of osteotomy (Ruf et al., 2009) (Figure 8).

Preoperative and postoperative radiographs, and the final follow-up after 13 years (Ruf et al., 2009).

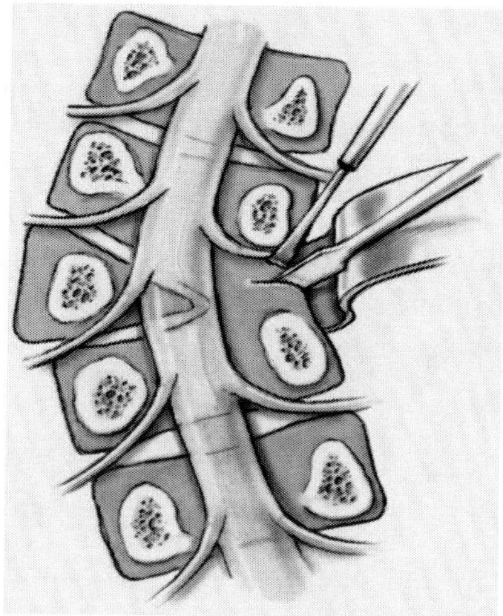

**Figure 7.** Exposing the concave side with the osteotomy of bar formation (Ruf et al., 2009).

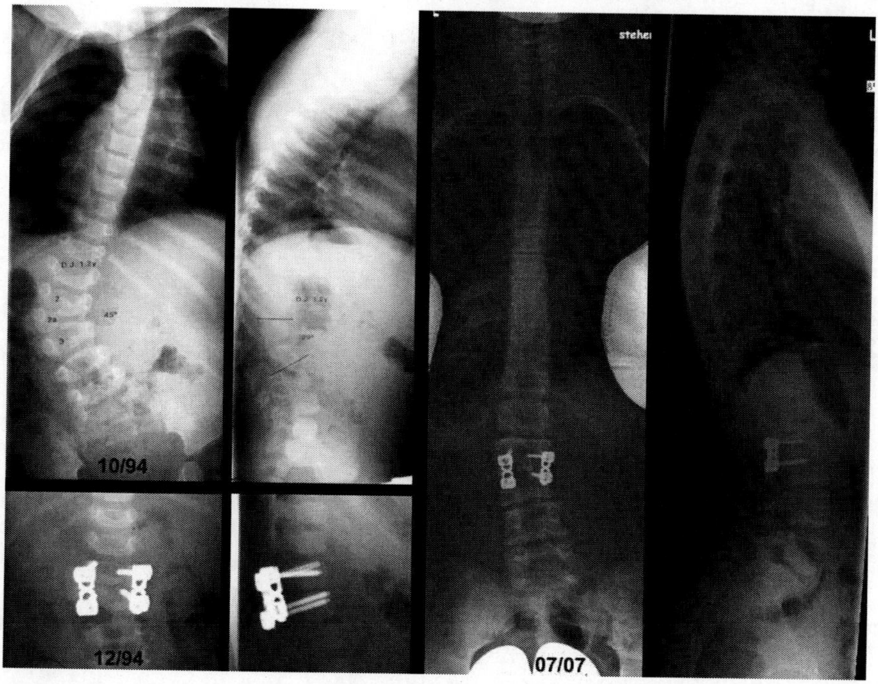


**Figure 8.** Resection of a complete segmented hemivertebra at 16 months of age (Ruf et al., 2009).

## Rehabilitation

In cases without complications, patients are usually assisted to stand up on the first postoperative day. The patients are followed with a thoracolumbosacral orthosis for 3 months in the postoperative period. Most of the time, there is no need to remove spinal implants; however, in some patients, the protrusion of implants may cause discomfort, and it can be necessary to remove them after one year.

## Complications

Complications such as inadequate correction, dural injury, neurological damage, implant failure, excessive blood loss, non-union, and infection in hemivertebra resection can be observed.

## Conclusion

Hemivertebra is one of the most common causes of scoliosis. A segmental hemivertebra can lead to progressive spinal deformities if left untreated because it has growth potential similar to that of a normal vertebra. Therefore, hemivertebra deformity should be treated before it progresses. Hemivertebra resection is a safe and effective treatment method for patients with early onset scoliosis. Approximately 70% of the patients have excellent correction of the curvature, and the fusion rates are close to 100%.

## References

Akalan, T (2014). *Adölesan idiyopatik skolyozun cerrahi tedavisinde posterior enstrümantasyon ve füzyon sonuçlarımız [Outcomes of Posterior Instrumentation and Fusion in Adolescent Idiopathic Scoliosis] (Sp. Thesis)*. Mersin University Faculty of Medicine.

Callahan, B. C., Georgopoulos, G., & Eilert, R. E. (1997). Hemivertebral excision for congenital scoliosis. *Journal of Pediatric Orthopaedics*, *17*(1), 96-99. https://doi.org/10.1097/00004694-199701000-00020.

Kawakami, N., Tsuji, T., Imagama, S., Lenke, L. G., Puno, R. M., Kuklo, T. R., & Spinal Deformity Study Group. (2009). Classification of congenital scoliosis and kyphosis: a new approach to the three-dimensional classification for progressive vertebral anomalies requiring operative treatment. *Spine, 34*(17), 1756-1765. https://doi.org/10.1097/BRS.0b013e3181ac0045.

McMaster, M. J., & Ohtsuka, K. (1982). The natural history of congenital scoliosis. A study of two hundred and fifty-one patients. *JBJS, 64*(8), 1128-1147. https://doi.org/10.2106/00004623-198264080-00003.

Nasca, R. J., Stilling 3rd, F. H., & Stell, H. H. (1975). Progression of congenital scoliosis due to hemivertebrae and hemivertebrae with bars. *JBJS, 57*(4), 456-466. https://doi.org/10.2106/00004623-197557040-00003.

Ruf, M., Jensen, R., Letko, L., & Harms, J. (2009). Hemivertebra resection and osteotomies in congenital spine deformity. *Spine, 34*(17), 1791-1799. https://doi.org/10.1097/BRS.0b013e3181ab6290.

Weinstein, S. L. (1994). Adolescent idiopathic scoliosis: prevalence and natural history. In: *Weinstein, SL (ed.): The pediatric spine: principles and practice*, New York, Raven Press.

Winter, R. B., Moe, J. H., & Eilers, V. E. (1968). Congenital Scoliosis A Study of 234 Patients Treated and Untreated: PART II: TREATMENT. *JBJS, 50*(1), 15-47. https://doi.org/10.2106/00004623-196850010-00002.

## Chapter 28

# Outcomes in Children with EOS

**Furkan Soy[1,*], MD**
**and Ozan Pehlivan[2], MD**
[1]Department of Orthopedics and Traumatology, Kahramankazan State Hospital, Ankara, Turkiye
[2]Department of Orthopedics and Traumatology, Beytepe State Hospital, Ankara, Turkiye

## Abstract

Early-onset scoliosis is a difficult and time-consuming deformity with fatal consequences if left untreated. For this reason, analyzing early-onset scoliosis well, managing possible complications well, and getting ideas from the literature, especially by following the current treatment principles, will contribute significantly to the development of the children we follow with this diagnosis. Early-onset scoliosis causes pulmonary developmental defects, especially when it accompanies deformities in the thoracic region. Therefore, it can cause death in later periods. This information shows how important the treatment of early-onset scoliosis is. When determining the treatment method, the advantages and disadvantages of the desired result should be well evaluated. In this regard, all available treatment methods should be known in detail, and the most appropriate treatment for the patient should be selected from among the available options, considering the indications and contraindications of all treatment options.

**Keywords:** early-onset scoliosis, outcomes, conservative treatment, surgical techniques, complication

---

* Corresponding Author's Email: dr.furkansoy@gmail.com.

In: Early Onset Scoliosis
Editor: Ahmed Majid Heydar
ISBN: 979-8-89113-600-7

## Introduction

Scoliosis patients may also have some physiological problems, the severity of which varies according to the vertebral segment where the curvature is located, the severity of the curvature, and the presence of anomaly accompanying the curvature. Thoracic curvatures may cause deterioration of shoulder-body balance, cervical spine pathologies, and cardiopulmonary dysfunction depending on the size of the deformity (Pehrsson et al., 1992; Swank et al.,1982). Likewise, varying degrees of pelvic obliquity, leg length difference, and gait disturbance may occur as a result of the deformity in the lumbar region. In early childhood, lung and thorax development progresses rapidly in proportion to skeletal development. Scoliosis deformities also show more progression during periods of rapid skeletal growth (Bjerkreim and Hassan, 1982). Life-threatening cardiopulmonary abnormalities, such as restrictive pulmonary disease, pulmonary arterial hypertension, and cor pulmonale, can be seen in progressive scoliosis that hinders the development of the thorax (Pehrsson et al., 1992; Swank et al.,1982). Especially in early-onset scoliosis in which the thoracic spine is affected, insufficient spinal cord length and, as a result, insufficient thoracic cavity formation causes thoracic insufficiency syndrome. For this reason, the aim of surgical techniques applied in the treatment of early-onset scoliosis is to allow the maximum growth of the lungs and thorax, to ensure the continuation of spinal elongation, and to prevent the progression of the curvature. The time of initiation of treatment and the extent to which the selected treatment options reduce these complications are the subject of new studies. Studies aiming to find which treatment options are superior are among the current topics in the literature.

## Main Body

Scoliosis deformities show more progression in the skeletal development process (Bjerkreim and Hassan,1982). While the concave side of the curve is subjected to growth-suppressing compression, the convex side of the curve is exposed to growth-stimulating distraction, leaving the spine outside of normal spinal development physiology. These additional forces place scoliosis patients in a vicious circle that causes an increase in deformity. Compression-distraction forces and the effects of these forces on bone growth were first described by the Hueter-Volkmann law and inspired many treatment methods for growing spinal deformities (Mehlman et al., 1997). Based on this law, surgical methods have been developed, such as applying compression to the convex side spine exposed to distraction or applying distraction to the concave side exposed to compression.

Early-onset scoliosis causes pulmonary developmental defects, especially because it accompanies deformities in the thoracic region. Therefore, it can cause death in later periods. Pehrsson et al. studied the rate of mortality in 115 women who did not receive scoliosis treatment. The mortality rate was 32% in 29 infantile-onset patients with untreated scoliosis in infancy, and this rate was higher than in juvenile-onset scoliosis patients. In 40% of the patients who died, the cause of death was respiratory failure. In 21 patients (90%) who died due to respiratory failure, scoliosis was diagnosed before the age of nine (Pehrsson et al., 1992). This information shows how important the treatment of early-onset scoliosis is. When determining the treatment method, the advantages and disadvantages of the desired result should be well evaluated.

Contrary to adolescent idiopathic scoliosis, correcting the curvature does not always mean curing early-onset scoliosis. The short torso, disproportionate body, and the "Crankshaft" phenomenon (Karol et al., 2008a) that occur in the spine of a young child with the fusion of more than one segment, especially in the thoracic region, in addition to the possibility of developing further deformity, may inhibit the normal growth of the spine and thorax (Karol et al., 2008b), leading to inadequate or even worse outcomes. As a result, the old view that a short but straight spine is better than a long and crooked spine is no longer accepted (Day et al., 1994; Winter et al., 1982). Due to the negative effects of premature fusion of the spine on cardiopulmonary function, it will not be able to prevent future spinal deformities as the child grows and matures (Karol et al., 2008a). Studies have shown that definitive spinal fusion prevents the enlargement of the rib cage in patients with early-onset scoliosis. In the study by Karol et al. (Karol et al., 2008b), thorax growth retardation was observed in early spinal fusion patients compared to the normal values published by Dimeglio (1992).

## Comparison of Outcomes of Treatment Options

### *Conservative Treatment*

According to the principles of Mehta (1972) and Akbarnia (2007), the Cobb angle is greater than 25°, the RVAD is greater than 20°, the phase II ribs, and the initial curve progression after 1 year of age. Ceballos et al. (1980) showed that patients with double curves are more likely to progress and should be closely followed. In patients with curves greater than 25°, treatment is initiated if the Cobb angle or RVAD increases from 5° to 10°.

Before the development of surgical methods, the standard treatment for all scoliosis treatments was casting. Various complications including pressure sores, superior mesenteric artery syndrome, and rib or mandible deformities were commonly seen in the Risser casting technique, which largely eliminated the derotational casting technique based on the three-point bending principle (Hutchinson and Bassett, 1990; Moe and Gustilo, 1964; Mehta, 2005).

The modern technique is called 'EDF' casting (extension, derotation, and flexion). Spinal deformities are 3-dimensional deformities. EDF plastering can also address these three dimensions. When checked it every 2 or 4 months, the cast is terminated when the curvature is <10-20° or the treatment is continued using a brace. Care should be taken to ensure that the children who will be cast have no sensory defects and that their lung functions are not weak.

Several modern studies document the positive results of casting treatment. In Mehta's series of 136 patients, outcomes were related to age and the severity of the curve when treatment was started. In children with a mean age of 1.6 years and children with a coronal deformity of 32° (group 1), scoliosis resolved towards the age of 4 years, and no additional treatment was required. The deformities of the children treated with a mean age of 2.5 years and a mean deformity of 52° (group 2) progressed, and 15 of these children required spinal fusion (Mehta, 2005). Similar results were reported by Sanders et al. (2009). They concluded that in 55 patients with documented or anticipated progression, sequential cast correction of infant scoliosis resulted mostly in complete resolution in infants with idiopathic curves of 60° lower when started before 20 months of age. In older pediatric patients with greater curvature or a diagnosis of non-idiopathic scoliosis, cast correction still results in curvature improvement, with improvement in chest and body shape. Therefore, while it plays an important role in the treatment of progressive infantile scoliosis at young age, it also plays a role in delaying surgery and reducing the degree of curvature in older and syndromic patients (Fletcher et al., 2012).

### *Surgical Treatment*

The goal of surgical treatment of early-onset scoliosis is to allow the continuation of spinal elongation while ensuring maximum growth of the lung and thorax, while at the same time preventing the progression of the curvature. Surgical treatment of infantile idiopathic scoliosis is recommended for children with advanced curves (Cobb ≥45°) and who have not reached maturity (Lenke, 2004). The patient's age and maturity during the progression of the curve will determine the type of surgical procedure chosen. Skaggs divides growth-friendly spinal implant systems into distraction-based, compression-based, and guided growth systems based on the correction forces exerted by the implant on the spine (Skaggs et al., 2014).

Distraction-based implants are growing rods that can be applied to the spine or ribs, vertically extensible titanium rib prosthesis (VEPTR), and externally extendable devices. Examples of compression-based systems are spine staples and binders (tether). Guided growth systems correct the spinal deformity by attaching multiple vertebrae (usually including the apical vertebra) to the rods through translation and other mechanical forces during initial implantation. Most anchors are not firmly attached to the rods, and thus slide over the rods over time, allowing for longitudinal growth. Guided growth systems are the Luque trolley and Shilla.

The staple technique is effective in congenital scoliosis, but its effectiveness in early-onset scoliosis has not been reported. Today, SMA (shape memory alloy) "Staple" (Betz et al., 2010) and "Tethers" (Newton et al., 2008) are used to perform epiphysiodesis. Although most of these techniques are experimental, clinical experience with SMA Staple treatment in older children has been reported (Betz et al., 2010, Stücker, 2009). Potential advantages of a compression-based approach are the preservation of motion and disc viability, as well as the ability to correct spinal deformity with a single surgical procedure (Newton et al., 2008). It is not the ideal method for children, as it can restrict growth.

In a series that Betz et al. treated using staples, there were a total of 41 children with 26 thoracic and 15 lumbar curvatures. The average age of children is 9. In the group with thoracic curvature, the success rate was 78% for curvatures lower than 35°, while there was a 75% improvement in the group with high curvature (greater than 50°). The success rate is the highest in the group with thoracic curvature under the age of 10, at 75%. Stapling in patients with hypokyphosis has also been found to be beneficial in correcting the sagittal contour. This method is contraindicated for thoracic kyphosis. While the success rate for lumbar curvatures is 87%, this rate is 100% under the age of ten.

Tethers inhibit growth on the convex side of the curve, similar to stapling. Theoretically, it causes less damage to the intervertebral discs. It has been demonstrated in an animal model study that it protects the discs (Newton et al., 2011). In the case report published by Crawford and Lenke, an 8-year-old male patient has 40° thoracic scoliosis and was treated with a 4-5 mm polypropylene tether by placing a T6-T12 screw (Crawford and Lenke, 2010). In the early postoperative radiograph, the curvature regressed from 40° to 26° and regressed to 6° after 4 years of follow-up. Thoracic kyphosis was 26° preoperatively, 14° in postoperatively, and 18° after 4 years of follow-up.

The most important disadvantage of guided growth systems is that repetitive surgical lengthening may be required. It does not cause any change in the patient's kyphosis, as growth occurs at the same rate at both endpoints. As a matter of fact, adjacent segment kyphosis may occur in distraction-based systems. Although the main goal of using these systems is to leave the patient without an implant at the end of the treatment, it cannot be predicted in advance which patient will require fusion after treatment or from which patient the implants will be removed. The Luque Trolley and Shilla techniques are examples of guided growth systems.

Luque and Cardosa described fusion-free segmental spinal correction and published a series in which they operated on 47 patients using Harrington rods and combined sublaminar wires (Luque, 1982). An average of 2.6 cm of elongation and a 78% improvement in curvature were obtained in the instrumented spine with the technique used in this series. Later, this technique was modified as the "Luque Trolley" technique by adding 'L' shaped rods and wires. In this technique, there is no need for repetitive surgical intervention, since the implants can slide over rods during elongation (Leatherman, 1988). Due to the fixation power of the technique, there is no need for postoperative immobilization. In the study by Pratt et al., it was stated that 32% of the expected growth was achieved in the 5-year follow-up of 18 patients who underwent the Luque trolley, the Cobb angle worsened in patients with the Luque alone, and the Cobb angle improved over time in 2 of 13 patients who underwent the Luque trolley and convex epiphysiodesis (Pratt et al., 1999). Studies conducted in many different centers show that the Luque trolley technique causes spontaneous fusion and growth restriction in implanted vertebrae within 5 years after surgery. Due to the necessity of extensive subperiosteal dissection, interlaminae ankylosis and adhesions can be seen. The advantage of this technique is that it is performed in a single session of surgery. Thus, new surgeries are not required for lengthening in these children with high comorbidity.

The Shilla technique, developed by McCarthy et al. (2010), is a system in which rod and pedicle screws are used to allow growth. First, the apical deformity is corrected to be neutral in all planes (coronal, sagittal, and axial). The effectiveness of this technique has been proven in the goat model. Currently, there are no long-term follow-up series on the Shilla technique.

There are 10 patients in the publication of McCarthy et al. (2015), the mean age of these patients is 7 years, and the minimum follow-up period is 2 years. The mean pre-operative curvature angle was 70°, the early post-operative curvature was 27°, and this correction was maintained at a 2-year follow-up. The length between C7-S1 increased by an average of 12% during surgery and follow-up.

Current examples of distraction-based implants are conventional growing rods, VEPTR, and magnetic growing rods. A new surgical technique was developed by Robert Campbell. This technique does not include the previously used spinal arthrodesis, instead, expansion thoracoplasty is performed via open wedge thoracostomy, and the thoracic reconstruction is stabilized by adding rib-to-spine or rib-to-pelvis VEPTR to treat spinal curvature and placing another rib-to-rib VEPTR to increase the volume of the restricted hemithorax (Campbell et al., 2003). This new procedure treats thoracic insufficiency syndrome by directly enlarging and lengthening the restricted hemithorax and improving the thoracic spine and thoracic development, indirectly treating congenital scoliosis without the need for spinal fusion (Campbell et al., 2003). Campbell et al. (2004) studied 27 children with 35 congenital scolioses associated with a fused rib, and the mean improvement in scoliosis decreased from 74° to 49°. Thoracic spine height increased by an average of 7.1 mm/year. 52 complications (193%) were seen in 22 patients. The most frequent complication was proximal migration of the device passing through the ribs in 7 patients. Hasler et al. (2010) studied 23 patients with non-congenital early-onset scoliosis. The Cobb angle decreased from 68° pre-operatively to 54° at the final follow-up. Wound complications were observed in 16 of 23 complications, and implant-related complications were observed in 7.

Current information has created some reservations about the use of VEPTR-type instrumentation on the chest wall. Specifically, the use of VEPTR has been associated with spontaneous rib and vertebral fusions, which can worsen spinal balance in addition to increasing the stiffness of the chest wall and deformity (Yilgor et al., 2012; Groenefeld and Hell, 2013). It has been shown that the risk of this ossification may increase 4 years after VEPTR treatment.

In children treated for early-onset scoliosis related to chest deformity, eventual arthrodesis of the spine is often required when adequate growth is achieved. Lattig et al. found that eventual arthrodesis of the spine was risky and challenging in patients treated with VEPTR secondary to the development of high thoracic hyperkyphosis, the autofusion of the ribs and vertebral bodies, and the progression of the curvature. However, VEPTR is still the most advanced surgical technique in the presence of an underdeveloped thorax in thoracic insufficiency syndrome. Currently, there is no better alternative treatment for children with spinal curvatures caused by the stretching effect of thoracic deformities and a thorax with a restricted range of motion. However, spinal implants should be preferred for thoracic deformities that occur secondary to spinal curvatures.

Harrington was the first to describe the modern growing rod technique in the treatment of scoliosis. He described this technique in 1962. Harrington described a subcutaneous, non-fusion surgical technique with a single distraction rod attached to laminal hooks placed at both ends of the concave side of the deformity. While performing this technique, the surgeon encountered complications such as rod fracture and hook separation from the applied area, but long-term follow-up results were not specified. Harrington said that progressive scoliosis under 10 years of age could be treated with this distraction rod without applying fusion, but he recommended that fusion be performed together with the first operation in a child older than 10 years of age (Harrington, 1962). It has become a cornerstone of modern early-onset scoliosis surgery.

After Harrington's technique, Moe et al. (1984) modified this technique by limiting the subperiosteal dissection to the area where the hook was inserted. No fusion was applied to the area where the hook was placed. The middle region has been modified to facilitate the placement of the rod, prevent scar formation, and allow the sagittal contour to be given at the same time. The results of this technique showed that instrumentation patients had an average growth of 2.9 cm at the instrumentation site. While the average growth was 3.8 cm in the patients who underwent fusion, the estimated growth was 4.5 cm in the same patients who did not undergo fusion. Moe et al. reported complication rates of 50%, involving the separation of the hook from the rod and lamina.

The dual-growing rod technique applied by Akbarnia works on the same principle as the single-growing rod (Thompson et al., 2005). The largest series using dual-growing rods was published by Akbarnia (2005). The mean amount of curvature increased from 82° pre-operatively to 38° after the first surgery and 36° at the last follow-up. The lengthening procedure was applied to the patients an average of 6.6 times, with an average increase in T1-S1 length of 1.2 cm/year. Complications were observed in 11 (48%) of 23 patients due to various reasons.

In a study by Bess et al. (2010), it was shown that complications occur 1.2 times more in patients treated with a single-growing rod than in patients with dual rods. It has been shown that the use of dual rods reduces mechanical stress compared to a single rod. This feature is very important for non-fusion techniques because the implant is subjected to loading and micromovement, which leads to metal fatigue and mechanical failure. Using a dual rod reduces the amount of stress per rod compared to a single rod. Furthermore, in the event of the failure of a rod, the intact rod provides stability and delays implant revision until the next scheduled lengthening procedure.

Surgical lengthening performed with an interval of 6 months or less causes significantly more growth and correction (Hardy and Curtis, 1971). However, in order to determine the optimal interval for lengthening, it should be considered that each additional surgery increases the risk of complications by 24% (Bess et al., 2010). It has been shown that repetitive distraction depends on the 'diminishing returns' rule. According to this rule, repetitive lengthening results in less lengthening each time. In a study involving 38 patients, the average gain in T1-S1 distance observed from the first lengthening was 1.04 cm, while this gain decreased to 0.41 cm in the 7th extension (Sankar et al., 2011). This study has caused concern that when distraction-based devices are used, it results in autofusion of the spine, possibly due to loss of motion of the facet joints over the years. A study of 28 patients at 6 centers found an increase in the Cobb angle, T1-S1 length, and usable space volume for the lung, as well as a 35% implant-related complication rate, with a mean follow-up of 37 months. Complications were seen primarily in those who had a single rod. No loss of fixation was observed when bilateral hooks and 3 or more hooks were used (Myung et al., 2010). The multiple extensions required for conventional grow rods expose patients to many complications (Bess et al., 2010). These repetitive surgeries are associated with an increased risk of skin problems, wound infections, and implant-related complications (Sankar et al., 2010). The high number of complications with conventional growing rods limits their use, and some surgeons prefer non-surgical methods, while others have begun to reduce surgical indications in patients with early-onset scoliosis (Fletcher et al., 2012). All of these developments have encouraged the search for alternative methods that reduce complications and achieve better results. From this point of view, the idea of non-invasive multiple lengthening without surgery or complications has become interesting. Rod technology that can grow with remote-controlled extension has opened a new era in the treatment of these patients. Takaso et al. showed that a remote-controlled pickup could be the driving force for a growing rod. In his animal study with 12 dogs, he showed that after 4 distractions over a 12-week period, the scoliosis created at 24° was corrected to an average of 3°. In 2004, the development of the remotely controlled magnetic rod called the Phenox rod was followed (Takaso et al., 1998), and it was the first magnetic rod used in humans (Wick and Konze, 2012). The clinical results of this device are limited; Wick and Miladi reported a limited human experience with short follow-up. Later, a new remote-controlled spinal distraction system called MAGEC (Magnetic Expansion Control) was developed. The first study was performed by Akbarnia et al. (2012) on 6 immature pigs. The mean distraction over a 7-week period was 39 mm without any implant-related complications. Loss of distraction, which is an early complication of this technique, was seen in first-generation designs, and this problem was solved by adding a locking mechanism to the magnetic distraction elements to prevent loss in the next generation of implantation or the next distraction (Dannawi et al., 2013). A few publications have been published on this technique in humans (Dannawi et al., 2013; Hickey et al., 2014). The MAGEC system has sterile titanium grow rods used as the single or double and a remote control for non-invasive extension. The magnetic inside the actuator is rotated non-invasively with a remote-controlled device. This remote-controlled device provides rod lengthening and spine distraction. Bess et al. reported that patients with double-growth rod application decreased from 82° pre-operatively to 38° post-operatively and up to 36° in their follow-up (Bess et al., 2010).

Akbarnia et al. (2008) divided the patients into two groups in a study. The patients in the first group were lengthened at intervals of ≤6 months, and the patients in the second group at intervals of >6 months. The results show that the amount of T1-S1 elongation and curvature correction was better in the group with traditional extendable rods and lengthening at short intervals than in the group with long-interval lengthening.

There is a high risk of encountering various complications during early-onset scoliosis treatment. McCarthy et al. (2015) reported many complications in their experience with growth-guided and compression-based systems. The most common complication with conventional extensible implants is wound dehiscence due to repeated lengthening procedures (Myung et al., 2010). Bess et al. (2010) concluded that the increase in the number of lengthening surgeries was associated with an increased risk of complications. Other important complications of extensible rods include posttraumatic stress disorder and depression (Akbarnia et al., 2013). Additionally, it imposes a significant economic burden on the patient's family. Repetitive surgical procedures are a burden on the patient and family as a result of time lost from work and school (Caldas et al., 2004).

The most common complications associated with the magnetic growing rod are the prominence of the implant under the skin, screw stripping, and junctional kyphosis. However, it has lower complication rates compared to traditional methods that require repetitive surgery.

Controversy continues regarding the placement of magnetic growing rods. Some studies have stated that the most accurate region to be selected during the placement of the rods is under the fascia, and methods such as the use of a thoracic drainage tube can be used for this (Munigangaiah et al., 2018). However, the number of studies suggesting intramuscular placement cannot be underestimated.

In a case series, metallosis was observed in the rod elongation zone in patients who were followed up for a long time and required revision surgery (Teoh et al., 2016). Magnetic growing rods are made of Ti-6Al-4V titanium alloy. While increased serum aluminum and titanium ions can be observed in patients using traditional growing rods, increased serum vanadium ion levels have been observed in patients using magnetic rods. There is also boron content in the actuator region of magnetic rods, but it was not detected in patient serums (Yilgor et al., 2018).

The main limitation of magnetic growing rods is the size of the rod and its distraction elements, called actuators. The thickness of the actuator causes wound problems and implant-related skin disorders in small patients. In order to minimize skin disorders, the patient's weight gain can be supported by a pediatrician and dietitian. For patients who are predicted to have skin problems, it may be beneficial to seek advice from nutrition-related branches. However, since the magnetic rods cannot provide sufficient sagittal contour due to their length, they distort the sagittal plane.

One of the disadvantages of magnetic rods is that repetitive scoliosis radiographs are required before and after distraction to see rod elongation (Dannawi et al., 2013). Radiological imaging may need to be performed up to 17 times a year (Hickey et al., 2014). It is not recommended to use the magnetic rod in patients who may require continuous MRI examination, such as syringomyelia. Although no side effects were observed using MRI imaging, it has been observed to cause image artifacts over 30cm. As a natural consequence of this, evaluation of medulla spinalis lesions has become quite difficult. Some recent studies have shown that ultrasonography has high reliability as an alternative to reducing radiation exposure (Stokes et al., 2014).

However, spot radiography may be necessary in the evaluation of scoliotic curvature alignment and balance in order to obtain adequate patient follow-up.

It is possible that the magnetic growing rod system will be improved in the future and thus have a lower complication rate. New designs can be developed with the aim of providing the contours more easily, providing and maintaining the sagittal balance. Making implants use more robust materials with a thinner profile will reduce their usability in small and weak children and reduce complications such as screw prominence.

## Conclusion

Early-onset scoliosis includes patients with different etiological bases. Each patient has unique medical conditions and additional morbidities and findings that should be considered during development and are important in treatment. In a diagnosis with such a wide variety of patients, it is not possible to impose a single treatment as the gold standard method for all patients. Among current treatment options, there are new techniques that have long-term results and have long-term clinical applications, in addition to techniques that have long-term results offered to us by the developing technology, but which theoretically have the potential for more promising results. Choosing the most suitable method for the patient among these techniques requires experience. The benefits of the treatment can be more clearly demonstrated by adding some parameters that show the thorax, pulmonary circulation, and lung development obtained by the patients, apart from the metric measurement values obtained during the follow-up period. As a result of these values, we hope that the early-onset scoliosis treatment principles of the next period will be more clearly shaped.

## References

Akbarnia, B. A. (2007). Management themes in early onset scoliosis. *JBJS*, 89(suppl_1), 42-54. https://doi.org/10.2106/JBJS.F.01256.

Akbarnia, B. A., Breakwell, L. M., Marks, D. S., McCarthy, R. E., Thompson, A. G., Canale, S. K., & Growing Spine Study Group. (2008). Dual growing rod technique followed for three to eleven years until final fusion: the effect of frequency of lengthening. *Spine*, 33(9), 984-990. https://doi.org/10.1097/BRS.0b013e31816c8b4e.

Akbarnia, B. A., Cheung, K., Noordeen, H., Elsebaie, H., Yazici, M., Dannawi, Z., & Kabirian, N. (2013). Next generation of growth-sparing techniques: preliminary clinical results of a magnetically controlled growing rod in 14 patients with early-onset scoliosis. *Spine*, 38(8), 665-670. https://doi.org/10.1097/BRS.0b013e3182773560.

Akbarnia, B. A., Marks, D. S., Boachie-Adjei, O., Thompson, A. G., & Asher, M. A. (2005). Dual growing rod technique for the treatment of progressive early-onset scoliosis: a multicenter study. *Spine*, 30(17S), S46-S57. https://doi.org/10.1097/01.brs.0000175190.08134.73.

Akbarnia, B. A., Mundis Jr, G. M., Salari, P., Yaszay, B., & Pawelek, J. B. (2012). Innovation in growing rod technique: a study of safety and efficacy of a magnetically controlled growing rod in a porcine model. *Spine*, 37(13), 1109-1114. https://doi.org/10.1097/BRS.0b013e318240ff67.

Bess, S., Akbarnia, B. A., Thompson, G. H., Sponseller, P. D., Shah, S. A., El Sebaie, H, Boachie-Adjei, O., Karlin, L., Canale, S., Poe-Kochert, C. & Skaggs, D. L. (2010). Complications of growing-rod treatment for early-onset scoliosis: analysis of one hundred and forty patients. *JBJS*, 92(15), 2533-2543. https://doi.org/10.2106/JBJS.I.01471.

Betz, R. R., Ranade, A., Samdani, A. F., Chafetz, R., D'Andrea, L. P., Gaughan, J. P., Asghar, J., Grewal, H. & Mulcahey, M. J. (2010). Vertebral body stapling: a fusionless treatment option for a growing child with moderate idiopathic scoliosis. *Spine*, 35(2), 169-176. https://doi.org/10.1097/BRS.0b013e3181c6dff5.

Bjerkreim, I., & Hassan, I. (1982). Progression in untreated idiopathic scoliosis after end of growth. *Acta Orthopaedica Scandinavica*, 53(6), 897-900. https://doi.org/10.3109/17453678208992845.

Caldas, J. C. S., Pais-Ribeiro, J. L., & Carneiro, S. R. (2004). General anesthesia, surgery and hospitalization in children and their effects upon cognitive, academic, emotional and sociobehavioral development–a review. *Pediatric Anesthesia*, 14(11), 910-915. https://doi.org/10.1111/j.1460-9592.2004.01350.x.

Campbell Jr, R. M., Smith, M. D., Mayes, T. C., Mangos, J. A., Willey-Courand, D. B., Kose, N., Pinero, R. F., Alder, M. E., Duong, H. L. & Surber, J. L. (2003). The characteristics of thoracic insufficiency syndrome associated with fused ribs and congenital scoliosis. *JBJS*, 85(3), 399-408. https://doi.org/10.2106/00004623-200303000-00001.

Campbell Jr, R. M., Smith, M. D., Mayes, T. C., Mangos, J. A., Willey-Courand, D. B., Kose, N., Pinero, R.F., Alder, M.E., Duong, H.L. & Surber, J. L. (2004). The effect of opening wedge thoracostomy on thoracic insufficiency syndrome associated with fused ribs and congenital scoliosis. *JBJS*, 86(8), 1659-1674. https://doi.org/10.2106/00004623-200408000-00009.

Ceballos, T., Ferrer-Torrelles, M., Castillo, F., & Fernandez-Paredes, E. (1980). Prognosis in infantile idiopathic scoliosis. *JBJS*, 62(6), 863-875. PMID: 7430174.

Crawford III, C. H., & Lenke, L. G. (2010). Growth modulation by means of anterior tethering resulting in progressive correction of juvenile idiopathic scoliosis: a case report. *JBJS*, 92(1), 202-209. https://doi.org/10.2106/JBJS.H.01728.

Dannawi, Z., Altaf, F., Harshavardhana, N. S., El Sebaie, H., & Noordeen, H. (2013). Early results of a remotely-operated magnetic growth rod in early-onset scoliosis. *The bone & joint journal*, 95(1), 75-80. https://doi.org/10.1302/0301-620X.95B1.29565.

Day, G. A., Upadhyay, S. S., Ho, E. K., Leong, J. C., & Ip, M. (1994). Pulmonary functions in congenital scoliosis. *Spine*, 19(9), 1027-1031. https://doi.org/10.1097/00007632-199405000-00004.

Dimeglio, A. (1992). Growth of the spine before age 5 years. *Journal of Pediatric Orthopaedics*, 1(2), 102-107. https://doi.org/10.1097/01202412-199201020-00003.

Fletcher, N. D., McClung, A., Rathjen, K. E., Denning, J. R., Browne, R., & Johnston III, C. E. (2012). Serial casting as a delay tactic in the treatment of moderate-to-severe early-onset scoliosis. *Journal of Pediatric Orthopaedics*, 32(7), 664-671. https://doi.org/10.1097/BPO.0b013e31824bdb55.

Groenefeld, B., & Hell, A. K. (2013). Ossifications after vertical expandable prosthetic titanium rib treatment in children with thoracic insufficiency syndrome and scoliosis. *Spine*, 38(13), E819-E823. https://doi.org/10.1097/brs.0b013e318292aafa.

Hardy, J. H., & Curtis, B. H. (1971, January). Neuromuscular Scoliosis. *Journal of Bone And Joint Surgery* (No. 5, P. 1021). https://doi.org/10.1016/j.otsr.2012.11.002.

Harrington, P. R. (1962). Treatment of scoliosis: correction and internal fixation by spine instrumentation. *JBJS*, 44(4), 591-634. PMID: 14036052.

Hasler, C. C., Mehrkens, A., & Hefti, F. (2010). Efficacy and safety of VEPTR instrumentation for progressive spine deformities in young children without rib fusions. *European spine journal*, 19, 400-408. https://doi.org/10.1007/s00586-009-1253-9.

Hickey, B. A., Towriss, C., Baxter, G., Yasso, S., James, S., Jones, A., Howes, J., Davies, P. & Ahuja, S. (2014). Early experience of MAGEC magnetic growing rods in the treatment of early onset scoliosis. *European Spine Journal*, 23, 61-65. https://doi.org/10.1007/s00586-013-3163-0.

Hutchinson, D. T., & Bassett, G. S. (1990). Superior mesenteric artery syndrome in pediatric orthopedic patients. *Clinical orthopaedics and related research*, (250), 250-257. PMID: 2293937.

Karol, L. A., Johnston, C., & Mladenov, K. (2008a). Pulmonary function, radiographic measures, and quality of life in children with congenital scoliosis: an evaluation of patient outcomes after early spinal fusion. *Spine*, 33, 1242-1249. https://doi.org/10.1097/brs.0b013e3181714536.

Karol, L. A., Johnston, C., Mladenov, K., Schochet, P., Walters, P., & Browne, R. H. (2008b). Pulmonary function following early thoracic fusion in non-neuromuscular scoliosis. *JBJS*, 90(6), 1272-1281. https://doi.org/10.2106/JBJS.G.00184.

Leatherman, K. D., Dickson, R. A. (1988) *The management of spinal deformities* (pp. 329-332). London: Wright.

Lenke, L., & Dobbs, M. (2004) *The adult and pediatric spine*. Lippincott Williams & Wilkins.

Luque, E. R. (1982). Paralytic Scoliosis in Growing Children. *Clinical Orthopaedics And Related Research*, 163, 202-209. PMID: 7067255.

McCarthy, R. E., Luhmann, S., & Lenke, L. (2015). Greater than two year follow-up Shilla growth enhancing system for the treatment of scoliosis in children. *In Proceedings of 2nd International Congress on Early Onset Scoliosis and Growing Spine*. Montreal, Quebec. https://doi.org/10.2106/JBJS.N.01083.

McCarthy, R. E., Sucato, D., Turner, J. L., Zhang, H., Henson, M. A., & McCarthy, K. (2010). Shilla growing rods in a caprine animal model: a pilot study. *Clinical Orthopaedics and Related Research*, 468, 705-710. https://doi.org/10.1007/s11999-009-1028-y.

Mehlman, C. T., Araghi, A., & Roy, D. R. (1997). Hyphenated history: the Hueter-Volkmann law. *American Journal Of Orthopedics*, 26, 798-800. PMID: 9402217.

Mehta, M. H. (1972). The rib-vertebra angle in the early diagnosis between resolving and progressive infantile scoliosis. *The Journal of bone and joint surgery. British volume*, 54(2), 230-243. PMID: 5034823.

Mehta, M. H. (2005). Growth as a corrective force in the early treatment of progressive infantile scoliosis. *The Journal of bone and joint surgery. British volume*, 87(9), 1237-1247. https://doi.org/10.1302/0301-620X.87B9.16124.

Moe, J. H., & Gustilo, R. B. (1964). Treatment of scoliosis: results in 196 patients treated by cast correction and fusion. *JBJS*, 46(2), 293-312. PMID: 14129680.

Moe, J. H., Kharrat, K., Winter, R. B., & Cummine, J. L. (1984). Harrington instrumentation without fusion plus external orthotic support for the treatment of difficult curvature problems in young children. *Clinical Orthopaedics and Related Research,* 185, 35-45. PMID: 6705397.

Munigangaiah, S., Brown, P., Mohamed, M., Bruce, C. E., Trivedi, J. M., & Davidson, N. T. (2018). A novel technique for the subfascial insertion of magnetically controlled growing rods–The Alder Hey technique. *Journal of Craniovertebral Junction & Spine*, 9(4), 250. https://doi.org/10.4103/jcvjs.JCVJS_105_18.

Myung, K. S., Skaggs, D. L., Yazici, M., Diab, M., Noordeen, H. H., Vitale, M. G., & Johnston, C. E. (2010, January). Hybrid growth rods using spinal implants on ribs: Paper# 85. *In Spine Journal Meeting Abstracts* (pp. 105-106). https://doi.org/00152232-201000002-00085.

Newton, P. O., Farnsworth, C. L., Faro, F. D., Mahar, A. T., Odell, T. R., Mohamad, F., Breisch, E., Fricka, K., Upasani, V., & Amiel, D. (2008). Spinal growth modulation with an anterolateral flexible tether in an immature bovine model: disc health and motion preservation. *Spine*, 33(7), 724-733. https://doi.org/10.1097/BRS.0b013e31816950a0.

Newton, P. O., Farnsworth, C. L., Upasani, V. V., Chambers, R. C., Varley, E., & Tsutsui, S. (2011). Effects of intraoperative tensioning of an anterolateral spinal tether on spinal growth modulation in a porcine model. *Spine*, 36(2), 109-117. https://doi.org/10.1097/BRS.0b013e3181cc8fce.

Pehrsson, K., Larsson, S., Oden, A., & Nachemson, A. (1992). Long-term follow-up of patients with untreated scoliosis a study of mortality, causes of death, and symptoms. *Spine*, 17(9), 1091-1096. https://doi.org/10.1097/00007632-199209000-00014.

Pratt, R. K., Webb, J. K., Burwell, R. G., & Cummings, S. L. (1999). Luque trolley and convex epiphysiodesis in the management of infantile and juvenile idiopathic scoliosis. *Spine,* 24(15), 1538. https://doi.org/10.1097/00007632-199908010-00007.

Sanders, J. O., D'Astous, J., Fitzgerald, M., Khoury, J. G., Kishan, S., & Sturm, P. F. (2009). Derotational casting for progressive infantile scoliosis. *Journal of Pediatric Orthopaedics*, 29(6), 581-587. https://doi.org/10.1097/BPO.0b013e3181b2f8df.

Sankar, W. N., Acevedo, D. C., & Skaggs, D. L. (2010). Comparison of complications among growing spinal implants. *Spine*, 35(23), 2091-2096. https://doi.org/10.1097/brs.0b013e3181c6edd7

Sankar, W. N., Skaggs, D. L., Yazici, M., Johnston, C. E., Shah, S. A., Javidan, P., Kadakia, R. V., Day, T. F., & Akbarnia, B. A. (2011). Lengthening of dual growing rods and the law of diminishing returns. *Spine*, 36(10), 806-809. https://doi.org/10.1097/BRS.0b013e318214d78f

Skaggs, D. L., Akbarnia, B. A., Flynn, J. M., Myung, K. S., Sponseller, P. D., & Vitale, M. G. (2014). A classification of growth friendly spine implants. *Journal of Pediatric Orthopaedics*, 34(3), 260-274. https://doi.org/10.1097/BPO.0000000000000073.

Stokes, O. M., O'Donovan, E. J., Samartzis, D., Bow, C. H., Luk, K. D., & Cheung, K. M. (2014). Reducing Radiation Exposure in Early-Onset Scoliosis Surgery Patients: Novel Use of Ultrasonography to Measure Lengthening in Magnetically-Controlled Growing Rods. *The Spine Journal*, 2014, 14.10: 2397-2404. https://doi.org/10.1016/j.spinee.2014.01.039.

Stücker, R. (2009). Results of treatment of progressive scoliosis with SMA staples. *Der Orthopade*, 38(2), 176-180. https://doi.org/10.1007/s00132-008-1364-8.

Swank, S. M., Winter, R. B., & Moe, J. H. (1982). Scoliosis and cor pulmonale. *Spine*, 7(4), 343-354. https://doi.org/10.1097/00007632-198207000-00004.

Takaso, M., Moriya, H., Kitahara, H., Minami, S., Takahashi, K., Isobe, K., Yamagata, M., Otsuka, Y., Nakata, Y., & Inoue, M. (1998). New remote-controlled growing-rod spinal instrumentation possibly applicable for scoliosis in young children. *Journal of orthopaedic science*, 3(6), 336-340. https://doi.org/10.1007/s007760050062.

Teoh, K. H., Von Ruhland, C., Evans, S. L., James, S. H., Jones, A., Howes, J., Davies, P. R., & Ahuja, S. (2016). Metallosis following implantation of magnetically controlled growing rods in the treatment of scoliosis: a case series. *The bone & joint journal*, 98(12), 1662-1667. https://doi.org/10.1302/0301-620X.98B12.38061.

Thompson, G. H., Akbarnia, B. A., Kostial, P., Poe-Kochert, C., Armstrong, D. G., Roh, J., Lowe, R., Asher, M. A., & Marks, D. S. (2005). Comparison of single and dual growing rod techniques followed through definitive surgery: a preliminary study. *Spine*, 30(18), 2039-2044. https://doi.org/10.1097/01.brs.0000179082.92712.89.

Wick, J. M., & Konze, J. (2012). A magnetic approach to treating progressive early-onset scoliosis. *Aorn journal*, 96(2), 163-173. https://doi.org/10.1016/j.aorn.2012.05.008.

Winter, R. B., & Moe, J. H. (1982). The results of spinal arthrodesis for congenital spinal deformity in patients younger than five years old. *JBJS*, 64(3), 419-432. PMID: 7061559.

Yilgor, C., Demirkiran, G., Ayvaz, M., & Yazici, M. (2012). Is expansion thoracoplasty a safe procedure for mobility and growth potential of the spine? Spontaneous fusion after multiple chest distractions in young children. *Journal of Pediatric Orthopaedics*, 32(5), 483-489. https://doi.org/10.1097/BPO.0b013e318257d3a9.

Yilgor, C., Efendiyev, A., Akbiyik, F., Demirkiran, G., Senkoylu, A., Alanay, A., & Yazici, M. (2018). Metal ion release during growth-friendly instrumentation for early-onset scoliosis: a preliminary study. *Spine deformity*, 6(1), 48-53. https://doi.org/10.1016/j.jspd.2017.06.005.

# Chapter 29

# Future Directions in the Management of EOS

**Ercan Bayar, MD**
**and Hüseyin Sina Coşkun***
Department of Orthopaedics and Traumatology, Ondokuz Mayıs University, Samsun, Turkiye

## Abstract

What we do not know about scoliosis is probably more than what we do know. This chapter aims to evaluate future treatment options for early-onset scoliosis. This chapter aims to review the current management of EOS, highlight its limitations and challenges, and explore potential future directions that may improve the outcomes of children with EOS.

**Keywords:** early-onset scoliosis, future directions, treatment

## Introduction

Early-onset scoliosis (EOS) can have a long-term detrimental impact on children's physical and psychological well-being. Over the past few decades, the management of EOS has evolved significantly, from early casting to growth-friendly implants and with the introduction of non-invasive devices like braces. However, the standard of care for EOS is still evolving, with constant technological advances and new techniques being developed. Although many new techniques have been used to treat EOS, there is still no consensus on the optimum treatment modality.

* Corresponding Author's Email: sina.coskun@hotmail.com.

In: Early Onset Scoliosis
Editor: Ahmed Majid Heydar
ISBN: 979-8-89113-600-7

## Review of Current Management Strategies

The management of EOS is a complex process that requires a comprehensive assessment of the patient's medical history, physical examination, and imaging studies. The current best-practice management of EOS involves a multidisciplinary team approach that includes pediatric orthopedic surgeons, pulmonologists, physical therapists, and psychologists. The main goals of management for EOS include correcting or stabilizing the spinal deformity, preventing future complications, and maintaining normal spinal growth and development.

## Conservative Management

Non-invasive management options include bracing and casting. This is the first step in the treatment of EOS by the conservative method. Bracing works on the principle of applying constant external pressure on the spine, which helps to straighten the curve gradually. In contrast, casting involves the use of an immobilizing full body cast to keep the spine in a fixed position. Both treatments can be effective when started early and need regular monitoring of the child's growth and spinal curve. While these non-invasive management strategies have proved effective in managing the curves in the short term, they can sometimes fail to provide adequate correction.

Historically, many braces have played a critical role in the treatment of scoliosis. The Milwaukee brace, also known as STLSO (cervical-thoracic-lumbo-sacral orthosis), is widely used. Still, the children did not tolerate it much because of its cervical component. The Boston (TLSO) brace replaced it with an absent design of the cervical component. This type of brace is much more comfortable than the STLSO but has some difficulties with rotational control. Therefore, all these requirements lead us to 3D bracing. 3D bracing is now one of the most trending brace treatments in EOS. There are many different techniques for applying the 3D brace. 3D printers are used in production, but not widely due to their cost. Some particular brace types also help correct axial plane deformity, which is not expected in conventional brace types (Rigo & Weiss, 2008). In the future, it seems that every brace will be individualized for every child, and custom design will be inevitable because of the different nature of the curves.

## Surgical Management of EOS

Surgical management for EOS, such as spinal fusion or growing implants, is invasive and can have many limitations. Implants and spine fusion surgery aim to prevent spinal deformities from worsening or recurring, but they can also have some complications. Spinal fusion is not the first consideration in the surgical treatment of EOS.

Standard medical implants that treat EOS include vertical expandable prosthetic titanium rib (VEPTR) and the magnetically controlled growing rod (MCGR). However, VEPTR may result in thoracic insufficiency syndrome (TIS), leading to severe respiratory complications. On the other hand, the magnetically controlled mechanism of the MCGR can improve and reduce the risks associated with implant revision (Obid et al., 2021; Peiro-Garcia et al., 2021). These techniques are cost-intensive; therefore, careful consideration must be taken to select the best option for the patient.

Anterior Vertebral Body Tethering (AVBT) is a recently developed surgical technique to treat progressive and severe scoliosis in patients with significant growth potential (Courvoisier et al., 2023). In a recent study, the authors showed satisfactory correction for deformity in most cases. However, the rates of complication and revision suggest the need for improved implants and patient selection (Rushton et al., 2021). The limitation of the AVBT tethering is the rigid curves, older children, and the upper thoracic curves due to surgical access problems. A recent meta-analysis concluded that AVBT effectively reduces the deformity in the coronal plane, and the maximum correction can be achieved in one year. However, the method should be optimized to reduce the rate of complications, such as overcorrection and tether breakage (Mariscal et al., 2023).

## Growth-Friendly Implants

The ultimate goal of managing EOS is to prevent spinal deformity while preserving spine growth. Consequently, most cases of EOS require surgical intervention, and growth-friendly implants have become more popular because of their long-term superior outcomes compared to traditional spinal fusion. Spinal fusion is not considered the first step of surgical treatment in the groups of patients with EOS .

Growing rods, magnetically controlled growth rods, vertical expandable prosthetic titanium ribs, and Shilla growth guidance systems are the commonly used growth-friendly implants to correct EOS (Skaggs et al., 2014). These implants allow continuous and customizable distraction and expansion, which correct spinal deformity and normal spine growth. However, some concerns remain with growth-friendly implants, including early implant-related complications such as device migration, wound infections, implant failure, and frequent surgical interventions to lengthen the devices.

## Challenges and Limitations of Current Management

One of the significant challenges of managing EOS is tracking the progression and recurrence of spinal deformities. Serial imaging studies, including X-rays and magnetic resonance imaging (MRI), are required to follow changes in the spinal curve. However, prolonged exposure to radiation in serial X-rays could potentially lead to malignant lesions in children. MRI is a viable alternative to X-rays but is more expensive and often requires general anesthesia in younger children. Additionally, growth-friendly implants have been associated with a higher rate of complications than traditional spinal fusion; thus, there is often uncertainty about the optimal timing of implant surgery, and surgeons must balance the risks and benefits of surgical intervention. Preventive medicine in EOS is the successful resolution between the disease and the physician; however, the entrance of the spine surgeon into the picture often occurs in the later stages of the disease (Yazici et al., 2022).

## Future Directions in the Management of EOS

As with most disciplines in medicine, rapidly advancing technologies have revolutionized the management of EOS, opening up new avenues to improve the outcomes and quality of life for affected children. The SRS Growing Spine Committee has published the following goals of treatment for patients with EOS:

- Minimize spinal deformity over the life of the patient with EOS
- Maximize thoracic function over the life of the patient with EOS
- Minimize the extent of any final spinal fusion

- Maximize motion of the chest and spine
- Minimize complications, hospitalizations, and burdens for the family.

These goals are standard for current and future treatment of EOS (El-Hawary & Akbarnia, 2015).

The following are some of the potential future directions in the management of EOS:

1. Advanced Imaging Technologies
   There has been much interest in using non-invasive imaging techniques in the management of spinal deformities. EOS Imaging, a French manufacturer of 3D medical imaging and software solutions for orthopedics, is one company that has developed a revolutionary imaging system called the EOS system (Garg et al., 2020). The system provides high-quality and low-dose 3D images of the spine and other orthopedic structures in a standing position, reducing the need for radiation exposure and general anesthesia in young children. The potential benefits of this technology for diagnosing and monitoring scoliosis are enormous. This cost-intensive technology can gain a larger field of use in the future.
2. Artificial Intelligence (AI)
   AI plays an increasingly important role in the medical field, and researchers are investigating its potential applications in the management of EOS. For instance, AI can help detect subtle changes in spine alignment, allowing clinicians to intervene earlier, reducing the need for radiation, and streamlining care. Currently, there are many software programs for that aim. Furthermore, AI could allow clinicians to predict the progression of spinal deformities, enabling early identification of children at high risk of developing spinal deformities. Furthermore, 3D-printed spine models produced before surgery may allow the surgeon to better visualize the deformity and help reduce intra-operative blood loss (Courvoisier et al., 2022).
3. Biologics and Gene Therapy
   There is growing interest in the application of biologics and gene therapy in the management of spinal deformities. Researchers are investigating the use of growth factors, such as BMP-2 and BMP-7, to stimulate bone growth. Today, there are several gene studies in the literature, but we do not know the exact genetic reason for EOS. In the future, it can be possible to genetically modulate the expression

of specific genes involved in spinal growth, development, and curvature.

4. Expandable Biomaterials and Bioengineering
   Expandable biomaterials are a promising intervention in the management of EOS. They are biocompatible materials that can be implanted in the spine and expand and promote spine growth in response to environmental stimuli, such as temperature and pH. Researchers are investigating multiple stimuli-responsive materials that have potential to provide a customized and dynamic approach to EOS management.
5. New Biomechanical Tools
   Biomechanical tools such as finite element analysis (FEA) can potentially improve the predictability of surgical outcomes in EOS. FEA, which simulates the mechanics of the spine, provides a more accurate prediction of stress and strain in spinal structures and allows for trial and error of various implant configurations before embarking on invasive surgery. FEA might significantly improve alignment, stability, and mobility outcomes.

## Conclusion

EOS is a complex and challenging condition that requires early detection, intervention, and long-term follow-up. The current management of EOS includes non-invasive techniques and growth-friendly implants. However, there are limitations and challenges associated with these methods, including difficulty in tracking progression and recurrence, the risk of radiation exposure with imaging, and a high rate of complications associated with implant surgery. Emerging technologies, such as artificial intelligence, biomaterials, and biologics, can revolutionize the management of EOS by detecting subtle changes and helping clinicians make precise decisions. Despite ongoing challenges, multidisciplinary teams of healthcare providers seek to use future technology and innovative surgical tools to improve outcomes and quality of life for children affected by EOS.

## References

Courvoisier, A., Baroncini, A., Jeandel, C., Barra, C., Lefevre, Y., Solla, F., Gouron, R., Métaizeau, J. D., Maximin, M. C., & Cunin, V. (2023). Vertebral Body Tethering in AIS Management-A Preliminary Report. *Children (Basel), 10*(2). https://doi.org/10.3390/children10020192.

Courvoisier, A., Cebrian, A., Simon, J., Désauté, P., Aubert, B., Amabile, C., & Thiébaut, L. (2022). Virtual Scoliosis Surgery Using a 3D-Printed Model Based on Biplanar Radiographs. *Bioengineering, 9*(9), 469. https://www.mdpi.com/2306-5354/9/9/469.

El-Hawary, R., & Akbarnia, B. A. (2015). Early Onset Scoliosis - Time for Consensus. *Spine deformity, 3*(2), 105-106. https://doi.org/10.1016/j.jspd.2015.01.003.

Garg, B., Mehta, N., Bansal, T., & Malhotra, R. (2020). EOS® imaging: Concept and current applications in spinal disorders. *J Clin Orthop Trauma, 11*(5), 786-793. https://doi.org/10.1016/j.jcot.2020.06.012.

Mariscal, G., Morales, J., Pérez, S., Rubio-Belmar, P. A., Bovea-Marco, M., Bas, J. L., Bas, P., & Bas, T. (2023). Meta-analysis on the efficacy and safety of anterior vertebral body tethering in adolescent idiopathic scoliosis. *Eur Spine J, 32*(1), 140-148. https://doi.org/10.1007/s00586-022-07448-9.

Obid, P., Yiu, K., Cheung, K., Kwan, K., Ruf, M., & Cheung, J. P. Y. (2021). Magnetically controlled growing rods in early onset scoliosis: radiological results, outcome, and complications in a series of 22 patients. *Archives of orthopaedic and trauma surgery, 141*, 1163-1174. https://doi.org/10.1007/s00402-020-03518-z.

Peiro-Garcia, A., Bourget-Murray, J., Suarez-Lorenzo, I., Ferri-De-Barros, F., & Parsons, D. (2021). Early complications in vertical expandable prosthetic titanium rib and magnetically controlled growing rods to manage early onset scoliosis. *International Journal of Spine Surgery, 15*(2), 368-375. https://doi.org/10.14444/8048.

Rigo, M., & Weiss, H. R. (2008). The Chêneau concept of bracing--biomechanical aspects. *Stud Health Technol Inform, 135*, 303-319.

Rushton, P. R. P., Nasto, L., Parent, S., Turgeon, I., Aldebeyan, S., & Miyanji, F. (2021). Anterior Vertebral Body Tethering for Treatment of Idiopathic Scoliosis in the Skeletally Immature: Results of 112 Cases. *Spine (Phila Pa 1976), 46*(21), 1461-1467. https://doi.org/10.1097/brs.0000000000004061.

Skaggs, D. L., Akbarnia, B. A., Flynn, J. M., Myung, K. S., Sponseller, P. D., & Vitale, M. G. (2014). A classification of growth friendly spine implants. *Journal of pediatric orthopaedics, 34*(3), 260-274. *DOI:* 10.1097/BPO.0000000000000073.

Yazici, M., Akbarnia, B. A., Thompson, G. H., El-Hawary, R., & Emans, J. B. (2022). A Journey from the Past to the Future. In *The Growing Spine: Management of Spinal Disorders in Young Children* (pp. 867-871). Springer. https://doi.org/10.1007/978-3-662-48284-1_57.

# Index

## O



## P



## R



## S